450 Single Best Answers in the

CLINICAL
SPECIALTIES

Dedications

To my parents and brother, who during the darkest nights have forever remained the brightest stars

Sukhpreet S Dubb

Dedicated to Abba and Mum for your loving support

Jeffrey Ahmed

To Arcadia and Indigo, and of course Bundle

Edward Maclaren

450 Single Best Answers in the

CLINICAL SPECIALTIES

Sukhpreet Singh Dubb, Foundation Year 1 Doctor

Alex Bailey, Teaching Fellow and Honorary Lecturer in Psychiatry

Charlene M.C. Rodrigues, Academic Clinical Fellow in Paediatric Infectious Disease

Margaret P. Rhoads, Academic Clinical Fellow in Paediatric Infectious Disease

Jeffrey Ahmed, Foundation Year 2 Trainee

Edward MacLaren, Specialist Registrar in Obstetrics and Gynaecology

Editors
Martin Lupton, Consultant in Obstetrics and Gynaecology

Gareth Tudor-Williams, Consultant in Paediatric Infectious Diseases

James Warner, Consultant in Older Adults Psychiatry

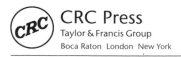

CRC Press
Taylor & Francis Group
Boca Raton London New York

CRC Press is an imprint of the
Taylor & Francis Group, an **informa** business

CRC Press
Taylor & Francis Group
6000 Broken Sound Parkway NW, Suite 300
Boca Raton, FL 33487-2742

© 2012 by Taylor & Francis Group, LLC
CRC Press is an imprint of Taylor & Francis Group, an Informa business

No claim to original U.S. Government works
Printed on acid-free paper
Cover image © Lisa Eastman - Fotolia

Printed and bound in India by Replika Press Pvt. Ltd.

International Standard Book Number: 978-1-4441-4902-9 (Softcover)

**Library of Congress Cataloging-in-Publication Data and
The British Library Cataloging in Publication Data are Available**

**Visit the Taylor & Francis Web site at
http://www.taylorandfrancis.com**

**and the CRC Press Web site at
http://www.crcpress.com**

Contents

PART I OBSTETRICS AND GYNAECOLOGY

PART II PAEDIATRICS

SECTION 32: PSYCHOSEXUAL, SLEEP AND EATING DISORDERS

SECTION 33: SUBSTANCE MISUSE DISORDERS

SECTION 34: PSYCHOPHARMACOLOGY

SECTION 35: CHILD PSYCHIATRY AND LEARNING DISABILITY

Foreword

Practice makes perfect? I'm not sure this is always the case, but practice certainly helps in knowledge acquisition and exam preparation. This book has been created by a group of enthusiastic young teachers and senior experts in their fields who both practise and teach these specialties as part of their weekly lives. As such the book not only represents an account of key features of contemporary clinical practice, but also offers an insight into the thinking of experienced educators who are continuously assessing whether those in their charge have reached the required standard to pass the dreaded assessments.

In my opinion, the clinical specialties covered in this book are fascinating and exciting areas of the medical curriculum. However, these specialties also represent some of the most intimidating areas of medicine. A student approaching their first sick child or entering the labour ward is surely always inwardly trembling. Furthermore, every qualified doctor also realises just how much specialties such as psychiatry play a part in their working lives, regardless of their particular area of practice. Thus, knowledge and understanding of these areas of medicine are essential, and what better way to check your knowledge than by answering questions on the subject? Use this book to help guide you, and good luck!

Professor Jenny Higham
Deputy Principal and Director of Education
Faculty of Medicine
Imperial College London

Preface

There has been a transition in the method used by medical schools to test the knowledge-based and clinical acumen of medical students. Although multiple choice questions (MCQs) were a commonly used test across a broad range of topics they have largely been abandoned in favour of extending matching questions (EMQs) and, more recently, the single best answer (SBA) question format. EMQs and SBAs overcome the ambiguity that occurs in MCQ exams as well as being able to provide more clinical question stems reflecting real life situations. The SBA format is highly favoured in examinations at both the undergraduate and postgraduate level since students must not only demonstrate their clinical knowledge and understanding but also make sound judgements that are more congruent with clinical practice.

There is often a shortfall in the resources available for the clinical specialties, including Obstetrics and Gynaecology, Paediatrics and Psychiatry, especially for SBAs. The Royal Colleges of Obstetricians and Gynaecologists, Paediatrics and Child Health and Psychiatrists have all now incorporated SBAs as part of their examination process to gain membership.

450 Single Best Answers in the Clinical Specialties provides a comprehensive examination of the typical medical undergraduate curriculum. Each question not only provides an opportunity to apply clinical knowledge and correctly identify the single best answer to a question but also to learn why the other answers are wrong, greatly increasing the learning opportunity of the reader. This book aims to provide medical students with a useful source for exam revision as well as supplementing the reader's knowledge such that they feel fully prepared for the undergraduate medical written examinations.

Acknowledgements

Neeral Patel
Final Year Medical Student
Imperial College London

Osayuki Nehikhare
Final Year Medical Student
Imperial College London

Dhupal Patel
Final Year Medical Student
Imperial College London

Abhijit Singh Gill
Final Year Medical Student
Imperial College London

Asiya Tafader
Third Year Medical Student
Barts and The London Medical School

Omair Shariq
Final Year Medical Student
Imperial College London

Martin Wong
Final Year Medical Student
Imperial College London

Upama Banerjee
Final Year Medical Student
Imperial College London

We would also like to thank Dr. Joanna Koster, Stephen Clausard and the rest of the Hodder Arnold team whose support and advice have made this project possible.

How to prepare for a single best answer examination

An important part of exam preparation is ensuring that you have addressed the learning objectives of the curriculum upon which the exam is based upon. Students can often become disheartened when using exam revision books if they have not adequately covered the knowledge base required for examinations. An equally important aspect of exam preparation is becoming familiar with the format of the exam that you are to sit. Relying on revision books that do not reflect the examination to be undertaken may provide useful knowledge but will not prepare you for the questions that you will face under exam stress.

HOW TO WRITE A SINGLE BEST ANSWER QUESTION

A single best answer (SBA) question format adopts three important facets: the question stem, question lead in and the answer options. A significant difference from multiple choice question (MCQ) formats is that SBA questions have longer question stems with short answer options. The question stem is usually a realistic clinical scenario that reflects a typical case that might be seen in clinical practice. An SBA question is not designed for the recall and regurgitation of knowledge, a hallmark of the MCQ, but the application of such knowledge. A well written SBA should have only one categorically correct answer for the given question stem although the other answers should be plausible.

HOW TO USE THIS BOOK

The authors, contributors and editor of this book have extensive experience of writing and sitting examinations and all acknowledge the importance of correct exam preparation for undergraduate medical examinations. The questions in this book aim to address the basic, intermediate and most advanced levels expected of medical students for undergraduate exams. The comprehensive answers for each question should provide adequate explanations for the correct answer but also maximize your learning opportunity by explaining in detail why the other answers are not correct. We hope you enjoy using this book for your revision and wish you the very best of luck with your exams.

Sukhpreet Singh Dubb, James Warner, Gareth Tudor-Williams and Martin Lupton

List of abbreviations used

AChEI	acetylcholinesterase inhibitor	CSF	cerebrospinal fluid
AD	Alzheimer's disease	CT	computed tomography
ADHD	attention deficit hyperactivity disorder	CTG	cardiotocograph
		CTPA	computed tomography pulmonary angiogram
AIDS	acquired immune deficiency syndrome	CVT	cerebral vein thrombosis
		DAT	direct antiglobulin test
AIS	androgen insensitivity syndrome	DCDA	dichorionic–diamniotic
AMHP	Approved Mental Health Professional	DIC	disseminated intravascular coagulation
AML	acute myeloid leukaemia	DKA	diabetic ketoacidosis
ANA	anti-nuclear antibody	DLB	dementia with Lewy bodies
aPTT	activated partial thromboplastin time	DOLS	Deprivation of Liberty Safeguards
ASD	atrial septal defect	DSM	Diagnostic and Statistical Manual of Mental Disorders
ASOT	antistreptolysin O titre		
ATLS	Advanced Trauma Life Support	DSPS	delayed sleep phase syndrome
		EAS	external anal sphincter
AVSD	atrioventricular septal defect	EBV	Epstein–Barr virus
BAC	blood alcohol concentration	ECG	electrocardiogram
bd	twice a day	ECT	electroconvulsive therapy
BE	base excess	ECV	external cephalic version
BMI	body mass index	EEG	electroencephalogram
bpm	beats per minute	ELISA	enzyme-linked immunosorbent assay
BV	bacterial vaginosis		
CAH	congenital adrenal hyperplasia	ERPC	evacuation of retained products of conception
CAMHS	Child and Adolescent Mental Health Services	EUA	examination under anaesthesia
CBT	cognitive behavioural therapy	FBS	fetal blood sampling
CCF	congestive cardiac failure	FEV1	forced expiratory volume in 1 second
CIN	cervical intraepithelial neoplasia		
		FGM	female genital mutilation
CJD	Creutzfeld–Jakob disease	FISH	fluorescence *in situ* hybridization
CK	creatinine kinase		
CMV	cytomegalovirus	FSH	follicle-stimulating hormone
CNS	central nervous system	FVC	fixed vital capacity
COCP	combined oral contraceptive pill	FY1	foundation year 1 doctor
		G6PD	glucose-6-phosphate dehydrogenase
COPD	chronic obstructive pulmonary disease		
		GA	general anaesthesia
CPR	cardiopulmonary resuscitation	GABA	gamma aminobutyric acid
CRP	C-reactive protein	GAD	generalized anxiety disorder

GBS	Group B *Streptococcus*	LBC	liquid-based cytology
GCS	Glasgow Coma Scale	LH	luteinizing hormone
GDM	gestational diabetes mellitus	LP	lumbar puncture
GMC	General Medical Council	MCA	Mental Capacity Act
GnRH	gonadotrophin-releasing hormone	MCV	mean corpuscular volume
		MG	myasthenia gravis
GP	general practitioner	MHA	Mental Health Act
GUM	genitourinary medicine	MMR	measles, mumps and rubella
HAART	highly active antiretroviral therapy	MMSE	Mini-Mental State Examination
Hb	haemoglobin	MRI	magnetic resonance imaging
HBA$_{1c}$	glycated haemoglobin	MRSA	methicillin-resistant *Staphylococcus aureus*
hCG	human chorionic gonadotrophin	MS	multiple sclerosis
HD	Huntingdon's disease	NAI	non-accidental injury
HG	hyperemesis gravidarum	NBM	nil by mouth
HIE	hypoxic ischaemic encephalopathy	NBSS	newborn blood spot screening
		NEC	nectrotizing enterocolitis
HIV	human immunodeficiency virus	NHS	National Health Service
		NICE	National Institute of Health and Clinical Excellence
HMB	heavy menstrual bleeding		
HPA	hypothalamic-pituitary axis	NMS	neuroleptic malignant syndrome
HPV	human papilloma virus		
HRT	hormone replacement therapy	NT	nuchal translucency
HSG	hysterosalpingogram	OCD	obsessive–compulsive disorder
HSP	Henoch–Schönlein purpura	OCP	oral contraceptive pill
HSV	herpes simplex virus	ODD	oppositional defiant disorder
HUS	haemolytic uraemic syndrome	OGTT	oral glucose tolerance test
IBD	inflammatory bowel disease	OHSS	ovarian hyperstimulation syndrome
IBS	irritable bowel syndrome		
ICD	International Classification of Diseases	*P*	partial pressure
		PCD	primary ciliary dyskinesia
ICP	intracranial pressure	PCOS	polycystic ovary syndrome
IIH	idiopathic intracranial hypertension	PCR	protein creatinine ratio
		PD	Parkinson's disease
IM	intramuscular	PDD	Parkinson's disease dementia
INR	international normalized ratio	PID	pelvic inflammatory disease
ITP	idiopathic thrombocytopenic purpura	PIH	pregnancy-induced hypertension
ITU	intensive therapy unit	PKU	phenylketonuria
IUD	intrauterine device	PMS	premenstrual syndrome
IUGR	intrauterine growth restriction	PPROM	preterm pre-labour rupture of membranes
IV	intravenous		
IVF	*in vitro* fertilization	PR	per rectum
JIA	juvenile idiopathic arthritis	PRN	pro re nata (take as needed)

PT	prothrombin time	TD	tardive dyskinesia
PTSD	post-traumatic stress disorder	TOP	termination of pregnancy
PUPP	pruritic urticarial papules and plaques of pregnancy	TOT	transobturator tape
		TSH	thyroid-stimulating hormone
RMI	risk of malignancy index	TTP	thrombotic thrombocytopenic purpura
RSV	respiratory syncytial virus		
SAH	subarachnoid haemorrhage	TVT	tension-free vaginal tape
SCID	subacute combined immunodeficiency disorder	UDCA	ursodeoxycholic acid
		UMN	upper motor neuron
SGA	small for gestational age	UPSI	unprotected sexual intercourse
SIADH	syndrome of inappropriate antidiuretic hormone		
		US	ultrasound
SIRS	systemic inflammatory response syndrome	UTI	urinary tract infection
		V/Q	ventilation/perfusion
SLE	systemic lupus erythematosus	VF	ventricular fibrillation
SNRI	serotonin and noradrenaline reuptake inhibitor	VLOSLP	very late-onset schizophrenia-like psychosis
SSRI	serotonin specific reuptake inhibitor	VSD	ventricular septal defect
		VTE	venous thromboembolism
STI	sexually transmitted infection	vWD	von Willebrand's disease
STOP	surgical termination of pregnancy	vWF	von Willebrand factor
		VZIG	varicella zoster immunoglobulin
STP	superficial transverse perineii		
SVT	supraventricular tachycardia	WCC	white cell count
TB	tuberculosis	WHO	World Health Organization
TCA	tricyclic antidepressant	YOD	young-onset dementia

Common reference intervals

Investigation/test	Range	Units
Alanine transaminase ALT	0–31	IU/L
Albumin	33–47	g/L
Alkaline phosphatase ALP	30–130	IU/L
Amylase	70–400	U/L
aPTT	22.0–29.0	secs
Aspartate transaminase AST	0–31	IU/L
Bicarbonate	22–29	mmol/L
Bilirubin	0–17	µmol/L
Calcium	2.15–2.65	mmol/L
Chloride	95–108	mmol/L
Cholesterol	<5	mmol/L
Cholesterol HDL ratio	0–5.00	
C-reactive protein	0–10	mg/L
Creatinine	60–110	µmol/L
Eosinophils	0.0–0.4	$\times 10^9$/L
Ferritin	10–120	µg/L
Free T4	9.0–26.0	pmol/L
Gamma GT	2.0–30	IU/L
Glucose fasting	3.0–6.0	mmol/L
Glucose random	3.0–8.0	mmol/L
Haemoglobin A_{1c}	4.3–6.1	%
HDL cholesterol	1.00–2.20	mmol/L
Hb	11.4–15.0	g/dl
Insulin	3.0–17.0	mU/L
Iron	7.0–27	µmol/L
LDL cholesterol	2.0–5.0	mmol/L
Lymphocytes	1.0–3.5	$\times 10^9$/L
MCH	26.7–32.9	pg
MCV	83.0–101.0	fl
Monocytes	0.3–1.0	$\times 10^9$/L
MPV	8.0–12.0	fl
Neutrophils	2.0–7.5	$\times 10^9$/L
Osmolality serum	275–295	mOsm/kg
Osmolality urine	50–1200	mmol/kg
$PaCO_2$	4.7–6	kPa
$PaCO_2$	35–45	mmHg
PaO_2	>10.6	kPa
PaO_2	75–100	mmHg
pH	7.35–7.45	
Phosphate	0.80–1.40	mmol/L
Platelets	120–400	$\times 10^9$/L

Potassium	3.8–5.5	mmol/L
Prolactin female	0–750	mU/L
Prolactin male	150–500	mU/L
Prothrombin time	9.0–12.0	secs
RBC	3.74–4.99	$\times 10^6/\mu L$
Serum vitamin B12	160–800	ng/L
Sodium	135–145	mmol/L
Total iron binding capacity	49–78	μmol/L
Total protein	64–83	g/L
Transferrin sat	20–45	%
Triglycerides	0.00–1.80	mmol/L
TSH	0.3–4.2	mU/L
Urea	2.5–7.0	mmol/L
WBC	4.0–11.0	$\times 10^9/L$

PAEDIATRIC REFERENCE INTERVALS

Albumin	36–48 g/dL
α1-antitrypsin	1.3–3.4 g/dL
Ammonium	2–25 μmL/L; 3–35 μg/dL
Amylase	70–300 u/L
Aspartate aminotransferase	<40 u/L
Bilirubin	2–16 μmol/L; 0.1–0.8 mg/dL
Blood gases, arterial	pH 7.36–7.42
PCO_2	4.3–6.1 kPa; 32–46 mmHg
PO_2	11.3–14.0 kPa; 85–105 mmHg
Bicarbonate	21–25 mmol/L
Base excess	−2 to +2 mmol/L
Calcium	2.25–2.75 mmol/L; 9–11 mg/dL
	neonates: 1.72–2.47; 6.9–9.9 mg/dL
Chloride	98–105 mmol/L
Cholesterol	≤5.7 mmol/L; 100–200 mg/dL
Creatine kinase	<80 U/L
Creatinine	25–115 μmol/L; 0.3–1.3 mg/dL
Glucose	2.5–5.3 mmol/L; 45–95 mg/dL (lower in newborn; fluoride tube)
IgA	0.8–4.5 g/L (low at birth, rising to adult levels slowly)
IgG	5–18 g/L (high at birth, falls and then rises slowly to adult level)
IgM	0.2–2.0 g/L (low at birth, rises to adult level by 1 year)
IgE	<500 U/mL
Iron	9–36 μmol/L; 50–200 μg/dL
Lead	<1.75 μmol/L; <36 μg/dL
Mg^{2+}	0.6–1.0 mmol/L

Osmolality	275–295 mosmol/L
Phenylalanine	0.04–0.21 mmol/L
Potassium	3.5–5.5 mmol/L
Protein	63–81 g/L; 6.3–8.1 g/dL
Sodium	136–145 mmol/L
Transferrin	2.5–4.5 g/L
Triglyceride	0.34–1.92 mmol/L (=30–170 mg/dL)
Urate	0.12–0.36 mmol/L; 2–6 mg/dL
Urea	2.5–6.6 mmol/L; 15–40 mg/dL
Gamma GT	<20 U/L
Hormones:	
Cortisol	9am 200–700 nmol/L midnight <140 nmol/L, mean
Dehydroepiandrosterone sulfate	
day 5–11	0.8–2.8 µmol/L (range)
5–11 yrs	0.1–3.6 µmol/L
17α-Hydroxyprogesterone	
days 5–11	1.6–7.5 nmol/L (range)
4–15 yrs	0.4–4.2 nmol/L
T4	60–135 nmol/L (not neonates)
TSH	<5 mu/L (higher on day 1–4)

NB: Figures in brackets are values for neonates; other figures are for infants aged 1 year and above.

Day	Hbg/dL	MCVfl	MCHC %	Retics%	WCC	Neutrophils	Eosins	Lymphs	Monos
1	19.0±2	119±9	31.6±2	3.2±1	9–30	6–26 (11)	0.02–0.8	2–11	0.4–3.1
4	18.6±2	114±7	32.6±2	1.8±1	9–40				
5	17.6±1	114±9	30.9±2	1.2±0.2					
Weeks									
1–2	17.3±2	112±19	32.1±3	0.5±0.03	5–21	1.5–10 (5)	0.07–0.1	2–17	0.3–2.7
2–3	15.6±3	111±8	33.9±2	0.8±0.6	6–15	1–9.5 (4)	0.07–0.1	2–17	0.2–2.4
4–5	12.7±2	101±8	34.9±2	0.9±0.8	6–15	(4)		(6)	
6–7	12.0±2	105±12	33.8±2	1.2±0.7	6–15	(4)		(6)	
8–9	10.7±1	93±12	34.1±2	1.8±1	6–15	(4)		(6)	
Months – all the following Hb values are medians/lower limit for normal									
3	11.5/9	88/88			6–15	(3)		(6)	
6	11.5/9	77/70			6–15	(3)		(6)	
12	11.5/9	78/72			6–15	(3)		(5)	
Year									
2	11.5/9	78/74			6–15	(3)		(5)	
4	12.2/10	80/75			6–15	(4)		(4)	
6	13/10.4	82/75			5–15	(4.2)		(3.8)	
12	13.8/11	83/76			4–13	(4.9)		(3.1)	
14B	14.2/12	84/77			4–13	(5)		(3)	
14G	14/11.5								
16B	14.8/12	85/78	30–36	0.8–2	4–13	2–7.5 (5)	0.04–.4	1.3–3.5	0.2–0.8
16G	14/11.5								
18B	15/13								

PART I
OBSTETRICS AND
GYNAECOLOGY

SECTION 1: ANTENATAL CARE AND MATERNAL MEDICINE

Questions

QUESTIONS

1. Antenatal screening

A nervous 42-year-old woman presents herself to your antenatal clinic very worried that she has missed the right time to have her combined test for Down's syndrome screening. She is now 17 weeks pregnant and is very concerned about her age. You counsel her about the appropriate alternative, the quadruple test and arrange to have this done. What assays make up the quadruple test?

A. AFP, PAPP-A, inhibin B and beta hCG
B. Unconjugated oestradiol, hCG, AFP and inhibin A
C. Beta hCG, PAPP-A, nuchal translucency and inhibin A
D. AFP, inhibin B, beta hCG and oestradiol
E. Unconjugated oestradiol, PAPP-A, beta hCG and inhibin A

2. Breast lumps in pregnancy

A 33-year-old nulliparous woman is 29 weeks pregnant. She was referred to the rapid access breast clinic for investigation of a solitary breast lump. Sadly, a biopsy of this lump revealed a carcinoma. After much counselling from the oncologists and her obstetricians a decision is reached on her further treatment. What option below may be available to her?

A. Tamoxifen
B. Computed tomography (CT) of the abdomen-pelvis
C. Radiotherapy
D. Chemotherapy
E. Bone isoptope scan to look for metastases in order to stage the disease

3. High risk antenatal care

A 38-year-old woman with type 2 diabetes attends the maternal medicine clinic. She has a body mass index (BMI) of 48 and is currently controlling her sugars with insulin. You have a long discussion about her weight. What should not be routinely offered to this woman?

A. Post-natal thromboprophylaxis
B. Vitamin C 10 mg once a day
C. Regular screening for pre-eclampsia
D. Referral to an obstetric anaesthetist
E. An active third stage of labour as increased risk of post-partum haemorrhage

4. Complications of pregnancy (1)

A nulliparous woman is seen at the antenatal clinic 27 weeks into her first pregnancy. Routine screening with a 75 g oral glucose tolerance test for gestational diabetes mellitus (GDM) is performed. Which of the following would confirm a diagnosis of GDM?

    A.   Fasting plasma venous glucose of greater than 5.0 μmol/L
    B.   2-hour plasma venous glucose of greater than 7.8 μmol/L
    C.   Random plasma venous glucose of greater than 4.8 μmol/L
    D.   2-hour plasma venous glucose of less than 7.0 μmol/L
    E.   2-hour plasma venous glucose of less than 7.8 μmol/L

5. Routine antenatal care

A 29-year-old woman is seen at her booking visit and has blood taken for screening. Which of these is the most appropriate set of booking tests?

    A.   Hepatitis C, human immunodeficiency virus (HIV), syphilis and toxoplasmosis
    B.   Rubella, hepatitis B, hepatitis C and syphilis
    C.   Syphilis, rubella, hepatitis B and HIV
    D.   HIV, cytomegalovirus, rubella and hepatitis B
    E.   HIV, syphilis, rubella and group B *Streptococcus*

6. Disorders of placentation

A 34-year-old woman attends antenatal clinic for a routine ultrasound scan. Abnormalities of placentation are detected and a magnetic resonance imaging (MRI) scan is organized by the fetal medicine consultant. The MRI report shows: 'The placenta is in the lower anterior uterine wall with evidence of invasion to the posterior wall of the bladder'. What is the most likely diagnosis?

    A.   Placenta accreta
    B.   Placenta percreta
    C.   Placenta increta
    D.   Placenta praevia
    E.   Ectopic pregnancy

7. Painless antenatal bleeding

A 30-year-old nulliparous woman is 29 weeks pregnant. She presented to hospital with a history of a minor, unprovoked painless vaginal bleed of about a teaspoonful. Her anomaly scan at 20 weeks showed a low-lying placenta. Her fetus is moving well and continuous cardiotocography (CTG) is reassuring. What is the most appropriate management?

A. Allow home since the bleed is small
B. Admit and give steroids
C. Admit, intravenous access, observe bleed-free for 48 hours before discharge
D. Admit, intravenous access, Group and Save and administer steroids if bleeds more →8mm
E. Group and Save, full blood count and allow home; review in clinic in a week

8. Rupture of membranes

A 28-year-old pregnant woman attends accident and emergency with a history of clear vaginal loss. She is 18 weeks pregnant and so far has had no problems. Her past medical history includes a large cone biopsy of the cervix and she is allergic to penicillin. She is worried because the fluid continues to come and there is now some blood. On examination it is apparent that her membranes have ruptured. What is the most appropriate initial management?

A. Discharge, ultrasound scan the next day
B. Offer her a termination as it is not possible for this pregnancy to continue
C. Admit, infection markers, ultrasound and steroids —2 weeks on.
D. Ultrasound, infection markers and observation
E. Discharge and explain that she will probably miscarry at home

9. Complications of pregnancy (2)

A 37-year-old woman in her fourth ongoing pregnancy presents to the labour ward at 34 weeks' gestation complaining of a sharp pain in her chest, worse on inspiration. An arterial blood gas shows: pH 7.51, PO_2 8.0 kPa, PCO_2 4.61 kPa, base excess 0.9. What is the most appropriate investigation?

A. Computed tomography pulmonary angiogram (CTPA)
B. MRI
C. D-dimer
D. Ventilation/perfusion scintigraphy
E. Ultrasound

10. Antenatal haemorrhage

A 32-year-old woman in her second pregnancy presents at 36 weeks gestation with a history of a passing gush of blood stained fluid from the vagina an hour ago, followed by a constant trickle since. The admitting obstetrician reviews her history and weekly antenatal ultrasound scans have shown a placenta praevia. What is the most appropriate management? She has a firm, posterior cervix and has not been experiencing any contractions.

A. Induction of labour with a synthetic oxytocin drip
B. Cervical ripening with prostaglandins followed by a synthetic oxytocin drip
C. Digital examination to assess the position of the fetus
D. Monitor for 24 hours and manage as for preterm pre-labour rupture of membranes (PPROM)
E. Caesarean delivery

11. Physiology of pregnancy

Maternal physiology changes throughout pregnancy to cope with the additional demands of carrying a fetus. Which of the following changes best represents a normal pregnancy?

A. Stroke volume increases by 10 per cent by the start of the third trimester
B. Plasma volume increases disproportionately to the change in red cell mass creating a relative anaemia
C. Plasma levels of fibrinogen fall, reaching a trough in the mid-trimester
D. Systemic arterial pressure rises to 10 mmHg above the baseline by term
E. Aortocaval compression reduces venous return to the heart, in turn increasing pulmonary arterial pressure

12. Contraception after pregnancy

A 30-year-old woman attends the antenatal clinic asking to be sterilized at the time of her elective caesarean. She is 34 weeks into her second pregnancy having had her first child 2 years ago via an emergency caesarean section. She is not sure that she wants any more children. Further more, she does not wish to try for a vaginal birth. She has tried the contraceptive pill in the past but does not like the side effects. You talk to her about other options, including the sterilization she is requesting. What is the best management option for this woman?

A. Mirena coil
B. Sterilization at the time of her caesarean section
C. T380 coil
D. Implanon
E. Vasectomy

13. Complications of pregnancy (3)

A 41-year-old multipara attends the antenatal clinic at 36 weeks gestation complaining of lower abdominal cramps and fatigue when mobilizing. Clinical examination is unremarkable save for a grade I pansystolic murmur, loudest over the fourth intercostal space in the midaxillary line. What is the most appropriate management?

A. Urgent outpatient echocardiogram and referral to a maternal–fetal medicine consultant
B. Reassurance and a 38-week antenatal clinic follow-up
C. Admission and work-up for cardiomyopathy
D. Post-natal referral to a cardiologist
E. Admission to the labour ward for induction of labour

14. Infection in pregnancy

A 32-year-old HIV positive woman who booked for antenatal care at 28 weeks gestation arrives on the delivery suite at 37 weeks with painful regular contractions and a cervix dilated to 4 cm. Ultrasonography confirms a breech singleton pregnancy with a reactive fetal heart rate. What is the most appropriate management option?

A. Await onset of labour, avoid operative delivery, wash the baby at delivery
B. Induce labour with synthetic prostaglandins
C. Await onset of labour, but have a low threshold for expediting vaginal delivery using forceps
D. Await onset of labour, avoid operative delivery, administer steroids to the infant immediately after birth
E. Caesarean delivery, wash the baby at delivery

15. Complications of pregnancy (4)

A 41-year-old multiparous woman attends accident and emergency at 32 weeks gestation complaining of sudden onset shortness of breath. A CTPA demonstrates a large saddle embolus. What is the most appropriate treatment regimen?

A. Load with warfarin to achieve a target international normalized ratio (INR) of 3.0
B. Load with warfarin to achieve a target international normalized ratio (INR) of 2.5
C. Load with warfarin to achieve a target international normalized ratio (INR) of 20
D. 80 mg enoxaparin twice daily
E. 7.5 mg fondaparinux once daily

16. Antepartum haemorrhage

A 21-year-old woman attends the labour ward with per vaginal bleeding of 100 mL. She is 32 weeks pregnant and has had one normal delivery in the past. An important history to note is that of an antepartum haemorrhage in her last pregnancy and she smokes 10 cigarettes a day. Her 20-week anomaly ultrasound revealed a posterior fundal placenta. She admits she and her partner had intercourse last night and is concerned by terrible abdominal pains. What is the most likely diagnosis?

A. Vasa praevia
B. Placenta praevia
C. Placenta accreta
D. Placental abruption
E. Cervical ectropion

17. Rhesus isoimmunization

At a booking visit a first time mother is told that she is rhesus negative. Which of these answers is the most appropriate advice for the mother?

A. It is important to have anti-D as it will make sure your baby does not develop antibodies
B. If you have any bleeding before 12 weeks be sure to get an injection of anti-D
C. Anti-D will stop your body creating antibodies to your baby's blood that may help protect the health of your next child
D. If your partner is rhesus negative you do not need to have anti-D
E. You need one injection that will cover your pregnancy even if you have episodes of vaginal bleeding

18. Antepartum haemorrhage

A 42-year-old para 4 with a dichorionic–diamniotic (DCDA) twin pregnancy at 31 weeks gestation presents to hospital with a painful per vaginam bleed of 400 mL. The bleeding seems to be slowing. She is cardiovascularly stable, although having abdominal pains every 10 minutes. There is still a small active bleed on speculum and the cervix appears closed. Both fetuses have reactive CTGs. She has had no problems antenatally and her 28-week ultrasound revealed both placentas to be well away from the cervix. What is your preferred management plan?

A. Admit to antenatal ward, ABC, IV access, Group and Save, CTG, steroids, consider expediting delivery
B. Reassure and ask to come back to clinic next week if there are any problems
C. Admit for observation, IV access
D. Admit to labour ward, ABC, IV access, full blood count, cross-match 4 units of blood, CTG, steroids, consider expediting delivery
E. As bleeding settled and placenta not low, offer admission but arrange follow-up if refused

19. Seizures in pregnancy

You are the FY1 covering the antenatal ward. A 27-year-old nulliparous woman who is 36 weeks and 5 days pregnant has been admitted to your ward with suspected pre-eclampsia. The emergency buzzer goes off in her room. You are the first to attend and find your patient flat on the bed having a generalized seizure – what do you do?

A. Call for help, ABC, nasopharyngeal airway, IV access and wait for fit to stop
B. Call for help, ABC, protect her airway, prepare for grade 1 caesarean section
C. Call for help, ABC, left lateral tilt, wait for seizure to end, listen in to fetus
D. Call for help, ABC, left lateral tilt, protect airway, prepare magnesium
E. Call for help, ABC, protect airway, prepare magnesium, check blood pressure

20. Thrombocytopenia

A 38-year-old woman in her first pregnancy is 36 weeks pregnant. She presents to the labour ward feeling dizzy with a mild headache and flashing lights. Her past medical history includes systemic lupus erythematosus (SLE), renal stones and malaria. Her blood pressure is 158/99 mmHg with 2+ protein in her urine. Her platelets are 55×10^9/L, Hb 10.1 g/dL, bilirubin 62 µmol/L, ALT 359 IU/L, urea 2.3 mmol/L and creatinine 64 µmol/L. What is the most likely diagnosis?

A. Thrombotic thrombocytopenic purpura (TTP)
B. HELLP syndrome
C. Idiopathic thrombocytopenic purpura (ITP)
D. Systemic lupus erythematosus (SLE)
E. HIV

21. Vertical infections

A 19-year-old woman in her first pregnancy presents to the GUM clinic with an outbreak of primary herpes simplex infection on her labia. She is 33 weeks pregnant. What is the best advice regarding her herpes?

A. Aciclovir from 36 weeks until delivery
B. Caesarean section should be performed if she labours within the next 8 weeks
C. Reassure as the infection will pass and pose no further concern
D. If she labours within 6 weeks, a caesarean should be recommended
E. Aciclovir for 10 days and an elective caesarean at 39 weeks

22. Antenatal care (1)

A 33-year-old woman presents to hospital with a 2-day history of itching on the soles of her feet and the palms of her hands. Her pregnancy has been straightforward and she has good fetal movements. Liver function tests reveal an alanine transaminase (ALT) of 64 IU/L and bile acids of 30 µmol/L. You suspect that she might have developed obstetric cholestasis. Which of the following bits of advice is true?

A. She could have intermittent monitoring in labour
B. Ultrasound and CTG surveillance help prevent stillbirth
C. Poor outcomes can be predicted by bile acid levels
D. Ursodeoxycholic acid (UDCA) helps prevent stillbirth
E. Meconium stained liquor is more common in labour

23. Headaches in pregnancy

A 24-year-old woman who is 32 weeks pregnant presents to the labour ward with a terrible headache that has not improved despite analgesia. It started 2 days ago and came on suddenly. She has stayed in bed as it hurts to be in sunlight and she vomited twice this morning. Her past medical history includes a macroprolactinoma (which has been removed) and occasional migraines. She is haemodynamically stable with no focal neurology or papilloedema. You arrange for her to have a CT of her head as an emergency, which adds no further information to aid your diagnosis. There are red cells on lumbar puncture but no organisms are isolated. What is the most likely diagnosis?

    A. Migraine
    B. Viral meningitis
    C. Cerebral vein thrombosis (CVT)
    D. Subarachnoid haemorrhage (SAH)
    B. Idiopathic intracranial hypertension (IIH)

24. Antenatal care (2)

A 19-year-old woman in her first pregnancy is admitted to the labour ward with a 4-hour history of lower abdominal pain – she is 22 weeks pregnant. She has not had any vaginal bleeding but describes a possible history of rupture of her membranes. Her past medical history includes an appendectomy and a large cone biopsy of her cervix. On examination she has palpable lower abdominal tenderness, her cervix is 2 cm dilated, she has an offensive vaginal discharge and her temperature is 38.9°C. Her white cell count is 19.0×10^9/L and her C-reactive protein is 188 mg/L. There are no signs of cardiovascular compromise. How would you manage this woman?

    A. Insert a cervical suture
    B. 12 mg betamethasone, atosiban for tocolysis and antibiotics
    C. Head down, bed rest, antibiotics and await events
    D. Antibiotics and induce labour
    E. Caesarean section

25. Antenatal care (3)

A 24-year-old multiparous woman is 23 weeks pregnant. She has not had chicken pox before. She goes to a collect her 3-year-old son from a birthday party and comes into contact with a child with an infective chicken pox infection. She is naturally very anxious. What is the best course of management?

    A. Wait and see if she develops a rash. If she does treat with aciclovir
    B. Test for varicella antibodies and give varicella zoster immunoglobulin (VZIG) within the first 24 hours
    C. Test for varicella antibodies and give aciclovir within the first 24 hours
    D. Test for varicella antibodies and give VZIG within 10 days
    E. Reassure that there is no significant risk at present as contact was so brief

26. Breech presentation

A 32-year-old woman in her third pregnancy is 37 weeks pregnant and has an extended breech baby on ultrasound. After discussion in the antenatal clinic, which of the following is not an absolute contraindication to an external cephalic version (ECV)?

- A. Multiple pregnancy
- B. Major uterine abnormality
- C. Antepartum haemorrhage within 7 days
- D. Rupture of membranes
- E. Small for gestational age with abnormal Doppler scan

27. Diabetes mellitus in pregnancy (1)

A 24-year-old type 1 diabetic woman has just had her first baby delivered by caesarean section at 35 weeks due to fetal macrosomia and poor blood sugar control. The operation is straightforward with no complications. She has an insulin sliding scale running when you review her on the ward 12 hours postoperatively. She has begun to eat and drink. How would you manage her insulin requirements?

- A. Continue the sliding scale for 24 hours
- B. Change her back to her pre-pregnancy insulin and stop the sliding scale
- C. Halve the dose of insulin with each meal for the next 48 hours
- D. Stop the insulin now that baby is delivered
- E. Sliding scale for 48 hours to prevent hyperglycaemia

28. Maternal medicine

A 19-year-old woman is referred to your pre-conception clinic. She has SLE and wants to fall pregnant. She is currently not on any treatment and has no symptoms. As part of your general counselling you should talk about the risks associated with pregnancy. Which of the following is not a particular risk to a woman with SLE?

- A. Fetal growth restriction
- B. Diabetes mellitus
- C. Pre-eclampsia
- D. Stillbirth
- E. Preterm delivery

29. Antenatal care (4)

A 44-year-old women who is 18 weeks pregnant presents to your clinic with a 2-day history of a viral illness. She is extremely anxious and is in floods of tears. She recently had some soft cheese in a restaurant and after an internet search she is convinced she has a particular infection. What infection is she concerned about?

    A.   Toxoplasmosis
    B.   Cytomegalovirus (CMV)
    C.   *Listeria monocytogenes*
    D.   Hepatitis E
    E.   Parvovirus B 19

30. Rashes in pregnancy

A 26-year-old woman is 37 weeks pregnant and consults you about a rash that started on her abdomen and has now spread all over her body. Interestingly her umbilicus is spared. The rash is very itchy and nothing is helping. The rash is her first problem in this pregnancy. Of interest, her mother has pemphigoid and her sister has psoriasis. What is the most likely cause of her rash?

    A.   Pemphigoid gestationis
    B.   Pruritic urticarial papules and plaques of pregnancy (PUPP)
    C.   Impetigo herpetiformis
    D.   Prurigo gestationis
    E.   Contact dermatitis

31. Medication in pregnancy

Which of the following drugs is not absolutely contraindicated in pregnancy?

    A.   Acitretin
    B.   Fluconazole
    C.   Mebendazole
    D.   Sodium valproate
    E.   Methotrexate

32. Hypertension in pregnancy

A 42-year-old woman is in her first pregnancy. She conceived with *in vitro* fertilization (IVF) and has had a straightforward pregnancy so far. At 25 weeks' gestation she is seen in clinic with a blood pressure of 142/94 mmHg and protein + in her urine. A protein creatinine ratio (PCR) comes back as 19. She says that her blood pressure is often up at the doctor's. With the information you have to hand what is the most likely diagnosis?

    A.   Pre-eclampsia
    B.   White coat hypertension
    C.   Essential hypertension
    D.   Conn's syndrome
    E.   Pregnancy-induced hypertension

33. Diabetes mellitus in pregnancy (2)

A 24-year-old woman attends the antenatal clinic. She has had a glucose tolerance test which is abnormal. A diagnosis of gestational diabetes is made. The primary purpose of this appointment is to explain to her what gestational diabetes means to her and her baby. You explain to her that sugar control is important and there are specific glucose ranges that she should try to adhere to. Which of the following would be correct advice for this woman?

    A.   Pre meal blood sugar <7.1 µmol/L
    B.   Post meal 1-hour sugar <11.1 µmol/L
    C.   Post meal 1-hour sugar <7.8 µmol/L
    D.   Post meal 2-hour blood sugar <7.8 µmol/L
    E.   Pre meal blood sugar <7.8 µmol/L

34. Gestational diabetes

A 24-year-old woman in her first pregnancy has a significantly raised glucose tolerance test at 28 weeks gestation: 4.6 fasting 12.1 at one hour 9.1 at 2 hours (µmol/L). She is given the diagnosis of GDM. You are asked to counsel her about the effects of gestational diabetes on pregnancy. Which of the following is not an additional effect of having GDM?

    A.   Shoulder dystocia with a macrosomic fetus
    B.   Stillbirth
    C.   Neonatal hypoglycaemia
    D.   10 per cent chance of developing type 2 diabetes over the next 10 years
    E.   Pre-eclampsia

35. HIV in pregnancy

A 24-year-old woman who is HIV positive is in her first pregnancy. She is 39 weeks pregnant and is seen by you in the antenatal clinic. She has just transferred to your care, with no other previous antenatal care. She reports that her pregnancy has been uncomplicated. Her CD4 count is 180/mm^3 and her viral load is 5500 copies/mL. She has come to find out what advice you have for her delivery.

    A.   Spontaneous vaginal delivery
    B.   Induction of labour to prevent CD4 decreasing
    C.   Caesarean section
    D.   Start highly active antiretroviral therapy (HAART) and await for labour to start
    E.   Start HAART, amniotomy and HAART for baby when born

ANSWERS

Antenatal screening

1 B Down's syndrome screening is offered to all pregnant women in the UK. She is 42 which gives you an age-related risk of one in 55 of having a child with Down's syndrome. Early in the second trimester the combined test is offered. This includes an ultrasound scan of the fetal neck looking at the nuchal translucency (NT) and two blood tests – PAPP-A and beta hCG. This can be reliably performed from 10 to 13 weeks. Ideally, an integrated test using the combined test and the quadruple test can be used to create a Down's risk. As she has missed the chance to have an NT, she would only be offered the quadruple test, which is unconjugated oestradiol, total hCG, AFP and inhibin A – Answer (B). The downside of the quadruple test is that it has a 4.4 per cent false-positive rate compared with 2.2 per cent for the combined test and only 1 per cent for the integrated test. In the event of a high risk result, this woman would be offered an amniocentesis to exclude Down's syndrome and other chromosome abnormalities.

Breast lumps in pregnancy

2 D This is difficult to answer as it depends on how aggressive the cancer is. There may be a need for delivery but it would not be immediate as she is only 29 weeks pregnant. You would give a course of betamethasone in order to promote fetal lung maturity prior to delivery. Tamoxifen (A) is not safe in pregnancy and breastfeeding because of the high risk of teratogenicity. Radiotherapy (C) is contraindicated in pregnancy unless it is as a life-saving option. All chemotherapy is potentially teratogenic in the first trimester but may used in the mid- and third trimesters. Ideally birth should be 2–3 weeks after the most recent chemotherapy session to allow bone marrow regeneration. Bone isotope scans (E) and CT of the abdomen and pelvis (B) are likely to provide insufficient clinical value to warrant the high dose of radiation that the fetus would be exposed to.

High risk antenatal care

3 B Obesity is an increasing problem for healthcare providers. The number of women falling pregnant who have a BMI >30 kg/m² (obese) is increasing year on year. The rate of increase of morbidly obese and super morbidly obese women falling pregnant is dramatic. The Confidential Enquiries into maternal deaths informs us that a disproportionate number of mothers who die are obese. Ideally, pre-conception advice is key for these women; this should include weight loss and high-dose (5 mg) folic acid supplementation. This woman is already diabetic but those who are not need to be screened for diabetes. Venous thromboembolism risk is high in pregnancy anyway due to the increased coagulability of the maternal blood. That risk increases massively in women who are morbidly obese **(A)** so all obese women should be offered mechanical and pharmaceutical thromboprophylaxis. Vitamin D 10 mg once a day is recommended for all women with a BMI >30, not vitamin C. Obese patients pose particular difficulties to the anaesthetist and the risks of failed regional anaesthesia and intubation, should a general anaesthetic be necessary, are much higher than for women of normal BMI: it is wise to offer obese women an antenatal anaesthetic review (D). Obese women have a higher risk of post-partum haemorrhage, so an actively managed third stage (the use of syntometrine and controlled cord traction at delivery) is routine (E).

Complications of pregnancy

4 B   Between 2 and 5 per cent of pregnancies in the UK are complicated by diabetes, of which 85 per cent are gestational. Diabetes is associated with maternal and fetal risks. Risk factors include high BMI, previous macrosomic baby, previous history of GDM, family history of diabetes and ethnicity. Routine antenatal screening in Britain follows NICE and WHO guidance. Those women at risk of GDM should be tested using a 75 g oral glucose tolerance test (OGTT), where the fasted woman is given a 75 g oral load of glucose and has a venous plasma glucose level tested at 2 hours. The WHO definition of gestational diabetes encompasses both impaired glucose tolerance (2-hour glucose greater than or equal to 7.8 μmol/L **(B)**) and diabetes (random glucose greater than or equal to 7.0 μmol/L or 2-hour glucose greater than or equal to 7.8 μmol/L). The other answer options are therefore not correct.

Routine antenatal care

5 C   The serum tests for infection that NICE recommend as an offer at booking are syphilis, HIV, hepatitis B and rubella (C). Cytomegalovirus (D) is a DNA virus that usually leads to asymptomatic infection. Transmission to the fetus leading to damage occurs in about 10 per cent of cases. Forty to 50 per cent of all women of childbearing age have not had cytomegalovirus infection so it is not cost effective to screen everyone. Toxoplasmosis is contracted from such things as undercooked/cured meat and cat faeces. It is not routinely tested for in pregnancy as the low risk of toxoplasmosis (A) becoming a florid infection rather than an indolent disease in a non-immunocompromised infection makes it not worthwhile. It is not cost effective to test for hepatitis C (B).

Disorders of placentation

6 B   Placenta praevia (D), where the placenta attaches to the uterine wall close to or overlying the cervical opening, afflicts one in 200 pregnancies. Placenta accreta (A) is firm adhesion of the placenta to the uterine wall without extending through the full myometrium, as occurs in placenta increta (C). If the placenta invades the full thickness of the myometrium and beyond it, it is called placenta percreta (B). Risk factors for placenta accreta (and increta and percreta) include the presence of uterine scar tissue, which may be seen in Asherman's syndrome after uterine cavity surgery, for example dilatation and curettage. It is postulated that a thin decidua – the uterine cavity lining in pregnancy which is formed under the influence of progesterone – can encourage abnormal placentation. Although the case in this question may represent one example of placenta praevia owing to the placenta's proximity to the cervical opening, it is more likely to be an example of placenta percreta here, given the invasion of the bladder. Ectopic pregnancy (E) may rarely carry to late pregnancy, leading to trophic invasion of the bladder, but in such cases an extrauterine pregnancy would be clearly demonstrated on ultrasound scanning.

Painless antenatal bleeding

7 D   Bleeding in pregnancy is a very common complaint. It can range from trivial to life threatening. The two main things to rule out are a placental abruption and placenta praevia. We know that this woman at 20 weeks had a placenta praevia. Abruptions tend to lead to painful bleeding. Small bleeds can precede very big bleeds so this woman should be admitted to hospital for observation and an ultrasound arranged the next day for placental localization. Therefore, (A) and (E) are incorrect. There is debate whether steroids should be given for small antepartum bleeds in a haemodynamically stable woman. In this case, it would be reasonable to wait to see if the bleeding returns before instigating a course of steroids, so (B) is not the most appropriate management. If the bleeding ceases and the woman otherwise remains well, there is no need to keep her in hospital for 48 hours (C) with the attendant risks (risk of hospital-acquired infections and venous thromboembolism associated with immobility).

Rupture of membranes

8 D   This is a very traumatic and frightening experience for any woman. Her large cervical cone biopsy is a risk factor for second trimester miscarriage. The outlook for this pregnancy is very poor if rupture of membranes is confirmed: most pregnancies at this gestation are lost if the membranes rupture. However, it would be inappropriate to offer termination (B) at this stage until there was definitive evidence of ruptured membranes, or if the mother requested it. This woman needs to be admitted to hospital for observation. She needs investigating to rule out infection – ensuring there is no leukocytosis, rising C-reactive protein or growth on a mid-stream urinary culture – along with regular observations. The main concern is that she is at risk of developing sepsis from the prolonged rupture of membranes. Owing to the risk to the mother of ascending infection, chorioamnionitis and thus generalized sepsis, this woman should not be discharged so options (A) and (E) are incorrect. It may well be that this woman will become septic and in order to save her life she will need to be induced, but while she remains well this is not the first step. She is ≤24 weeks gestation so she should not be given steroids (C) for fetal lung maturity. An ultrasound will help add weight to your clinical diagnosis if no liquor is seen but ultrasound alone is not diagnostic. Very occasionally women with preterm rupture do not become septic or spontaneously miscarry. If she gets to 24 weeks there may be a case for steroids although there may well be additional factors for lung hypoplasia with the fetus having developed in an environment without much liquor.

Complications of pregnancy

9 D This patient has a respiratory alkalosis and is hypoxic. Coupled with her clinical presentation, it is imperative to immediately rule out a pulmonary embolism. Venous thromboembolism remains one of the largest causes of maternal mortality in the developed world, and preventing it remains a focus of modern obstetric practice. Imaging in pregnancy aims to deliver the highest diagnostic value for the lowest dose of ionizing radiation. Ultrasound (E) has little value in the investigation of pulmonary embolism and MRI scanning is unhelpful in showing the vascular abnormalities present in pulmonary embolism. D-Dimer (C) is normally raised after the first trimester of pregnancy, and in any case is only of predictive value and not diagnostic importance. This patient requires urgent definitive diagnosis, and only CTPA (A) or ventilation/perfusion (V/Q) (D) scanning will suffice. Of these, a V/Q scan exposes the patient to by far the lowest radiation dose, and is thus the preferred investigation in pregnant women.

Antenatal haemorrhage

10 E The gush of fluid followed by a steady trickle suggests ruptured membranes. At 36 weeks gestation she is technically preterm, and this combined with an absence of contractions indicates PPROM. This woman also has a placenta praevia, which indicates that the placenta is low-lying. As soon as the candidate realises this, it is clear that a vaginal delivery is not possible. Therefore, options (A) and (B) are immediately incorrect as these management options aim for an end-result of vaginal delivery. Digital assessment of a patient with antepartum haemorrhage is contraindicated (C) unless a diagnosis of preterm labour has been made; this is to reduce the risk of infection. We are therefore left with either caesarean delivery or managing conservatively as PPROM (D). Management of PPROM involves the use of a 10-day course of antibiotic prophylaxis against chorioamnionitis, steroids to aid fetal lung maturation before the 34th week, and expectant management until 34 weeks gestation. The RCOG recommends that a patient with PPROM should be delivered between 34 and 36 weeks gestation. This woman's pregnancy is in its 36th week and so delivery should be expedited. With a placenta praevia, the only feasible mode of delivery is caesarean section (E).

Physiology of pregnancy

11 B Understanding the physiological changes of pregnancy is vital to the recognition of pathology. There is a marked increase in fibrinogen, as well as factors VII, X and XII throughout pregnancy (C). Stroke volume increases from the first trimester and is over 30 per cent higher than in the non-pregnant state by the third trimester (A). Although there are often changes in the maternal blood pressure in pregnancy, largely due to changes in peripheral vascular resistance, neither the systemic (D) nor the pulmonary arterial pressures (E) alter. The gravid uterus does cause aortocaval compression, but this does not affect the pulmonary circulation. Haemodilution, caused by a relative increase in the plasma volume compared to the red cell mass, causes a reduction in haemoglobin concentration (B).

Contraception after pregnancy

12 C This woman has come to you asking for a permanent solution to not falling pregnant. It is important to find out why she wants a sterilization at 30 years old. It is imperative to explain that it is permanent, irreversible, has a failure rate of one in 200 and, if it fails, an increased risk of ectopic pregnancy. You must explore all long-acting reversible contraceptive methods with her, these being the Mirena coil, copper coil (T380) implanon and depoprovera IM injections. If she is sure that hormones (A, D) have a bad effect on her then the copper coil would be appropriate for her. This would leave her with the chance to have further children if she changes her mind or there is an unforeseen change in her circumstances. A vasectomy (E) is a very successful contraceptive method but it is a decision her partner would need to be here to discuss and to make, so in these circumstances it is not the most appropriate option. If she understands all the options and still wants a sterilization (B) it would be worth her having a second opinion before agreeing to it as it should be viewed as an irreversible procedure and one not without risk.

Complications of pregnancy

13 B This question tests the candidate's ability to distinguish physiological sequelae of normal pregnancy from more worrying features. In pregnancy, a soft systolic flow murmur is frequently audible on auscultation of the praecordium due to dilatation across the tricuspid valve causing mild regurgitant flow. Such a flow murmur is physiological and will disappear after delivery. Furthermore, the increasing size of the gravid uterus displaces the heart upwards and to the left. Mild abdominal pains and fatigue are common, particularly in the later stages of pregnancy. The woman in this case is experiencing normal pregnancy, and no specific treatment is necessary (B). Induction is not indicated in normal pregnancy at this gestation (E). Preterm induction of labour is offered to women for whom the maternal and fetal risks of continuing pregnancy outweigh the benefits associated with delivery at a later gestation (e.g. fetal maturation). Investigating physiological murmurs which pose no maternal or fetal risk may cause the mother unnecessary alarm (A, C, D). Maternal echocardiography (A) may be relevant if there was suspicion of structural heart disease (e.g. cardiomyopathy) or valvular disease (e.g. aortic steonsis in order to assess the patient's capacity to cope with the stress on the heart during labour, and in particular the second stage of labour.

Infection in pregnancy

14 E Although knowledge of managing HIV positive pregnant women is beyond the scope of most undergraduate curricula, in this question the presence of HIV infection is largely a distractor. Delivery of HIV positive women aims to lower the risk of vertical transmission and reduce morbidity. Washing the baby shortly after delivery is a part of that strategy. Induction of labour (B) is not indicated unless there is a benefit to expediting delivery, which in the vignette above there is not. Interventions which increase the risk of maternal/fetal blood transfusion (and therefore vertical transmission), such as amniocentesis, fetal blood sampling or forceps delivery, are avoided in HIV positive women so (C) is incorrect. Giving neonates steroids (D) is not warranted here for any reason. (A) and (E) could both be correct if the woman had a cephalic singleton delivery. However, this woman is at term, not in established labour and has a breech singleton pregnancy. Following publication of the planned vaginal versus caesarean delivery trial in 2000, which demonstrated improved fetal outcomes with caesarean delivery, most centres now exclusively offer elective caesarean section for these mothers. Hence, even if the woman was not HIV pregnancy, (E) would remain the single best answer.

Complications of pregnancy

15 D This woman requires treatment for pulmonary embolism. She is in the third trimester of pregnancy, which is when wafarin is contraindicated (A, B, C). Warfarin is a teratogen, although its use has different effects depending on the gestation of the fetus. Use in the first trimester confers the most risk of teratogenicity, and is associated with fetal warfarin syndrome, a constellation of symptoms comprising nasal hypoplasia, vertebral calcinosis and brachydactyly. The risk of teratogenicity with warfarin use in the mid- and third trimesters is reduced but evidence exists to show a chance of cerebral malformations and ophthalmic disorders.

Although both enoxaparin (Clexane) (D) and fondaparinux (Arixtra) (E) are both indicated in the treatment of pulmonary embolism, evidence of efficacy and safety in pregnancy only exists for enoxaparin: this is the agent used in the UK for the treatment of pulmonary embolism in pregnancy. Recognizing and treating pulmonary embolism in pregnancy is particularly important since it is one of the largest killers of mothers, as reported in the Confidential Enquiry into Maternal and Child Health.

Antepartum haemorrhage

16 D This woman gives a worrying history of painful vaginal bleeding. Vasa praevia (A) is rare and occurs at the time of rupture of membranes, presenting as a painless bleed associated with sudden fetal compromise and not infrequently intrauterine demise. Placenta praevia (B) characteristically presents as a painless bleed. In this case we know the placenta is not low so this is not the answer. Placenta accreta (C) is a diagnosis of an adherent placenta which may be made on attempting to deliver the placenta post-partum. Placenta accreta is commonly associated with a previous caesarean section scar but can be present in an unscarred uterus. Intercourse can lead to vaginal bleeding as a result of contact with the cervix. A cervical ectropion (E), which is common in pregnancy, is a cause of vaginal bleeding but would not lead to abdominal pains. This woman is most likely having a placental abruption (D) – a separation of the placenta from the wall of the uterus. Risk factors include a previous abruption, smoking, a growth restricted baby and hypertension. Classically, the presentation is of a painful vaginal bleed. Abruptions can be life threatening to both mother and child.

Rhesus isoimmunization

17 C The basis of this question is rhesus isoimmunization. If a rhesus negative mother is carrying a rhesus positive baby and then has a feto-maternal transfer of blood, the mother's immune system will respond to the fetal cells (sensitization). The mother will create anti-D antibodies. The problem arises in any subsequent pregnancy if she has a rhesus positive fetus. The anti-D antibodies will cross the placenta and attack the fetal red blood cells causing a haemolytic anaemia. (A) is wrong as it has no effect on this pregnancy. There is no need to have anti-D before 12 weeks gestation (B). Theoretically, if the woman's partner is rhesus negative their child will be rhesus negative (D). However, with possibly one in 10 partners not being the real father it would be prudent to advise all women to have the anti-D (avoiding accusing them of infidelity). National guidance now is to have one injection of 1500 IU at 28 weeks gestation but if there are sensitizing events such as vaginal bleeding, abdominal trauma or an external cephalic version the mother will need further doses (E). By elimination, (C) is therefore the best option.

Antepartum haemorrhage

18   D   There are serious concerns about this woman. She continues to have a significant per vaginam bleed in keeping with a placental abruption. She is not in labour and both twins have normal CTGs. It would be wrong to let this woman go home. She may well need to be delivered urgently by caesarean section. Answers (A) and (D) provide the most logical course of management, the only difference being that, in (D), that you are anticipating the very real prospect of this woman needing a blood transfusion and delivery. She should be admitted to your high risk area (i.e. labour ward). Initial assessment should involve a cardiovascular review, IV access, full blood count and cross-match for 4 units of blood. Continuous CTG should be in place and antenatal steroids should be commenced as while the patient bleeds the fetuses are at risk. If delivery is imminent, the steroids will not have enough time to affect fetal lung maturity. It is imperative that you involve the consultant obstetrician, anaesthetist, paediatricians and senior midwife as early as possible. Answers (B) and (C) confirm that the doctor has not grasped the seriousness of the situation. Twin pregnancies are at an increased risk of abruption. This woman should not be allowed to go home (E) as her life is in danger. (D) would be the most appropriate answer from the above.

Seizures in pregnancy

19   D   Your first suspicion should be that this woman is having an eclamptic fit. This is a potentially life-threatening situation. You will need help as soon as possible. Calling for help, lying the woman flat and tilting her onto her left are the first steps; therefore (C) and (D) are the best answers in an obstetric emergency. You need to protect her airway but insertion of an additional airway (A) in an actively fitting woman would be difficult and potentially dangerous. Also, obtaining IV access while someone is fitting is not safe. Option (B) may well be what happens but in the first instance you need to stabilize the mother and not be preparing to operate yourself. The airway, breathing, circulation approach is a sensible reliable method of leading through this emergency. Tilting onto the left will relieve any aortocaval compression and stop the woman choking if she vomits. The mother must be your primary concern so until the seizure has stopped and the cause of her seizure – likely a raised blood pressure – is controlled, it is prudent not to try and monitor the fetus. This is why answer (C) is not the best course of action as the mother should have her BP checked before checking the fetal heart. This is because even if there is evidence of fetal distress it is not possible to deliver the fetus until the mother is stable. Magnesium sulphate is used as a cerebral membrane stabilizer and should be given as soon as possible. Once the seizure has finished you will need to re-check her airway, breathing and circulation and then monitor the fetus. Option (E) is in fact a good answer but it is important not to forget to put a pregnant woman into a tilt with a wedge or a pillow, even when fitting. Answer (D) is the most appropriate answer.

Thrombocytopenia

20 B TTP can occur at any time in pregnancy and is characterized with a pentad of microangiopathic haemolytic anaemia, thrombocytopenia, fever, neurological involvement and renal impairment (A). There is evidence of haemolysis here but her renal function is normal. ITP is caused by autoantibodies against platelet surface antigens and is a diagnosis of exclusion (C). SLE (D) is a multisystem connective tissue disorder that can show haemolytic anaemia and thrombocytopenia. HIV (E) can cause a thrombocytopenia. It is likely that this woman has been tested for HIV as it forms part of the routine tests offered to mothers at booking. This woman appears to have developed HELLP syndrome (B) – a variant of pre-eclampsia. It is characterized by haemolysis, elevated liver enzymes and low platelets. She has symptomatic pre-eclampsia so answer (B) is the most likely cause.

Vertical infections

21 D If primary herpes develops in pregnancy it is imperative to consider risk of vertical transmission. If the herpes presents at the time of delivery or within 6 weeks of the due date a caesarean is the safest mode of delivery (D). If she labours within 6 weeks (not 8 weeks) of developing primary herpes she should consider a caesarean (B). If she refuses to have a caesarean then IV aciclovir during labour and close liaison with the neonatologist is recommended. Neonatal herpes is rare at one in 60000 but can lead to encephalitis, hepatitis and disseminated skin lesions. There is no evidence that aciclovir in the antenatal period decreases the chance of fetal infection – (A) and (E). You can reassure the woman (C) but only if she delivers after 6 weeks when the herpes should have cleared. It would be wrong to tell her that all will be well regardless of the timing of delivery.

Antenatal care

22 E Obstetric cholestasis is characterized by itching and deranged liver function, especially an elevated bile acid level (above 20 µmol/L). Once diagnosed, liver function should be checked weekly. The main concern is that of stillbirth so most clinicians recommend inducing patients between 37 and 38 weeks gestation. There is no way of predicting stillbirth (B). Preterm labour is more likely as well as meconium stained liquor in labour (E). UDCA is unlicensed but has been used for a long time and has no apparent side effects. It helps to treat the pruritis and reduce the bile acid level but there is no data to suggest it helps reduce stillbirths (D). There is no direct link between the level of bile acids and the outcome of the pregnancy (C). Obstetric cholestasis may increase fetal risk CTCG, so continuous CTG, not intermittent (A), is advised.

Headaches in pregnancy

23 A This in fact is very difficult as all five could be the cause for this headache. Migraines (A) are common, especially in pregnancy, even without a history of previous migraines. The concern here is that, although the symptoms could fit with a migraine, you need to consider other diagnoses. Subarachnoid haemorrhage (D) has a very sudden onset. In addition to the presenting symptoms there is often papilloedema and focal neurology. The negative CT result does not completely exclude SAH. A lumbar puncture would help diagnosis, looking for blood, bilirubin or xanthochromia in the cerebrospinal fluid. A CVT (C) classically presents post-partum. It has similar symptoms but up to two-thirds will have neurological deficit. MRI is generally a better imaging modality but is often not available out of hours. IIH (E) characteristically occurs in young obese women. It is a headache associated with papilloedema and raised intracranial pressure without CT or MRI evidence of hydrocephalus or a space occupying lesion. Viral meningitis (B) would classically give a fever as well as headache, vomiting, photophobia and neck stiffness. It is likely that a migraine is the most likely cause of her symptoms but it is important to remember that people with an acute onset of headache could have much more serious pathology.

Antenatal care

24 D This woman is unwell with sepsis. The history of possible ruptured membranes, offensive vaginal discharge, abdominal pain and a temperature point towards a diagnosis of chorioamnionitis. Inserting a rescue cerclage (A) is contraindicated in the presence of infection. She is 22 weeks pregnant and thus the fetus is not viable, which means she should not receive antenatal steroids (B). Tocolysis is contraindicated as she has septic chorioamnionitis. This woman needs to have antibiotics (D) to treat her infection and more importantly needs to have labour induced in order to remove the nidus of infection – the pregnancy. This is a very difficult scenario to deal with as obviously this is the last thing that the mother wants to do. In light of the gestation and how unwell the mother is, induction is the most appropriate course of action. Watchful waiting under antibiotic cover would not be appropriate (C). A caesarean section (E) or hysterotomy at this gestation should be avoided.

Antenatal care

25 D Mothers who have not had chicken pox are at risk of developing the disease in pregnancy. Pregnant women tend to be affected much worse if they contract chicken pox. Also, if chicken pox is contracted before 28 weeks gestation there is the risk of fetal varicella syndrome (eye defects, hypoplasia of limbs and neurological defects). This woman has had a significant contact with chicken pox and the fact that her child has been with the infected child means that he may well now be about to develop chicken pox. Waiting is simply not a sensible option (A) as she is at risk of developing chicken pox herself and potentially developing fetal varicella syndrome. Although the mother thinks that she has never had chicken pox she may have had a previous subclinical or unknown childhood infection, so if she has antibodies no further action is necessary. Aciclovir can be used to treat chicken pox within 24 hours of the rash appearing so does not need to be started straight away (C). The appropriate management here is for VZIG to be administered (on consultation with the blood products laboratory as it may be in short supply) (D) if her antibody screen is negative. This situation will make mothers very anxious and they will want VZIG straight away, which is not appropriate as her antibodies will not be back yet (B). The Health Protection Agency advises that VZIG may be given within 10 days of exposure. Answer (E) is not appropriate as you are not taking any steps to find out whether this mother is at risk.

Breech presentation

26 E ECV is offered from 36 weeks in first time mothers and from 37 weeks in multiparous women. Answer (E) is only a relative contraindication along with pre-eclampsia, a scarred uterus and oligohydramnios. At term, 3–4 per cent of all babies are breech. The success of ECV is dependent on case selection and operator experience. The success ranges from 30 to 80 per cent. If the baby turns cephalic there is a 95 per cent chance that it will stay there. In multiple pregnancy (A) ECV is contraindicated due to the risk of abruption and the fact that there is little or no room to turn the fetus. A major uterine abnormality (B) such as bicornuate uterus is a cause of breech presentation. The pregnancy has usually implanted in one of the horns of the uterus and there is no space to turn. You will not be able to turn the baby and may use excessive force. If there has been an antepartum haemorrhage (C) you should not be putting pressure on the uterus as this may increase the chance of an abruption. When the membranes have ruptured (D) the fetus is unlikely to turn as there is less space as the liquor has been drained.

Diabetes mellitus in pregnancy

27 B Once she is eating and drinking, which will usually be about 6 hours after the operation, she can have the sliding scale taken down. She can now be put back on her pre-pregnancy doses of insulin. Naturally you will need to monitor her blood sugars to ensure that this is adequate insulin replacement. Stopping the insulin (D) all together is not correct as she is a type 1 diabetic who needs exogenous insulin. Continuing the sliding scale for 24 (A) or even 48 (E) hours is unnecessary if the patient is eating. It subjects them to frequent finger prick testing, including at night when they are trying to sleep. Halving her pre-pregnancy dose of insulin (C) is likely to give her less than she requires and provoke hyperglycaemia.

Maternal medicine

28 B SLE is a systemic connective tissue disorder that is more common in black African and black Caribbean women with an overall incidence of one in 1000. It may manifest as arthritis, renal impairment, neurological involvement, haematological complications, serositis–pericarditis or as various permutations of the above. Pregnancy increases the likelihood of a flare by 40–60 per cent. There is an increased risk of spontaneous miscarriage, fetal death (D), pre-eclampsia (C), preterm delivery (E) and fetal growth restriction (A). There is no specific link to diabetes.

Antenatal care

29 C *Listeria monocytogenes* (C) can cause listeriosis and pregnant women are at particular risk as they are immunocompromised. It is a food-borne infection and can be present in unpasteurized cheese and pâté. In pregnancy it can cause mid-trimester loss, early meconium and preterm labour. It typically presents as a flu-like illness. Toxoplasmosis (A) is caused by the parasite *Toxoplasma gondii* and characteristically is contracted via contact with cats and their faeces. CMV (B) is usually subclinical and 50–60 per cent of women in the UK are already immune having had exposure prior to pregnancy. It is not associated with food. Hepatitis E (D) is a non-chronic hepatitis transmitted by the faeco-oral route but it can have a fulminant course in pregnancy. Parvovirus B 19 (E) causes a facial rash called fifth disease/slapped cheek syndrome or erythema infectiosum. It has a respiratory droplet route of transmission.

Rashes in pregnancy

30 B Rashes in pregnancy are relatively common but there are very few that need medical attention. PUPP (B) classically starts on the abdomen in stretch marks and has peri-umbilical sparing. It can then move all over the body. It normally occurs after 34 weeks of pregnancy and disappears after birth. Pemphigoid gestationis (A) is a blistering condition that starts in the umbilicus and spreads. Prurigo gestationis (D) is usually a rash of the trunk and upper limbs with abdominal sparing. Impetigo herpetiformis (C) is a blistering condition that always presents with a febrile illness and if not treated early can lead to maternal and fetal death. (E) is a possibility as she may have had a reaction to a topical lotion, i.e. stretch mark cream. However, you would not find peri-umbilical sparing.

Medication in pregnancy

31 D The anti-convulsant sodium valproate (D) should ideally be avoided in pregnancy as it is associated with the highest risk of congenital malformations among the anti-convulsants. However, if it is the most appropriate agent to control the patient's seizures it should be used. The others are all to be avoided at all costs. Acitretin (A) and methotrexate (E) are teratogenic. Mebendazole (C), the anti-worming tablet, has been shown to be toxic in animal studies. Multiple congenital abnormalities have been reported with the anti-fungal fluconazole (B).

Hypertension in pregnancy

32 E This woman is at risk of developing hypertension in her pregnancy. She is 42, in her first pregnancy and has had IVF. Blood pressure in pregnancy normally falls with its lowest point reached between 22 and 24 weeks. Blood pressure then starts to rise for the rest of the pregnancy. Pre-eclampsia (A) is diagnosed with a raised blood pressure and proteinuria. A common cut off for normal urinary protein levels is a PCR of <30. It is always possible to diagnose her with white coat hypertension (B) but this is potentially a very dangerous label to give someone unless all other causes have been excluded. There is no evidence to diagnose Conn's syndrome (D) from the information given. Conn's syndrome arises when there is excess aldosterone production from the adrenal glands. This leads to hypertension and often lethargy and muscle fatigue as hypokalaemia can develop. This occurs due to the effect of excess aldosterone on the renal system leading to a potassium losing state. It is quite likely that this woman had a high essential blood pressure (C) at the beginning of pregnancy as it has risen so early in the pregnancy but we do not have that information. Importantly for this woman the risk of develops pregnancy-induced is around 40 per cent if she develops pregnancy-induced hypertension (E) under 30 weeks' gestation – she will need close monitoring throughout her pregnancy.

Diabetes mellitus in pregnancy

33 C In diabetes in pregnancy the reference ranges for sugar control are slightly different. Ideally before every meal the blood sugar should be less than 5.5 μmol/L and 1 hour after a meal less than 7.8 μmol/L. Outside of pregnancy 2-hour post meal readings are taken. So (C) is the correct answer. The appointment will involve referral to the dietician, the diabetes nurse (to learn how to test and record her blood sugars) and counselling about the risks of diabetes in pregnancy. These risks involve neonatal hypoglycaemia, pre-eclampsia, preterm labour, polyhydramnios, macrosomia and shoulder dystocia.

Gestational diabetes

34 D Women who develop GDM have a 35–60 per cent chance of developing type 2 diabetes over the next 10–15 years (D). All the others are true statements. Women who develop GDM should have growth scans to ensure the fetus is not growing excessively, in particular looking at the abdominal circumference as babies who are over 4.5 kg and born to a diabetic mother are at significant risk of shoulder dystocia (A). NICE recommends delivery after 38 weeks unless glycaemic control is very poor in order to reduce the risk of stillbirth (B). As soon as the cord is clamped the hyperglycaemic environment that the fetus has lived in for 9 months disappears so hypoglycaemia is a risk (C). Pre-eclampsia (E) is more common in diabetic mothers so urine dipsticks and blood pressure monitoring will form part of every clinic visit.

HIV in pregnancy

35 C You have very little information about this woman. The main aim is to prevent mother to child transmission of HIV. This woman has had little or no care. Her CD4 count is low (below 200/mm^3) and she is at risk of developing an AIDS defining illnesses. In addition her viral load is high (over 50 copies/mL). If a mother needs HAART she should start it and continue throughout her pregnancy and into the puerperium. If she does not need HAART to treat her HIV then she should start antiretroviral treatment between 20 and 28 weeks in order to prevent vertical transmission. If her viral load is less than 50 copies/mL she may choose to have a normal delivery (A and D). Ideally, prolonged rupture of membranes and artificial rupture of membranes should be avoided. For this reason induction of labour is not appropriate (B and E). This woman is at high risk of transmitting HIV to her baby so a caesarean section is the most appropriate management as there is evidence it reduces the risk of vertical transmission.

SECTION 2:
EARLY PREGNANCY

Questions

QUESTIONS

1. Early pregnancy loss

A 24-year-old woman attends accident and emergency 4 weeks after having a positive urinary pregnancy test. She has had 3 days of painless vaginal bleeding and is passing clots. Over the past 2 days the bleeding has settled. An ultrasound scan shows an empty uterus. What is the correct diagnosis?

    A. Threatened abortion
    B. Missed miscarriage
    C. Septic abortion
    D. Complete abortion
    E. Incomplete miscarriage

2. Complications of pregnancy

A 51-year-old woman in her 12th week of an assisted-conception triplet pregnancy presents to accident and emergency with severe nausea and vomiting. She has mild lower abdominal and back pains. Urine dipstick shows blood –ve, protein –ve, ketones ++++, glucose +. What is the most appropriate management plan?

    A. Intravenous crystalloids and doxycycline, urgent ultrasound assessment
    B. Discharge with 1 week's course of ciprofloxacin
    C. Referral to the medics for investigation of viral gastroneteritis
    D. Intravenous crystalloids, oral antiemetics
    E. Referral to the surgeons for investigation of appendicitis

3. Threatened miscarriage

A 19-year-old woman is referred to your early pregnancy unit as she is having some vaginal bleeding. This is her first pregnancy, she has regular menses and the date of her last menstrual period suggests she is 8 weeks gestation today. She is well apart from her bleeding and is naturally concerned. A transvaginal ultrasound reveals an intrauterine gestational sac of 18 mm with a yolk sac. What is the most likely explanation of these findings?

    A. A viable intrauterine pregnancy
    B. A pseudosac
    C. A blighted ovum
    D. A pregnancy of uncertain viability
    E. An anembryonic pregnancy

4. Pre-termination assessment

A 31-year-old woman is seen in the termination of pregnancy (TOP) clinic requesting a termination. She is 5 weeks pregnant in her first pregnancy. She is otherwise well but does have some lower abdominal pain on the right hand side. On examination her abdomen is soft and non-tender. An ultrasound reveals a small sac in the uterus which might be a pseudosac. What would be your next management step?

    A. Urgent referral to hospital to rule out ectopic pregnancy
    B. Rescan in 10 days time
    C. Blood test for beta human chorionic gonadotrophin (hCG) now and in 48 hours time
    D. Arrange for her to come in for a medical termination
    E. Arrange a surgical termination of pregnancy

5. Emergency gynaecology (1)

A 28-year-old woman with a history of pelvic inflammatory disease is 6 weeks into her third pregnancy. She previously had two terminations. She presents with lower abdominal pain and per vaginam bleeding. Her beta hCG is 1650 mIU/mL, progesterone 11 nmol/l. An ultrasound reveals a small mass in her left fallopian tube with no intrauterine pregnancy seen. There is no free fluid in the Pouch of Douglas. She is diagnosed with an ectopic pregnancy and is clinically stable but scared of surgery. How would you manage this case?

    A. Laparoscopic salpingectomy
    B. Methotrexate
    C. Laparotomy + salpingectomy
    D. Laparoscopic salpingotomy
    E. Beta hCG in 48 hours

6. Dyspareunia

A 24-year-old woman attends her GP complaining of deep dyspareunia and post-coital bleeding. She has crampy lower abdominal pain. Of note, she has been treated in the past for gonorrhoea on more than one occasion. On speculum examination there is no visible discharge, but the cervix bleeds easily on contact. What is the most appropriate management?

    A. IM cefotaxime, oral doxycycline and metronidazole
    B. 1 g oral metronidazole stat
    C. Urgent referral to the gynaecology clinic
    D. Referral to a sexual health clinic
    E. Admission to hospital under the gynaecologists

7. Investigation in emergency gynaecology

A 16-year-old girl attends accident and emergency complaining of mild vaginal spotting. Her serum beta hCG is 4016 mIU/mL. She is complaining of severe left iliac fossa pain and stabbing sensations in her shoulder tip. What is the most appropriate definitive investigation?

    A.   Diagnostic laparoscopy
    B.   Serial serum beta hCG measurement
    C.   Computed tomography of the abdomen and pelvis
    D.   Clinical assessment with speculum and digital vaginal examination
    E.   Transvaginal ultrasonography

8. Early pregnancy

An 18-year-old woman presents to accident and emergency having fainted at work. She is complaining of pain in the lower abdomen. A serum beta hCG performed in the emergency department is 3020 mIU/mL. The on-call gynaecologist performs transvaginal ultrasonography in the resuscitation area which shows free fluid in the Pouch of Douglas and no visible intrauterine pregnancy. Her pulse is 120 bpm and blood pressure 90/45 mmHg. What is the most likely diagnosis?

    A.   Ruptured ovarian cyst
    B.   Cervical ectopic pregnancy
    C.   Ruptured tubal pregnancy
    D.   Perforated appendix
    E.   Ovarian torsion

9. Menopause

A 50-year-old woman comes to your clinic with a 2-year history of no periods. Her GP has confirmed that her luteinizing hormone and follicle-stimulating hormone levels are menopausal. Her night sweats and hot flushes are unbearable and are preventing her from going to work. She would like to start hormone replacement therapy (HRT) but is very worried about the side effects. Which of the following is incorrect?

    A.   There is evidence that HRT prevents coronary heart disease
    B.   There is a small increase in the risk of strokes
    C.   There is an increased risk of breast cancer
    D.   There is an increase in the risk of ovarian cancer
    E.   There is an increase in the rate of venous thromboembolism

10. Emergency gynaecology (2)

A 24-year-old woman who is 9 weeks pregnant is brought to accident and emergency by ambulance with left iliac fossa pain and a small vaginal bleed. An abdominal ultrasound scan performed at the bedside demonstrates a cornual pregnancy and free fluid in the pelvis. Her observations are: pulse 119 bpm, blood pressure 74/40 mmHg, respiratory rate 24/minute. What is the most appropriate definitive management?

    A.   Transvaginal ultrasound scan
    B.   Serum beta hCG estimation

    C.   Diagnostic laparoscopy

    D.   Admission to the gynaecology ward and fluid resuscitation

    E.   Urine pregnancy test

11. Pain in early pregnancy

A 26-year-old woman presents to accident and emergency with left-sided lower abdominal pain and a single episode of vaginal spotting the day before. A urinary beta hCG is positive, and her last period was 6 weeks ago. A transvaginal ultrasound shows two gestational sacs. What is the most likely diagnosis?

    A.   Ruptured theca lutein cyst

    B.   Appendicitis

    C.   Diverticulitis

    D.   Complete miscarriage

    E.   Urinary tract infection

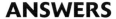

ANSWERS

Early pregnancy loss

1 D The terms abortion and miscarriage have historically been used interchangeably in gynaecology, which is as confusing to students as it is to patients. Most clinicians use miscarriage to mean a spontaneous fetal loss before 24 weeks' gestation and termination of pregnancy to use what the layman may call an 'abortion' – that is a deliberate termination of the pregnancy. Threatened abortion (A) refers to any vaginal bleeding before viability (traditionally 24 weeks, though this is decreasing) whereas after this point vaginal bleeding is referred to as antepartum haemorrhage. Missed miscarriage (B) is loss of the pregnancy without the passage of products of conception or bleeding. Often erroneously referred to in the media as a miscarriage 'that you didn't know happened', many women in fact experience the fetal loss as the sudden decline of pregnancy-related symptoms: early morning nausea, breast tenderness and vomiting. Septic abortion (B) refers to the loss of an early pregnancy complicated by infection of a retained conceptus. It is a serious complication of termination or miscarriage and must be managed actively: around the world, many women still die from this treatable condition. Incomplete miscarriage (E) is the loss of an early pregnancy with bleeding and/or passage of some but not all products of conception. It can be managed conservatively, medically (with misoprostol to expedite expulsion of the products) or surgically (with suction evacuation of the uterus). Complete abortion (D) refers to loss of the pregnancy where all products of conception have been expelled from the uterus.

Complications of pregnancy

2 D This woman is suffering from hyperemesis gravidarum (HG), a condition affecting around 2 per cent of pregnancies where vomiting in pregnancy becomes so severe that a woman may develop signs and symptoms of dehydration and may not be able to keep any fluid down. The ketonuria and triplet pregnancy are clues to this diagnosis as multiple fetuses are associated with hyperemesis. Mild lower abdominal and back pains are common at this stage in the pregnancy when the uterus grows out of the pelvis and stretches attached ligaments, and are usually of no consequence. The management of HG involves restoring fluid volume and preventing further nausea and vomiting (D). Diarrhoea and/or signs of sepsis might point in the direction of a gastroenteritis (C) or appendicitis (E). The latter would normally present with a more pronounced pain and less significant vomiting. Quinolones (e.g. ciprofloxacin) (B) and tetracyclines (e.g. doxycycline) (A) should be avoided in pregnancy as they are teratogenic.

Threatened miscarriage

3 D Abdominal pain and vaginal bleeding are very common in early pregnancy, with a miscarriage rate near one in five (20 per cent). This woman is having vaginal bleeding and has an intrauterine gestational sac, so is having a threatened miscarriage. There is no fetal pole and no fetal pulsation so we cannot say that this is viable (A). Although by 6 weeks we should see a fetal pole and a fetal heart, it may be that her dates are indeed wrong and that she is less pregnant than assumed. A blighted ovum (C) and an anembryonic pregnancy are the same thing, showing a gestational sac with no developing embryonic pole or yolk sac development. As there is a yolk sac this is unlikely. In view of uncertainties relating to status of pregnancy, it is imperative that people with suspected anembryonic pregnancies (E) have two scans 10-14 days apart to increase certainty that there is no embryo development. A pseudosac (B) is seen in 10–20 per cent of ectopic pregnancies. It is a decidual reaction rather than an embryonic sac – hence there would be no yolk sac. This is a pregnancy of uncertain viability that is in the uterus (D). This woman needs to have a repeat vaginal ultrasound scan in 10–14 days to confirm whether the pregnancy is viable.

Pre-termination assessment

4 C The concern is that the sac in the uterus may not be an early gestational sac but may be a pseudosac which would suggest an ectopic pregnancy. A pseudosac represents decidualized reactive tissue. Although she is only 5 weeks pregnant, with this scan result you are committed to ruling out an ectopic pregnancy. If the woman is well, is haemodynamically stable and understands what the symptoms are, that should prompt her immediate hospital attendance, then she can be managed as an outpatient. If this is not the case she should be referred to hospital. This woman needs a beta hCG and ideally a progesterone level, with a repeat beta hCG 48 hours afterwards. If there is more than a 67 per cent rise in beta hCG it is likely that the sac seen on the scan is that of a normal viable intrauterine pregnancy. If this is the case she will need an ultrasound in 10 days to confirm the diagnosis and then her TOP can be arranged if she still does not wish to continue her pregnancy. If there is a suboptimal rise in beta hCG she should be seen at hospital for further assessment. Surgical terminations should be performed after 7 weeks while medical terminations can be performed up to 9 weeks. The important message here is that you must always confirm the diagnosis of an intrauterine pregnancy before offering a TOP.

Emergency gynaecology

5 B Risk factors for ectopic pregnancies include a previous ectopic pregnancy, previous tubal surgery, intrauterine use, pelvic infection and *in vitro* fertilization. The main concern with an ectopic is that as it grows it may rupture and lead to intra-abdominal bleeding, acute collapse and occasionally death. We know that some people will undergo a tubal miscarriage and avoid rupture. A laparoscopic salpingectomy (A) would be a definitive procedure but would leave a young girl with only one fallopian tube. However, this may not significantly after her fertility as it may be that as a result of her pelvic inflammatory disease the tube is damaged already. She does not need a laparotomy (C) as she is stable. A salpingotomy (D) involves opening the affected tube and removing the ectopic pregnancy. This would leave the tube *in situ* but there is the concern of a another ectopic in the future. This woman is an ideal candidate for methotrexate (B). Methotrexate is given IM as an anti-metabolite, and a further dose may need to be given a week later. There are strict criteria about its use, including a small ectopic, no fetal pulse, no clinical compromise and no free fluid in the Pouch of Douglas. Another option is to keep her in hospital and repeat her beta hCG in 48 hours (E). If the hCG falls, a tubal miscarriage is a possibility. The benefits of methotrexate compared to surgery are that there is an increased chance of future fertility.

Dyspareunia

6 C The important part of this woman's presentation is that her cervix bleeds easily on contact. She has a significant history of (albeit treated) sexually transmitted infections. Although her presentation today could represent another sexually transmitted infection or pelvic inflammatory disease, the history of deep dyspareunia and post-coital bleeding, coupled with a cervix which bleeds on contact in a woman who is sexually active, should immediately raise suspicion of cervical cancer. She is 24 so it is unlikely that she will previously have had a cervical smear. Answers A, B, D and E are all potential management options in suspected pelvic inflammatory disease, and although it is likely that a competent clinician would initiate treatment immediately (most likely with option A) only option C reflects and addresses the urgent requirement to investigate and rule out cervical cancer.

Investigation in emergency gynaecology

7 E Apart from (C) all the options are potential diagnostic tools in assessing this woman: computed tomography is avoided if at all possible in pregnancy as it exposes the fetus to unacceptably high doses of ionizing radiation, the teratogenicity of which is highest in the first trimester. This woman is pregnant with vaginal bleeding and abdominal pain. Such patients should be treated as having an ectopic pregnancy until otherwise proven. Clinical assessment (D) and serial beta hCG measurements (B) would be the routine initial measures in assessing this woman, but they are by no means definitive in providing a diagnosis. In addition, meaningful information can only be drawn with a second beta hCG measurement, some 48 hours later. At this level of serum beta hCG an intrauterine pregnancy should be visible on transvaginal ultrasound (E), so it offers in this case the highest chance of providing a definitive answer to the ectopic pregnancy question. Diagnostic laparoscopy (A) may be employed if an ectopic pregnancy is suggested by the ultrasound scan, but it is not appropriate to perform this on a stable patient without first performing imaging. An early pregnancy is usually visible on transvaginal ultrasound if the serum beta hCG is above 1000 mIU/mL, and certainly above 1500 mIU/mL. Women with this level of hCG in whom no pregnancy can be detected on ultrasound scan should be managed as having a pregnancy of unknown location, which may included inpatient admission until ectopic pregnancy is definitively excluded.

Early pregnancy

8 C   This woman has lower abdominal pain and a positive pregnancy test with signs of haemodynamic instability: an ectopic pregnancy (C) should therefore be excluded urgently. Ovarian torsion (E) and ruptured ovarian cysts (A) classically present with a sudden onset abdominal pain, and are not commonly associated with a significant tachycardic hypotension. Differentiating between them can be difficult. However, the natural history of the pain is often helpful. Both may present with sudden onset pain, but usually the pain of ovarian torsion will be out of keeping with the clinical findings and will not improve with simple analgesia. Indeed it does not normally decrease significantly at all. By contrast, the pain of cyst rupture, while being of sudden onset, is often reduced by simple analgesia and may decrease gradually as the peritoneal lining (having been irritated by leaking fluid or blood from the cyst, causing pain) absorbs intraperitoneal free fluid. A woman with a perforated appendicitis (D) would often show signs of sepsis, including fever and peritonitis, and pain is normally localized initially to the central abdomen or right iliac fossa. At this level of beta hCG, an intrauterine pregnancy would normally be visible on transvaginal ultrasonography. Of the two ectopic pregnancy options available, cervical ectopics (B) would normally be demonstrable on transvaginal ultrasound. Ruptured ectopic pregnancy is a surgical emergency requiring prompt assessment, resuscitation and urgent surgery. The urgency of the situation is even more pronounced if there are signs of haemodynamic instability, such as in this case where there is evidence of hypovolaemic shock.

Menopause

9 A   All of the above are true except (A). There is no evidence that HRT prevents heart disease. In fact there is an increased risk of heart disease in women who start HRT 10 years after the menopause. In addition to the above there is a risk of endometrial cancer in oestrogen-only HRT which is related to duration of treatment. In general, if the woman still has her uterus progestogens must be given to prevent endometrial cancer developing. The risk of stroke (B) depends on age but there are additional 1–4 cases per 1000 women on HRT. The risk of breast cancer (C) is higher for patients in their 60s taking combined HRT. The risk with combined HRT taken over the age of 60 for 10 years will lead to an extra 36 cases of breast cancer per 1000 women. The risk of ovarian cancer (D) increases very slightly with an extra case per 1000 women. The risk of venous thromboembolism (E) is larger in the combined HRT group with an additional 7–10 cases per 1000 women.

Emergency gynaecology

10 C This woman is clearly in extremis. She has a tachycardic hypotension, which in the presence of a sonographically demonstrated ectopic pregnancy must be assumed to be due to a ruptured ectopic pregnancy causing significant haemorrhage. Emergency management is required to stop the woman bleeding to death. The woman has a visible pregnancy, so neither serum beta hCG (B) nor urinary confirmation of pregnancy (E) are required. Transvaginal ultrasound (A) would give a clearer picture of the pregnancy's location and the amount of pelvic blood, but in a pregnancy this far along, abdominal sonographic detection of an ectopic pregnancy coupled with the clinical findings confirm the diagnosis. Admission to a ward (D) is inappropriate for a woman who is so unwell: this woman requires concurrent resuscitation and transfer to theatre for stabilization and surgical management (C).

Pain in early pregnancy

11 A Functional ovarian cysts are common in women of childbearing age. A theca lutein cyst is a kind of ovarian cyst made of multiple luteinized follicular cells and is most common when the ovary is exposed to raised levels of beta hCG, as in multiple pregnancy. These cysts, like any other ovarian cyst, can rupture and bleed slowly onto the peritoneum where they cause irritation manifested as lower abdominal pain. Appendicitis (B) classically produces central pain localizing to the right iliac fossa. It is less common in pregnant women than non-pregnant women. Urinary tract infection (E) can cause lower abdominal pain, although this is usually central and associated with dysuria and frequency, which are not present here. Diverticulitis can cause left-sided pain, but patients are often febrile and commonly have a raised C-reactive protein and leukocytosis. Diverticulitis is an uncommon presentation at this age.

SECTION 3:
RESEARCH, ETHICS AND
CLINICAL GOVERNANCE

QUESTIONS

1. Consent and the Mental Health Act

A 32-year-old woman with paranoid schizophrenia is admitted for antenatal assessment at 36 weeks' gestation with twins. Her pregnancy is complicated by intrauterine growth restriction and impaired placental flow. She has had no psychotic symptoms in this pregnancy. Her obstetricians recommend an early caesarean section and argue it is in the best interests of the mother and her babies and to prevent further fetal insult. She has repeatedly said that despite the significant risks, which she understands, she refuses caesarean delivery. What is the most appropriate action?

    A. Detain under Section 5 of the Mental Health Act and deliver by caesarean section
    B. Detain under Section 2 of the Mental Health Act and deliver by caesarean section
    C. Determine that the patient lacks mental capacity and, acting in her best interests, delivery by caesarean section
    D. Determine that the patient lacks mental capacity and, acting in her fetus' best interests, deliver by caesarean section
    E. Encourage volunatary admission to the antenatal and repeatedly explain the benefits of caesarean delivery

2. Consent

Which of the following would be incorrect advice to give a woman requesting a caesarean section for non-medical indications?

    A. You are twice as likely to have a stillbirth in a subsequent pregnancy
    B. The risk of damaging the bladder is one in 20   1:1000
    C. There is an increased risk of placenta praevia in future pregnancies
    D. 1–2 per cent babies suffer lacerations
    E. The risk of infection is 6 per cent

3. Ethics of life-saving care

A 24-year-old Jehovah's Witness is brought to accident and emergency with a Glasgow coma scale (GCS) score of 3, BP 90/30 mmHg and pulse 110 bpm. Her husband reports that her last menstrual period was 8 weeks ago and she complained this morning of lower abdominal pain and vaginal spotting. Ultrasonography suggests a ruptured ectopic pregnancy. As part of the resuscitative measures employed before emergency laparotomy, a transfusion of group O-negative blood is prepared. Her husband interrupts and says that as a Jehovah's Witness she would absolutely refuse all blood products even at risk of death, and has previously signed an advance directive stating this. What is the most appropriate option?

A. Avoid transfusion and volume-replace with colloids before emergency transfer to theatre
B. Avoid transfusion and use a Cell Saver auto-transfuser in theatre
C. Avoid transfusion and immediately transfer to theatre
D. Stabilize the woman in accident and emergency before transfer to theatre
E. Transfuse the woman with group-O negative blood and immediately transfer to theatre

4. Abortion care ethics

An unbooked 26-week pregnant woman sees you at the hospital to request a termination of pregnancy. She says that if she leaves here today without a termination she will try and do it herself by stabbing her abdomen. Your consultant arranges an urgent psychiatric review which finds no grounds under which to detain this woman in regards to her mental health. Under these circumstances, if a termination was performed, which part of the Abortion Act would it fall under?

A. The continuance of the pregnancy would involve risk to the life of the pregnant woman greater than if the pregnancy were terminated
B. The termination is necessary to prevent grave permanent injury to the physical or mental health of the pregnant woman
C. The pregnancy has not exceeded its 24th week and continuance of the pregnancy would involve risk, greater than if the pregnancy were terminated, of injury to the physical or mental health of the pregnant woman;
D. The pregnancy has not exceeded the continuance of the pregnancy and would involve risk, greater than if the pregnancy were terminated, of injury to the physical or mental health of any existing child(ren) of the family of the pregnant woman
E. There is a substantial risk that if the child were born it would suffer from such physical or mental abnormalities as to be seriously handicapped.

5. Ethics in obstetrics

A 24-year-old woman in her first pregnancy presents to the labour ward in labour. She and her partner express an overwhelming desire to avoid a caesarean section. Her labour does not progress and after 9 hours her cervix is still only 3 cm dilated. Unfortunately, the fetal heart slows to 60 beats and does not recover after 5 minutes. Your senior registrar explains the situation to the woman and recommends an immediate caesarean section. She refuses and her partner tells you to stop harassing them. You explain that their unborn child will die if this continues. What options do you have?

    A.   Caesarean section under general anaesthesia (GA) under Section 3 of the
         Mental Health Act
    B.   Caesarean section under GA under Section 2 of Mental Health Act
    C.   No action. Allow fetus to die
    D.   Caesarean section without Mental Health Act application
    E.   Caesarean section under GA under Section 5(2) of the Mental Health Act

6. Ethics in gynaecology

A 16-year-old Muslim woman attends accident and emergency department with
her father. She complains of a 1-day history of left iliac fossa pain and mild
vaginal spotting. A urinary beta hCG test is positive. As part of your assessment
the patient consents to a vaginal examination. She insists you do not tell her father
that she is pregnant, and you consider her to be competent in her judgement. Her
father becomes angry and says you must not perform a vaginal examination. How
should you proceed?

    A.   Perform the examination with a chaperone present and tell the father
         that it is a routine examination
    B.   Perform the examination with a chaperone present and explain that
         parental consent is not necessary in this situation
    C.   Defer performing the examination and document the situation fully
    D.   Perform the examination with a chaperone present having assessed the
         girl's Gillick Competence
    E.   Perform the examination with a chaperone present having assessed the
         girl's Fraser Competence

7. Ethics in the emergency setting

A 32-year-old woman is rushed to accident and emergency as the viction of a
high speed vehicle collision. She is 35 weeks pregnant and unconscious. There
is evidence of blunt abdominal trauma and she is showing signs of grade 3
hypovolaemic shock. The consultant obstetrician on call immediately attends
the resus call and recommends immediate perimortem caesarean delivery in a
resuscitative effort to improve the management of her shock. Her husband has
been brought into resus by the police, and insists that she would refuse caesarean
section under any circumstances. What is the most appropriate management?

    A.   Rapid fluid resuscitation until the situation regarding the patient's
         wishes becomes clear
    B.   Replacement of the lost circulating volume with blood products
    C.   Admit to the intensive care unit and begin infusing inotropes to restore
         the cardiac output
    D.   Immediate caesarean delivery
    E.   Resucitation and transfer to the obstetric theatre for emergency
         caesarean delivery

8. Valid consent

A 59-year-old woman has been admitted for a hysterectomy for endometrial cancer. She has not yet given her consent and the rest of the team is in theatre. You have performed a hysterectomy before so feel confident in taking her through what will happen and the risks involved. The General Medical Council (GMC) says that you should tailor your discussion to all of the options except which of the following?

A. Their needs, wishes and priorities
B. Their level of knowledge about, and understanding of, their condition, prognosis and the treatment options
C. The onset of their condition
D. The complexity of the treatment
E. The nature and level of risk associated with the investigation

9. Improving patient care

A quality improvement process that seeks to improve patient care and outcomes through systematic review of care against explicit criteria and the implementation of change. This is an accepted definition of what?

A. Audit
B. Clinical governance
C. Clinical research
D. Clinical effectiveness
E. Integrated governance

10. Paediatric and adolescent gynaecology

A 15-year-old girl attends the gynaecology clinic with her boyfriend, also 15, requesting the morning after pill 4 months after being circumcised during a family trip to Somalia. She understands your advice and the implications of her decisions to engage in sexual activity, is using condoms regularly and refuses to inform her parents. What is the most appropriate management?

A. Decline to prescribe the morning after pill and refer the patient back to her GP
B. Decline to prescribe the morning after pill, and inform her parents that she is having underage sex
C. Prescribe the morning after pill, give contraceptive advice and recommend that the girl informs her parents
D. Prescribe the morning after pill, give contraceptive advice and immediately alert your consultant and the Safeguarding Children Team
E. Prescribe the morning after pill, give contraceptive advice and inform her parents

ANSWERS

Consent and the Mental Health Act

1 E Demonstrating that ethics and law are truly alive in obstetrics and gynaecology, this case is drawn from the one author's own experience (modified to protect confidentiality). There are two principal issues: one, the ethics and legality of treating a patient detained under the Mental Health Act and two, acting in the best interests of a patient who lacks capacity. It is not lawful to detain someone under the Mental Health Act for treatment of any disease other than a psychiatric condition. Therefore options (A) and (B) are incorrect. Section 5 orders are emergency holding powers to detain patients who are already inpatients and for whom there is no time to apply for another more appropriate detention order. Section 2 orders are usually used for patients in the community who require detention in hospital for assessment, although in practice they may also receive treatment (for the disease necessitating detention) as part of an assessment. In this case, the patient has not shown psychotic symptoms and it is unlikely that she would require formal admission. Options (C) and (D) imply that the patient lacks capacity. The question makes clear that this patient: (1) understands the information she is being given about risk, (2) retains the information, as she is repeatedly refusing care despite understanding the consequences of waiting, and (3) can weigh that information in the balance and communicate her choice. These three tests are met and the patient has capacity to make the decision about caesarean section. A patient with capacity can refuse treatment, even if that decision is irrational or against the advice of family or friends. The only option left is for the clinician to encourage engagement with the care team and recommended plan (E). She may require treatment – perhaps under detention – for the schizophrenia, but formal admission for this might deter her from accepting advice from all doctors and therefore reduce the likelihood of her accepting a caesarean section.

Consent

2 B The 2009 Royal College of Obstetricians and Gynaecologists' caesarean consent guidelines provide guidance on how to counsel a women undergoing emergency and elective caesarean delivery. The only incorrect answer here is (B). The risk of damage to the bladder is one in 1000: it is highly unlikely that caesarean section would have become accepted modern day obstetric practice were there a risk that 5 per cent of all women had iatrogenic bladder injury at operation. Other risks include venous thromboembolism (4–16 in 10000), significant haemorrhage (≈five in 100) and the need for hysterectomy (eight in 1000). The risk of death for caesarean section is around one in 12000.

Ethics of life-saving care

3 E   There are two principal ethical issues here. First is the concept of best interests in relation to a patient who is unable to consent themselves (in this case due to unconsciousness), and second is the idea of advance directives. This woman has been brought to accident and emergency in a life-threatening condition. It is likely that the transfusion of blood would be part of life-saving management of her condition. In an emergency, patients must always be given life-saving treatment unless they have made a valid advance directive declining such treatment. To be valid, an advance directive must be viewed by the treating clinician, signed by the patient who had capacity to make the decision at the time of signing, and be witnessed. The advance directive is not present in accident and emergency in this case, nor is there evidence of any discussion with her treating clinician. Therefore, in this case, a normative assessment of the patient's best interests would err on the side of giving life-saving treatment, e.g. blood (E). Given this is the case, avoiding volume replacement entirely (B, C) or delaying surgery by filling with colloids in a patient with catastrophic haemorrhage is inappropriate. Anaesthetists are unlikely to be willing to anaesthetize an unstable patient without preoperative resuscitation (C).

Abortion care ethics

4 B   Straight away answers (C) and (D) are not appropriate as they refer to pregnancies under 24 weeks. Answer (E) is not appropriate. If the child was born at 26 weeks there is a risk that it would have abnormalities but that is no different to any other case. Answers (A) and (B) seem to be the most appropriate. The psychiatrist is happy that she has capacity and is not suffering from any mental illness. You could argue that if she went home and stabbed her abdomen her life would be at risk. You could also argue that if she went home and carried out her threats this would have long-term effects on her mental health and possibly on her physical health. For this reason section (B) is probably more appropriate. This case is an ethical minefield. A lot of doctors would not be happy terminating a healthy fetus after 24 weeks. Theoretically, a termination is possible throughout pregnancy if the criteria on the Abortion Act form are met.

Ethics in obstetrics

5 C   The Mental Health Act does not provide legal justification for operating or providing treatment for a woman who has capacity but who declines on that treatment. There is nothing to suggest that this woman lacks capacity. Section 2 (B) is a 28-day section that allows a period of admission for assessment. Section 3 (A) allows up to 6 months of detention for treatment. Section 5(2) (E) is a temporary holding order that lasts for 72 hours in which time a patient can be assessed for Section 2 or 3. It can be exercised by the doctor in charge of the patient's care or 'his nominated deputy', which in practice refers to any hospital doctor attending a patient. It would, of course, always be prudent to involve the patient's consultant with such decisions. It only refers to patients who do not have capacity. Even if you have to watch this fetus die it would be legally unjustifiable to perform a caesarean section without consent. Options A,B, D and E would amount to a battery and would put the doctor at risk of criminal prosecution.

Ethics in gynaecology

6 B   The patient is 16 years old, and may therefore be considered competent, in which case parental consent is not required to perform any procedure or examination (B), although it is always preferable to have family members on board. Not performing a necessary clinical examination for a consenting patient would be negligent (C). You must respect the young woman's request to maintain confidentiality regarding her pregnancy, so (A) is incorrect. Gillick competence (D) is irrelevant here, as the patient is 16 years of age and competent. Fraser Guidelines (E) are a result of English case law and originally related to the legality of a doctor to provide contraceptive advice to minors without parental knowledge. The Fraser Guidelines do not apply to those over the age of 16. A female chaperone should always be present for intimate pelvic examinations, regardless of the gender of the examiner.

Ethics in the emergency setting

7 D   In this case, the wishes of the husband are largely irrelevant. The patient is in a life-threatening condition and lacks capacity due to unconsciousness. In such circumstances, life-saving treatment must be given if it is in the patient's best interests as judged by the attending clinician. This woman is likely to be bleeding into her abdomen from a ruptured viscus: she is gravely ill and close to cardiac arrest. A young woman can compensate significantly for blood loss, and the fact that she has significant signs of hypovolaemic shock indicates the likely massive loss of circulating volume. Replacement with fluids (A) or (B) will not stop the haemorrhage, though they will buy time. Transferring this peri-arrest patient (E), even to ITU (C), is unwise as she may arrest en route, for example, in a lift, where facilities are not available. In addition, inotropes may increase the cardiac output but they do not compensate for the lack of circulation caused by continuing haemorrhage. A senior obstetrician here has advised that delivery of the fetus in accident and emergency (D) would help with her resuscitation. Perimortem caesarean section is usually performed as a means of saving the life of the mother rather than the fetus. The gravid uterus reduces venous return and therefore preload on the heart, in turn reducing stroke volume and cardiac output.

Moreover, the placental oxygen requirement is huge and reduces the ability of what little circulating volume she has left to perfuse her vital organs. Perimortem caesarean would remove these obstacles to effective resuscitation of this critically ill trauma patient. It is usually performed through a midline incision: such an incision would also then give access to the abdomen for a general surgeon to perform a trauma laparotomy.

Valid consent

8 C The GMC have published extensive guidance about consent, in particular how to inform someone appropriately when asking for their consent. All of the above apart from (C) are crucial in relation to consent. (C) should read 'the nature of their condition'. These are five very useful pointers to remember when asking for consent, even verbal consent for a blood test. Assess the patient's understanding (B) of their disease, which enables the gynaecologist to tailor further information, and language, to the patient's needs and can augment the patient's understanding. Discuss a patient's needs, wishes and priorities (A), which involves the patient in their care and allows them to take a lead in its direction. Explain the complexity of the treatment (D) and the risks associated with it (E), which is vital for consent to be valid: without the above the patient may be successful in proving in a court of law that they had not been properly informed in relation to the procedure.

Improving patient care

9 A This is the National Institute for Health and Clinical Excellence (NICE) definition of audit. Audit is an integral part of NHS care, allowing clinical and non-clinical staff to evaluate what they are doing and bench marking it against the best care possible. Clinical governance (B) is an umbrella term that can be defined as a framework through which NHS organizations are accountable for continually improving the quality of their services and safeguarding high standards of care by creating an environment in which excellence in clinical care will flourish. Audit is part of this, along with research, education and risk management. Research (C) is a process to answer a clinical question. At its heart is the scientific method: a method of enquiry based on examining measurable evidence that can be tested. Integrated governance (E) is a term that refers to the combination of clinical and corporate governance. Clinical effectiveness (D) takes clinical research a step further by examining not only whether a particular intervention works but whether it is useful, acceptable to the patient and represents value for money.

Paediatric and adolescent gynaecology

10 D There are two significant issues here: a patient under 16 years requesting contraception, and her circumcision. The girl meets the Fraser Guidelines for giving contraceptive treatment or advice to those under 16: she understands the advice; she cannot be persuaded to tell her parents; she is likely – given that she has a boyfriend – to continue having sex and her health will suffer if contraceptive treatment is not provided (pregnancy is inherently more dangerous than non-pregnancy). Prescribing the morning after pill is an appropriate correct course of action, so (A) and (B) are wrong. Informing her parents would be a breach of confidence and is not permitted under the GMC's Good Medical Practice, so (E) is incorrect. Both (C) and (D) would be correct, but only (D) takes the further action that would be required given that she has had a female circumcision* abroad, a serious offence in the UK, contrary to the Female Genital Mutilation Act 2003.

* Female circumcision is referred to in the UK as female genital mutilation (FGM). It involves some or all of: removal of the clitoral hood, clitoris and labia and closure of the vaginal introitus. It is often performed under unhygienic conditions by unqualified women, it is common in sub-Saharan Africa, involves major psychosocial and physical trauma to the woman and has significant sequelae. Performing FGM in the UK or performing or assisting FGM on a UK national abroad is illegal.

SECTION 4:
GENERAL GYNAECOLOGY

QUESTIONS

1. Dyspareunia

A 59-year-old woman attends the gynaecology clinic complaining of worsening pain during penetrative sexual intercourse. She went through the menopause 9 years before, with very few problems, and did not require hormone replacement therapy (HRT). She has been with the same partner for 4 years since the death of her husband with whom she had four children. What is the most likely diagnosis?

    A. Ovarian malignancy
    B. *Chlamydia trachomatis* infection
    C. Discoid lupus erythematosus
    D. Atrophic vaginitis
    E. Bacterial vaginosis

2. Lower abdominal pain

A 19-year-old woman is referred to accident and emergency with a fluctuant lower right abdominal pain which started over the course of the morning, associated with vomiting. There is rebound tenderness on examination. She is afebrile. Serum beta human chorionic genadotrophin (hCG) is negative. An ultrasound shows free fluid in the peritoneal cavity but no other pathology to account for the pain. White cells are 14×10^9/L and the C-reactive protein (CRP) is 184 mg/L. What is the most likely diagnosis?

    A. Acute appendicitis
    B. Early ectopic pregnancy
    C. Pelvic inflammatory disease (PID)
    D. Tubo-ovarian abscess
    E. Ovarian torsion

3. Polycystic ovaries

A 39-year-old woman is seen in the gynaecology clinic having been diagnosed with polycystic ovarian syndrome (PCOS). She has lots of questions in particular about the associated long-term risks. Which of the following is not a risk of PCOS?

    A. Endometrial hyperplasia
    B. Sleep apnoea
    C. Diabetes
    D. Breast cancer
    E. Acne

4. Venous thromboembolism

A 54-year-old menopausal woman comes to your clinic desperate for hormone replacement therapy (HRT) as her vasomotor symptoms are very troubling. Her next door neighbour recently developed a deep vein thrombosis while on HRT. She is concerned about the risks of venous thromboembolism (VTE) and wants your advice. Which of the following would you not advise?

    A.   The risk of VTE is highest in the first year of taking HRT
    B.   She should have a thrombophilia screen prior to starting HRT
    C.   There is no evidence of a continuing VTE risk after stopping HRT
    D.   Personal history of VTE is a contraindication to oral HRT
    E.   If she develops any VTE while on HRT it should be stopped immediately

5. Heavy menstrual bleeding

A 34-year-old woman with long-standing menorrhagia attends accident and emergency having fainted at home. She is on the third day of her period, which has been unusually heavy this month. She insists she cannot be pregnant as she has not had sexual intercourse for a year. She is haemodynamically stable. A point-of-care test venous full blood count in the emergency department shows:

Hb 5.2 g/dL
WCC 8.9×10^9/L
Hct 0.41% L
MCV 80 fL

What should the initial management be?

    A.   Establish large-bore venous access, commence fluid resuscitation and cross-match four units of packed red cells
    B.   Call for senior help, establish large-bore venous access and prepare the patient for urgent laparotomy
    C.   Call for senior help, establish large-bore venous access and give group O rhesus negative blood
    D.   Establish large-bore venous access and begin transfusing group-specific blood as soon as it is available
    E.   Await the result of a beta hCG test before deciding further management

6. Ovarian cysts

A 66-year-old post-menopausal woman is referred to you urgently by her general practioner (GP). She had been complaining of some lower abdominal pain. An ultrasound arranged by the GP shows a 4 cm simple left ovarian cyst. A CA 125 comes back as 29 U/ml (normal 0-35 U/ml). What is the most appropriate management?

    A.   Referral to a specialist cancer unit
    B.   Laparoscopic ovarian cystectomy
    C.   Laparotomy and oophrectomy
    D.   Conservative management
    E.   Total laparoscopic hysterectomy and bilateral salpingo-oophorectomy

7. Atrophic vaginitis

A 79-year-old woman attends your clinic with some vaginal bleeding. Her last period was 16 years ago. She has had two children both via caesarean section, has a normal smear history and is currently sexually active. On examination the vagina appears mildly atrophic with some raw areas near the cervix. What is the most important next step in her management?

    A.   Vagifem nightly for 2 weeks and then twice a week after that
    B.   Triple vaginal swabs for sexually transmitted infection
    C.   Pelvic ultrasonography
    D.   HRT to help the vaginal raw areas
    E.   Smear test

8. Endometriosis

At laparoscopy a 21-year-old woman is found to have severe endometriosis. There are multiple adhesions and both ovaries are adherent to the pelvic side wall. The sigmoid colon is adherent to a large rectovaginal nodule. The nodule is excised and the bowel and ovaries freed. Which of the following medications would be appropriate to help treat her endometriosis?

    A.   Danazol
    B.   Triptorelin
    C.   Microgynon 30
    D.   Tranexamic acid
    E.   Medroxyprogesterone acetate

9. Vasomotor symptoms

A 54-year-old woman comes to your clinic complaing of hot flushes and night sweats that are unbearable. Her last mentrual period was 14 months ago. She has had a levonorgestrel releasing intrauterine system (Mirena) *in situ* for 2 years as treatment for extremely heavy periods. What treatment would you consider for her symptoms?

    A.   Elleste Solo
    B.   Elleste Duet
    C.   Vagifem
    D.   Oestrogen implants
    E.   Evorel

10. Progestogens

A 19-year-old biochemistry student is seen in your clinic worried about her hormone levels. She has been told by her GP that her progesterone is low. You enter into a long discussion about the effects of progesterone on the body. Progesterone:

    A.   Enhances endometrial receptivity
    B.   Stimulates endometrial growth

C. Increases uterine growth
D. Increases fat deposition
E. Increases bone resorption

11. Heavy menstrual bleeding

A 41-year-old mother of two presents to the GP with long-standing heavy menstrual bleeding which has become worse over the past year. She is otherwise well and has no significant medical history. She requests treatment to alleviate the impact of her heavy bleeding on her social life. Pelvic examination reveals a normal sized uterus. What is the most appropriate first line treatment?

A. Levonorgestrel-releasing intrauterine system
B. Tranexamic acid
C. Mefenamic acid
D. Tranexamic acid and mefenamic acid combined
E. Vaginal hysterectomy

12. Premenstrual syndrome

A 42-year-old woman is seen in the gynaecology clinic. She has been suffering from severe premenstrual symptoms all her life. They have now significantly affected her relationship and her husband is filing for divorce. She comes to your clinic in tears regarding the future of her children. She demands a hysterectomy and bilateral salpingoophrectomy. After taking her history you talk about other less radical treatments. Which management option is inappropriate?

A. Antidepressants
B. Vitamin C
C. Exercise
D. Cognitive behavioural therapy
E. Yasmin – combined oral contraceptive pill

13. Pelvic inflammatory disease

A 22-year-old woman is seen in accident and emergency with lower abdominal pain and some vaginal discharge. She has had PID once in the past and was treated for it. She is otherwise well. Her temperature is 36.9°c, pulse 90, blood pressure 105/66 mmHg. She is passing good volumes of urine. On clinical examination she has diffuse lower abdominal tenderness. There are no signs of peritonism on examing her abdomen. On vaginal examination she has adnexal tenderness and an offensive discharge. Her CRP is 28 mg/L and her white blood count is 12.2×10^9/L. Her pregnancy test is negative. She is reviewed by your senior and is diagnosed with PID. What would be an appropriate antibiotic regime?

A. IV ceftriaxone and IV doxycycline
B. IV ofloxacin and IV metronidazole
C. IM ceftriaxone, oral doxycycline and oral metronidazole
D. IV clindamycin and gentamicin
E. Oral azithromycin and benzylpeniciilin

ANSWERS

Dyspareunia

1 D   Dyspareunia is the sensation of pain before, during or after penetrative sexual contact with the vagina. It is most commonly associated with pain *during* penetration. It should not be confused with vaginismus which is the inability to engage in penetrative sex due to involuntary spasm of the pubococcygeus muscle. In younger (although not exclusively young) patients for whom there is new dyspareunia it is important to exclude sexually transmitted infections and acute intrapelvic conditions (such as ovarian cysts or appendicitis) and to ensure there is no cervical pathology (for example, cervical carcinoma *in situ*). The vaginal lining of women who have gone through the menopause progressively atrophies with age as the residual level of circulating estrogens decreases. Estrogens ensure the vaginal lining remains moist and expansile, comfortably permitting sexual penetration. Without exposure to these estrogens, the lining can become atrophied. Friction to an unlubricated atrophic vagina (D) can cause extreme discomfort. Sexually transmitted infections (B), although increasingly common in older couples, are rare in those beyond the menopause. Bacterial vaginosis (E) is uncommon in post-menopausal women also. Although these two diagnoses would be unlikely, it is still important to exclude them by careful vaginal examination and swabs. Ovarian malignancy (A) is not suggested by this clinical presentation here. In addition, she has no risk factors for ovarian cancer (including HRT) and has the protective factor of having had four pregnancies. Discoid lupus erythematous (C) is a complex atrophying lesion of the skin similar in aetiology to systemic lupus erythematosus but without the systemic features. Although it may result in dyspareunia, through atrophy of the vaginal lining, there are no other features here to suggest an autoantibody-mediated disease, and the usual age of onset for discoid lupus is 30 years.

Lower abdominal pain

2 A   Differentiating between pain caused by gynaecological or by surgical pathology is a difficult but important and common problem. Knowing the natural history of the diseases can help. Ovarian torsion (E) classically presents with a sudden onset pain on one side which does not improve and is constantly there. It often requires opiate analgesia. Ovarian torsion is an important diagnosis as the risk of compromising the ovarian blood supply is high, with ovarian compromise and possible infarction. In this case the pain is fluctuant not constant, and although torsion may cause an inflammatory response accounting for the raised CRP, it would not cause a leukocytosis which is present here. Tubo-ovarian abscess (D) and PID (C) would normally lead to a fever, with a high white cell count. Tubo-ovarian abscesses can be a sequel of untreated PID and their early courses may be similar. However, a woman with a frank abscess in the pelvis (D) would likely be much more seriously ill than the patient here (or a patient with PID) and the fever would usually be swinging. Serum beta hCG can detect the earliest of pregnancies, so an ectopic pregnancy (B) is highly unlikely here given the negative serum hCG. A normal ultrasound unfortunately cannot completely rule out adnexal or gastrointestinal pathology, not least because transabdominal ultrasound often cannot visualize the appendix.

Polycystic ovaries

3 D   PCOS is a condition diagnosed by the presence of two out of three of oligo/amennhorea, polycystic ovaries and clinical and/or biochemical signs of hyperandrogenism. Long-term risks include the development of endometrial hyperplasia (A), sleep apnoea (B) and diabetes (C). Diet, exercise and weight control are key to preventing long-term complications. Acne (E) is often present and is a clinical sign of hyperandrogenism. Endometrial hyperplasia should be treated with progestogens, and a withdrawal bleed should be induced every 3–4 months. There is no evidence of an increase in breast (D) or ovarian cancer in PCOS.

Venous thromboembolism

4 B   HRT can be very beneficial to ladies who are going through the menopause. Vasomotor symptoms can be debilitating and can seriously affect quality of life. The risk of developing a VTE is highest in the first year (A). It is not routine to offer thrombophilia screening to all patients (B) as it is not cost effective. If there was a suggestion of a family history of VTE this might however be sensible. There is no evidence of a continuing VTE risk after stopping HRT (C). If a woman has had a VTE she should not have oral HRT (D). HRT should be stopped immediately if the woman has a VTE (E) as the risk of further VTE is significantly increased if she continues taking replacement therapy.

Heavy menstrual bleeding

5 A   This woman has a significant normocytic anaemia as a result of blood loss, sufficient to cause a faint earlier in the day. The most likely cause is her menorrhagia. Initially she should be appropriately resuscitated (A). Although she is haemodynamically stable, with continuing blood loss she may decompensate rapidly. Therefore, large-bore venous access is warranted. Fully cross-matched blood is the safest option of the three transfusion options presented and will usually take around 45 minutes to prepare compared to 20 minutes for group-specific blood. As this patient is currently stable, one cannot justify the potential complications* associated with giving group-specific (D) or even ungrouped (O-negative, or universal donor) blood (C). A laparotomy (B) is not indicated here as the patient is haemodynamically stable and has a medically treatable cause for the (albeit severe) anaemia.

* When transfusion of packed red cells is necessary, the urgency of the situation dictates how it is tested before being given. The risk of transfusion reactions, particularly acute haemolytic reactions where there is ABO incompatability, is increased with the use of donor blood which has not been fully cross-matched with the recipient's. Cross-matching takes about 45 minutes and involves physically mixing the donor and recipient blood and testing for transfusion reactions. The next safest, and second quickest, transfusion option is group-specific blood. The recipient's blood is tested for ABO group and antibodies and a compatible blood is selected from the blood bank. This grouping process takes around 15 minutes. Group O-negative (universal donor) blood is given in life-threatening emergencies only as it carries the greatest risk of transfusion reactions. When O-negative blood is used, no tests on the recipient blood are performed before administration of the donor red cells.

Ovarian cysts

6 D   Ovarian cysts in post-menopausal ladies can be managed conservatively if they meet certain criteria. A risk of malignancy index (RMI) can be calculated using the CA 125 value, the characteristics of the cyst on ultrasound and the menopausal status. The features of concern on ultrasound are bilateral cysts, multiloculated cysts, solid components, ascites and metastases. RMI <50 has a 3 per cent chance of cancer. RMI between 50 and 250 has a 20 per cent chance of cancer and an RMI >250 has a 75 per cent chance of cancer. If the cyst is simple and less than 5 cm in diameter with a CA 125 <30 U/ml then conservative management (D) would be appropriate with 4-monthly scans and CA 125 levels for 1 year. Immediate referral to a specialist (A) is therefore not required in this case. Similarly, surgical management to remove an ovary (C) or both ovaries and the uterus (E) is unwarranted in a woman with no significant pathology. Laparoscopic cystectomy ((B) removal of the cyst, normally by aspirating the cyst contents and excising the cyst capsule to prevent recurrence) would be a potential management option if the patient was sufficiently symptomatic and all other therapies had failed. A cyst this small is unlikely to cause significant symptoms.

Atrophic vaginitis

7 C   This woman is post-menopausal. Whenever you see a woman with post-menopausal bleeding it is imperative to exclude cancer of the cervix or endometrium. She has had a normal smear history and there is normal cervical appearance on examination so carcinoma of the cervix is unlikely and repeat testing (E) is not required. She is still sexually active and may well have a sexually transmitted infection so triple swabs (B) would be a sensible part of an overall management plan. She has no other menopausal symptoms and is now 79 so starting HRT is not advisable (D). Topical vaginal oestrogen like Vagifem (A) may be appropriate. However, before prescribing oestrogens, an ultrasound of her pelvis (C) should be arranged to make sure that her endometrial thickness is <4 mm. This is the most important investigation as it would confirm or deny the most serious differential diagnosis (endometrial cancer). A normal ultrasound would be reassuring and make the diagnosis of endometrial cancer far less likely.

Endometriosis

8 B   This woman's disease is severe and it is most likely that the specialist will want to treat her with medication and then perform a second-look laparoscopy to remove any disease that remains. Danazol (A) has anti-oestrogenic and anti-progestogenic effects and is licensed for 3–6 months. Triptorelin (B) is a gonadotrapin-releasing hormone agonist that creates a temporary artificial menopause by reducing the follicle-stimulating hormone and luteinizing hormone levels. This is an excellent option for up to 6 months. After that there is the risk of loss of bone mineral density. Microgynon 30 (C) is a combined oral contraceptive pill. Tranexamic acid (D) is an antifibrinolytic used in the management of mennorhagia. Medroxyprogesterone acetate (E) is a progestogen. The answer to this question depends on the patient but triptorelin followed by another laparoscopy probably gives this woman the best chance of disease clearance.

Vasomotor symptoms

9 A   This woman is menopausal. When considering HRT a full history is important to highlight any important past medical history, including venous thromboembolism or cancer. The next step is to assess for the uterine function. If the woman has not had a hysterectomy you must always make sure she has constant or cyclical progestogens to reduce the risk of endometrial hyperplasia and endometrial cancer. In this case the woman already has a source of progestegens – the Mirena – so prescribing oestrogen alone would be appropriate (A). Elleste Solo contains estradiol alone while Elleste Duet (B) also contains norethisterone (a progestogen, which is not required here). Evorel (E) is another combined oestradiol and norethisterone preparation. Again, the progestogen component is unnecessary here. Vagifem (C) is used as a local treatment for atrophic vaginitis, not for systemic vasomotor symptoms. Oestrogen implants (D) can be very helpful at dealing with symptoms but supraphysiological levels of oestrogen can lead to a rapid recurrence of vasomotor symptoms when levels begin to fall.

Progestogens

10 A Progesterone is released by the corpus luteum following ovulation. Its main function is to enhance endometrial receptivity (A) in the event that an embryo should need to implant. If a pregnancy is successful then the developing embryo will release human chorionic gonadotrophin which will maintain the corpus luteum function. Increased uterine growth (C), increased fat deoposition (D), bone resorption (E) and endometrial growth stimulation (B) are all effects of oestrogens. Other progestogenic effects include an increase in respiratory rate, increase in sodium excretion, reduction in bowel motility and an increase in body temperature – some people will monitor their temperature as a measure of ovulation.

Heavy menstrual bleeding

11 A This woman requests symptom relief from heavy menstrual bleeding (HMB) which is interfering which her life. For women who have no structural uterine abnormality and present for treatment for the first time, NICE guidance recommends the use of levonorgestrel-releasing intrauterine systems (A) (e.g. Mirena coil) which in addition to reducing or stopping menstrual bleeding are contraceptive. Fertility returns soon after removal of the Mirena coil, so it is appropriate for women who have not undergone the menopause. Tranexamic acid (B) and mefamanic acid (D) and their concomitant use (D) are now second line treatments for HMB: tranexamic acid alone is most commonly prescribed (and recommended by NICE) as the principal pharmaceutical agent given the harsher side effects (nausea, vomiting and diarrhoea) of mefamanic acid. Hysterectomy (E) is reserved for those women who have tried other measures without success and have completed their family. Vaginal hysterectomy is the preferred approach in the absence of contraindications.

Premenstrual syndrome

12 B Premenstrual syndrome (PMS) is defined as a condition that is associated with distressing physical, behavioural and psychological symptoms, in the absence of organic or underlying psychiatric disease, which regularly recurs during the luteal phase of each menstrual (ovarian) cycle and which disappears or significantly regresses by the end of menstruation. First line measures for severe PMS include selective serotonin reuptake inhibitors (A), Vitamin B6, improved diet and physical exercise (C), cognitive behavioural therapy (D), and a trial of Yasmin or Cilest combined oral contraceptive pills (E). There is no evidence that Vitamin C (B) has any effect on symptoms. There are many other complementary treatments that many patients use in conjunction with pharmacological treatments. These include St. John's Wort, Ginkgo Biloba and Evening Primrose Oil.

Pelvic inflammatory disease

13 C Symptoms that suggest a diagnosis of PID include bilateral adnexal tenderness, abnormal vaginal discharge, fever over 38°C, vaginal bleeding, deep dyspareunia, bilateral adnexal tenderness and cervical motion tenderness. In addition there may be microbiological evidence of infection and raised white cells and inflammatory markers. Options (A), (B) and (D) are all intravenous antibiotic options for severe pelvic infection and sepsis. Systemic (intravenous) antibiotics should be used if there is evidence of clinically severe disease or sepsis, evidence of a tubo-ovarian abscess exists, the woman is pregnant* or there is a lack of response to oral therapy. This woman's case is mild to moderate (abscence of peritonism, fever, systemic infection or abscess) so option (C) would be appropriate. Option (E) is not a recognized treatment regimen for PID in the UK.

*   Note that tetracyclines such as doxycycline should be avoided in pregnancy: an alternative intravenous regimen should be offered to these women.

SECTION 5:
MANAGEMENT OF LABOUR AND DELIVERY

QUESTIONS

1. Analgesia in labour

A 24-year-old woman is in her first pregnancy. She has no significant medical history. She is 40 weeks and 2 days pregnant and has been contracting for 4 days. She is not coping with the pain. She has been given intramuscular pethidine. On examination she is found to be 4 cm dilated (fetus in the occipito-posterior position) having been the same 4 hours previously. What analgesia would you recommend?

    A.   Remifentanil
    B.   Pethidine
    C.   Diamorphine
    D.   Epidural injection
    E.   Entonox

2. Intrapartum care (1)

A 36-year-old woman is 41 weeks pregnant and is established in spontaneous labour. She is contracting three times every 10 minutes and has ruptured her membranes. She is draining significant meconium stained liquor. Her cervix is 7 cm dilated. Her midwife has started continuous electronic fetal monitoring using a cardiotocograph (CTG). The baseline rate has been 155, with variability of 2 beats per minute, for the past 60 minutes. There are no accelerations and no decelerations. What is the most appropriate management?

    A.   Pathological CTG – needs delivery
    B.   Suspicious CTG – needs delivery after fetal blood sampling (FBS)
    C.   Suspicious CTG – change maternal position, intravenous fluids and reassess in 20 minutes
    D.   Suspicious CTG – perform fetal blood sampling and deliver if abnormal
    E.   Normal CTG – do nothing

3. Intrapartum care (2)

A 19-year-old woman is giving birth to her first baby. She has been pushing for an hour and the fetal head has been on the perineum for 6 minutes. There seems to be a restriction due to resistance of her tissues. Her midwife carries out a right mediolateral episiotomy. Which of the following structures should not be cut with the episiotomy?

    A.   Bulbospongiosus
    B.   Superficial transverse perineii (STP)
    C.   Vaginal mucosa
    D.   Perineal membrane
    E.   Ischiocavernosus

4. Intrapartum care (3)

A 25-year-old woman in her first pregnancy has a pathological CTG. Her cervix is 5 cm dilatated. Which of the following might increase the risk to the fetus if the doctor performed a fetal blood sample?

- A. Human immunodeficiency virus (HIV)
- B. Human papilloma virus (HPV)
- C. Maternal immune thrombocytopenia
- D. Factor IX deficiency
- E. Hepatitis C

5. Cord prolapse

A multiparous woman is admitted to the labour ward with regular painful contractions. On examination she is 9 cm dilated with intact membranes and is coping well with labour pains. Forty minutes later her membranes rupture while she is being examined and you see the umbilical cord hanging from her vagina. You inform the woman what has happened. She is now fully dilated, the fetal position is Direct occipitoanterior, and the presenting part is below the ischial spines. What do you do next?

- A. Gain intravenous access, call for help and stop the woman pushing
- B. Perform a grade 1 emergency caesarean section
- C. Call for help, perform an episiotomy and commence pushing
- D. Call for help and prepare for an instrumental delivery
- E. Elevate the presenting part by inserting a vaginal pack

6. Active management of labour

A 34-year-old para 0 has been admitted for a post-dates induction of labour at 42 weeks. She has received 4 mg PGE_2 (prostaglandin) vaginally. After 72 hours her cervix is 5 cm dilated. Four hours later she is still 5 cm dilated. On abdominal examination the fetus appears to be a normal size. The fetal head position is left occipito-transverse, and the station is −1. There is no moulding but a mild caput. She is contracting two times in every 10 minutes and has an epidural *in situ*. You are asked to review and make a management plan. What would be the most appropriate plan?

- A. Re-examine in 4 hours provided the baby is not distressed
- B. Discuss the situation with the patient and offer her a caesarean section
- C. Start an oxytocin infusion and intermittent monitoring and reassess in 4 hours
- D. Insert another 1 mg PGE_2 as she is not contracting and reassess in 2 hours
- E. Start an oxytocin infusion, commence continuous monitoring and reassess within an appropriate time span

7. Intrapartum care (4)

A mother comes to labour ward who is low risk, in labour at term. The unit is short staffed and there are not enough midwives to provide intermittent auscultation of the fetal heart. You decide to start continuous electronic monitoring (CTG). She is an epidemiologist and asks you about the CTG and how it will help her labour and prevent her baby suffering harm. Which of the following would you tell her? Continuous monitoring has a:

    A.   High sensitivity and low specificity
    B.   High sensitivity and high specificity
    C.   Low sensitivity and low specificity
    D.   Low sensitivity and high specificity
    E.   High sensitivity and high positive predictive value

8. Fetal loss

A 29-year-old woman comes to the labour ward complaining that her baby has not been moving for 72 hours. She is 36 weeks pregnant. Otherwise her pregnancy has been complicated with gestational diabetes for which she is taking insulin. On examination you fail to pick up the fetal heart. You confirm the diagnosis of an intrauterine death. The scan shows no liquor and the baby is transverse. After a long discussion you explain that she unfortunately needs to deliver her baby. What is the best way for her to deliver her baby?

    A.   Induction with oral mifepristone and oral misoprostol
    B.   Induction with oral mifepristone and vaginal misoprostol
    C.   Induction with oral misoprostol
    D.   Induction with vaginal dinoprostone
    E.   Caesarean section

9. Complications of delivery

A 24-year-old woman with gestational diabetes has been progressing normally through an uncomplicated labour. The midwife delivers the head but it retracts and does not descend any further. What should the midwife do next?

    A.   Pull the emergency bell and place the woman in McRobert's position
    B.   Place the woman on all fours and instruct her not to push
    C.   Pull the emergency bell and commence rotational manoeuvres for shoulder dystocia
    D.   Pull the emergency cord and ask your helper to apply fundal pressure
    E.   Pull the emergency bell and prepare for emergency caesarean delivery

10. Complications of labour

A 29-year-old multiparous woman is in established labour contracting strongly. She is 4 cm dilated and had been having regular painful contractions for 6 hours before they stopped abruptly, heralded by a sudden onset of severe, continuous lower abdominal pain. The fetal heart trace is difficult to identify, and the tocometer does not register a signal. What is the most appropriate management?

A. Fetal assessment with formal ultrasound scan
B. FBS
C. Immediate trial of delivery in theatre, with resuscitation facilities on standby
D. Immediate caesarean delivery
E. Expedite delivery with synthetic oxytocin infusion

11. Obstetric anaesthesia

A 23-year-old woman is in her first labour. Her cervix is 6 cm dilated and she is in distress. She is asking for an epidural. Before you call the anaesthetist you check her history. Which of the following would be an absolute contraindication to an epidural?

A. Previous spinal surgery
B. Hypotension
C. Mitral stenosis
D. Multiple sclerosis
E. Aortic stenosis

12. Management of the second stage

A 38-year-old nulliparous woman has had an uncomplicated pregnancy. She has laboured very quickly and is 10 cm dilated. The fetal heart falls to 60 for 4 minutes. She is pushing effectively and the head is 1 cm below the ischial spines. You prepare for forceps delivery in the room. She has had no analgesia so you quickly insert a pudendal nerve block and deliver the baby 4 minutes later in good condition. Which of the following is not a branch of the pudendal nerve?

A. Inferior anal nerve
B. Perineal nerve
C. Dorsal nerve of the clitoris
D. Posterior labial nerve
E. Genital branch of the genitofemoral nerve

13. Obstetric emergencies

The obstetric team is alerted to a blue-light trauma call expected in accident and emergency. A 28-year-old woman who is 37 weeks pregnant has been involved in a high-speed road traffic collision. On arrival, where the obstetric team is on standby, her Glasgow Coma Scale score is 5 and she has a tachycardic hypotension. What is the most appropriate management sequence?

    A.   Resuscitation according to Advanced Trauma Life Support (ATLS) guidelines and transfer to the labour ward

    B.   Transfer to the CT scanner in preparation for immediate trauma laparotomy

    C.   Resuscitation according to ATLS guidelines and fetal assessment with the patient in left lateral tilt

    D.   Resuscitation according to ATLS guidelines with immediate caesarean delivery

    E.   Resuscitation according to ATLS guidelines and corticosteroids for fetal lung maturation

14. Third degree tears

A 24-year-old woman is seen after her normal vaginal birth. The midwife who delivered the baby is concerned that there is a third degree tear. Having examined the woman the obstetrician confirms a third degree tear. The woman is taken to theatre to repair the external anal sphincter. Which of the following is not a risk factor for third degree tear?

    A.   Forceps delivery

    B.   Second stage of labour lasting over an hour

    C.   Shoulder dystocia

    D.   Ventouse delivery

    E.   Maternal age

ANSWERS

Analgesia in labour

1 D   This woman has had a very long latent phase of labour (the latent phase usually being no longer than 24 hours). Her cervix is now 4 cm and she is in the active phase of labour. Unfortunately, the fetal position of occipito-posterior is associated with slower labours. She has not made progress over a 4-hour period so an assessment into whether there is a problem with the powers (contractions), passage (shape of pelvis) and passenger (size and position) needs to be undertaken. There is likely to be a significant amount of time left before baby is born. All question choices are analgesia options in labour. Remifentanil (A) is given through an infusion pump and tends to be used where there is a contraindication to having an epidural or a spinal. Pethidine (B) has been given before but had little effect so she is unlikely to want this again. Some hospitals use diamorphine (C) instead of pethidine. There is little difference between the two with some units preferring one or the other. All opiates primarily have a sedative effect rather than an analgesic effect in labour. Entonox (E) can be a helpful adjunct to pain relief but it is unlikely that this will be enough to ease her through the remainder of the labour. An epidural (D) would be the most appropriate analgesia to offer this woman. This is based on the expected length of labour ahead and also the likelihood of augmentation with syntocinon as she has made little progress in the active stage of labour.

Intrapartum care (1)

2 D   Classification of CTGs is an important part of intrapartum care and it is imperative that interpretation is uniform. There are four features to a CTG: baseline rate, variability, accelerations and decelerations.

	Baseline	Variability	Accelerations	Decelerations
Reassuring	110–160	>5 beats per minute	Present	None
Non-reassuring	161–180 to 100–109	<5 beats per minute	The absence of accelerations with otherwise normal trace is of uncertain significance	Typical variable decelerations with over 50% of contractions, occurring for over 90 minutes
		40–90 minutes		Single prolonged deceleration for up to 3 minutes
Pathological	>180 or <100	<5 beats per minute for 90 minutes	Either atypical variable decelerations with over 50% of contractions or late decelerations, both for over 30 minutes	Single prolonged deceleration for more than 3 minutes

A suspicious CTG has one non-reassuring feature. A pathological CTG has either two non-reassuring features or one abnormal feature. This woman has non-reassuring variability so has a suspicious trace. Furthermore, there is meconium in the liquor so the fetus is at risk of meconium aspiration. Answer (D) is correct.

Intrapartum care (2)

3 E   If the episiotomy is performed correctly it should avoid the ischiocavernosus (E). This muscle goes from the crus of the clitoris to the ischial tuberosity. The episiotomy should be at least 45° from the midline. The episiotomy creates extra space for delivery of the fetal head. Bulbospongiosus (A) inserts into the fascia of the corpus cavernosa and originates from the perineal body. STP (B) goes from the ischial ramus and tuberosity to the perineal body. The vaginal mucosa (C) will be involved as the inside blade of the scissors will be in the vagina. The perineal membrane (D) has two parts, the dorsal and ventral. The ventral part consists of the urethra and surrounding structures. The dorsal part consists of the attachment of the lateral wall of the vaginal and perineal body to the ischiopubic rami. The episiotomy will disrupt this.

Intrapartum care (3)

4 B   CTGs are a sensitive screening tool but have a high false-positive rate. For this reason whenever you are faced with a pathological CTG a fetal blood sample can help to reassure you that the fetus is coping with labour. HIV (A), and hepatitis C (E) are blood-borne viruses and invasive tests (such as FBS) increase the risk of vertical transmission. FBS should be avoided in women with factor IX deficiency (D) (haemophilia B) as there is a risk that the fetus may also be affected. In maternal immune thrombocytopenia (C) there is a risk that the fetus may also have a low platelet count. HPV (B) is the correct answer as FBS does not increase the risk to the fetus. HPV is associated with cervical cancer, especially HPV types 16, 18, 31 and 33.

Cord prolapse

5 D   If the cord is felt below the presenting part with ruptured membranes, there is a cord prolapse. This is an obstetric emergency since the cord can either become obstructed or go into spasm and starve the fetus of oxygen. Delivery needs to be expedited. Answer (A) is partially correct as you will need help and probably need IV access. Help is very important here. You will need trained obstetric, anaesthetic and midwifery staff. Generally, women with cord prolapse should be delivered immediately, in theatre. If the cervix is not fully dilated, they should be delivered by grade 1 caesarean section (B). In this case however, a vaginal delivery is the quickest option. She is a multiparous woman with a favourable fetal head position which is low in the pelvis. Answer (C) is inappropriate as delivery needs to be as quick as possible and an episiotomy alone will not guarantee delivery of the fetus. Elevating the presenting part is very important as this will relieve pressure on the cord, but not with a pack (E). In the community the midwife should either use their hand to move the fetal head from the cord, or a catheter can be inserted into the bladder and filled with 500 mL normal saline to elevate the presenting part. Answer (D) would be the best option in this case as it is most likely to effect the quickest delivery.

Active management of labour

6 E   This question focuses on delay in the first stage of labour. We know that she is in active labour as her cervix is 5 cm dilated (active labour is usually believed to have commenced once the cervix is more than 3 cm dilated). When considering labour we must think about the 'passage, passenger and powers'. This woman's labour has arrested, and she is only contracting twice every 10 minutes. It is technically difficult to assess the 'passage' but one can gauge obstruction when performing a vaginal examination by assessing the degree of caput or moulding of the head. The 'passenger' can be similarly difficult to assess but abdominal examination is mandatory to assess the size of the baby and gauge how much fetal head remains in the abdomen. Putting this together it would appear that the reason for the arrest of labour is a suboptimal contraction pattern. Option (A) is not appropriate as this woman's labour has not progressed in the last 4 hours. This woman may end up requiring caesarean delivery (B) but at this point it is more appropriate to offer augmentation. It is not appropriate to intermittently monitor a labour augmented by oxytocin so (C) is also incorrect: augmentation of labour carries a risk of hyperstimulation and thus requires continuous fetal monitoring. This woman is now in labour so there is no place for further PGE$_2$ (D) to dilate the cervix. Option (E) is the best answer. There may be debate about the timing of the subsequent examination but the aim is to achieve a vaginal delivery.

Intrapartum care (4)

7 A   The CTG was introduced as a way to reduce the number of babies born with fetal acidosis, and poor Apgar scores. In reality, the only proven benefit is a reduction in neonatal seizures. Currently, there is no clear evidence of a reduction in perinatal mortality or hypoxic brain injuries. However, the CTG is very sensitive so if the fetus becomes acidotic then it will pick this up as change becoming suspicious/pathological. However, it is not very specific, with a high false-positive rate. Nearly 50 per cent of babies delivered because of a pathological CTG will have normal blood gases. A monitoring tool which had low sensitivity and low specificity (C) would be of no use. A monitoring tool with low sensitivity and high specificity (D) would seldom have a false-positive result; however, it would miss patients with the condition you were looking for. A tool that was highly sensitive and specific monitoring or one with high positive predictive values (B, E), but these are unfortunately at present unavailable in relation to fetal monitoring.

Fetal loss

8 E Stillbirth is a tragic and often unpredictable event. There is an increase in stillbirths with diabetes. In this case, stillbirth may have been avoidable if the woman had attended hospital sooner than 72 hours after noticing a loss of fetal movements. Induction of labour for an intrauterine death normally involves using mifepristone for cervical ripening and misoprostol (A, B) to bring about the onset of contractions. Dinoprostone (D) is also used routinely in many institutions for induction of labour. Induction with misoprostol alone (C) in a woman with an unripe cervix is unlikely to be successful. In this scenario, however, the complicating factor is that there is no liquor and this baby is transverse at term. This baby will not deliver vaginally and the only option available therefore is caesarean delivery. Moreover, inducing a labour for transverse lie increases the risk of uterine rupture.

Complications of delivery

9 A This woman's delivery is complicated by shoulder dystocia, a risk factor for which is gestational diabetes. It is often heralded by the 'turtleneck' sign, where the head delivers but then appears to retract. It is an obstetric emergency. A series of manoeuvres are performed in a set order, the most important of which is placing the woman into McRobert's position (A) (knees and legs maximally flexed) to give the pelvic outlet its maximum possible diameter. In the majority of cases, the baby will deliver spontaneously with this manoeuvre. Placing the woman on all fours (B) and internal rotational manoeuvres (C) may all be attempted, and suprapubic pressure if McRobert's position have failed to disimpact the shoulder, but they are not the first step. Caesarean delivery is a last-ditch attempt to deliver the baby if all other methods have failed (E); in addition it requires Zavanelli's manoeuvre, where the baby is manually replaced into the uterine cavity. Fundal pressure increases the risk of brachial plexus injuries, causing Erb's or Klumpke's palsies.

Complications of labour

10 D This woman is likely to have suffered a uterine rupture, a potentially catastrophic event for both her and her baby. Although signs and symptoms are often subtle, the presentation here would strongly suggest rupture. Often there is significant fetal heart rate abnormality following rupture, and the tocometer will not register any contractions. Immediate surgical intervention (D) is necessary to save the life of the baby and mother, who is at risk of haemorrhagic shock. A 'crash' caesarean delivery is normally performed with subsequent repair, if possible, of the uterus, although a caesarean hysterectomy is sometimes necessary. In this case formal ultrasound offers little more useful information than can be garnered from the CTG (other than clarification of the presence of a fetal heart rate) (A). This should never replace emergency delivery if rupture is clearly present. FBS (B) is useful in labour when a CTG trace has become suspicious but in this case it has no place. Using an oxytocin infusion (E) would be contraindicated in the presence of suspected uterine rupture as it increases the strength and frequency of contractions and could exacerbate the rupture. Trial of vaginal delivery in theatre (C) is not appropriate as the cervix is only 4 cm dilated.

Obstetric anaesthesia

11 B Epidural anaesthesia is commonplace on a labour ward. Care must be taken when offering patients epidurals to consider conditions that might make the procedure more difficult. Absolute contraindications include patient refusal, allergies to anaesthetic agents, systemic infection, skin infection over the intended epidural site, bleeding disorders, platelet count less than 80 000/mL and uncontrolled hypotension. Hypotension (B) is of vital importance: the epidural will cause a peripheral vasodilation and worsen any pre-existing hypotension. This peripheral vasodilation is the reason why most obstetric anaesthetists preload the patient with 1 L of intravenous fluid before giving the epidural agent. Relative contraindications include conditions where the heart cannot adapt easily to circulatory changes such as hypertrophic obstructive cardiomyopathy, aortic stenosis or mitral stenosis (C). Anatomical abnormalities like spina bifida or previous spinal surgery (A) may make an epidural technically difficult but are not contraindications. Neurological conditions such as multiple sclerosis may be exacerbated by an epidural but again this is not a contraindication. Most hospitals now run anaesthetic clinics prior to labour, which is the optimum time for an assessment to be made about the woman's suitability for regional anaesthesia.

Management of the second stage

12 E The pudendal nerve arises from the ventral rami of the 2nd, 3rd and 4th nerves of the sacrum. It then passes between piriformis and coccygeus leaving the pelvis through the greater sciatic foramen. It then crosses the ischium and re-enters via the lesser sciatic foramen. It runs forward in the pudendal canal with the pudendal vessels. The inferior anal (A) and inferior haemorrhoidal nerves are the first to leave the pudendal nerve. The main benefit of the pudendal block for operative obstetrics is the effect it has on the perineal nerve (B). The dorsal nerve of the clitoris (C) is a terminal branch of the pudendal nerve that should not be involved in your delivery if you have to perform an episiotomy. Option (D) is another branch of the pudendal nerve. The block will help analgesia if there is any trauma to the labia. The genital branch of the genitofemoral nerve (E) does not innervate the perineum; instead it arises from L1 and L2 and descends over psoas major before entering the deep inguinal ring. It terminates with the round ligament in the female.

Obstetric emergencies

13 C Although obstetric major trauma is uncommon, this question tests the candidate's ability to apply basic obstetric and emergency medicine knowledge to unusual circumstances. By the process of elimination, only one answer is appropriate. The transfer of an unstable polytrauma patient is dangerous, particularly if as in this case there is evidence of haemorrhagic shock, so options (A) and (B) are incorrect. Steroids (E) for lung maturation are not required at this gestation. Corticosteroids promote fetal lung maturity and are used, if time permits, if a woman presents in early preterm labour before 34 weeks gestation. Although perimortem caesarean section may be performed in accident and emergency, this woman, although unwell, has a cardiac output which may respond to resuscitative measures, so immediate caesarean delivery (D) is unwarranted and may put her at further risk. Placing the woman in a left lateral tilt (C) is important to permit increased venous return, while fetal assessment will determine the fetal state following the accident and may contribute to the management plan.

Third degree tears

14 D One per cent of all vaginal births result in a third degree tear. It is imperative that the tear is identified at the time of delivery so that it can be repaired appropriately. A 3a tear involves less than 50 per cent of the external anal sphincter (EAS), while a 3b tear involves more than 50 per cent of the EAS. A 3c tear involves both EAS and the internal anal sphincter. All of the options are risk factors except maternal age. Others include being primiparous, induction of labour, a large (greater than 4 kg) baby, occipitoposterior position and midline episiotomy. Once repaired the patient needs to be debriefed, be prescribed antibiotics and stool softeners and be offered a 6-week review.

SECTION 6:
POST-PARTUM PROBLEMS

QUESTIONS

1. Post-partum coagulopathies

A 34-year-old woman is brought straight to intensive care from the obstetric theatre after an emergency caesarean section for fetal distress. The attending obstetrician remarks that she is showing haematological signs of disseminated intravascular coagulation. Which blood profile is she most likely to have?

	A	B	C	D	E
Prothrombin time (PT)	↓	↓	↑	↑	→
Activated partial thromboplastin time (aPTT)	→	→	↑	↑	↑
Bleeding time	↑	↑	↑	↑	↑
Platelets	→	↑	↓	↑	→
Active haemorrhage	Yes	No	Yes	No	No

2. Intraoperative complications

A 31-year-old undergoes a planned caesarean section for a breech presentation. After delivery of her healthy baby there is difficulty in delivering the placenta, as it is adhered to the uterus. She has lost 5 L of blood as a result of the placenta accreta. The placenta has been removed but she is still bleeding and is cardiovascularly unstable despite blood product replacement. What would be the most management to definitively arrest haemorrhage?

A. Syntocinon infusion
B. B-Lynch suture
C. Internal artery ligation
D. Hysterectomy
E. Intrauterine balloon

3. Post-partum complications (1)

A 39-year-old woman is 6 days post-partum and has come back to hospital with shortness of breath. She is struggling to breath at rest, has a respiratory rate of 28, pulse 115, BP 105/60 mmHg, temperature 37.4° C. On examination she has an audible wheeze and cough. Investigations reveal a PO_2 of 9.5 kPa on arterial blood gas and a PCO_2 3.7 kPa, pH 7.36, base excess -3.4. A chest x-ray shows some upper lobe diversion and bilateral diffuse shadowing with an enlarged heart. Her haemoglobin is 8.9 g/dL, white blood count 11.1×10^9/L and C-reactive protein 21 mg/L. What is the most likely cause of her symptoms?

A. Lower respiratory tract infection
B. Pulmonary embolism
C. Peri-partum cardiomyopathy
D. Systemic inflammatory response syndrome (SIRS)
E. Post-partum anaemia

4. Post-partum complications (2)

A 17-year-old girl is seen in accident and emergency 14 days after an emergency caesarean delivery of a healthy infant, her first. Her neighbours became concerned and called the police. She had been seen prostrate in the garden chanting verses from the Bible and shouted at them accusing them of being spies when they asked if she was ok. They say her problem has worsened over the past fortnight. What is the most likely diagnosis?

A. Post-partum depression
B. Bipolar affective disorder
C. Puerperal psychosis
D. Schizophrenia
E. Acute confusional state (delirium)

5. Fetal physiology

At birth, which of the following does not occur in the fetal circulation?

A. Right ventricular output increases
B. A decrease in venous return
C. Closure of the foramen ovale
D. Pulmonary artery vasoconstriction
E. Closure of the ductus arteriosus

6. Assessment of the newborn

A woman on the labour ward has just had a normal birth. At birth there was a lot of meconium present. The newborn did not respond initially but did after subsequent resuscitation. The midwife records the Apgar score as 5. Which of the following best describes the categories an Apgar score is created from?

A. Tone, colour, noise, pulse and blood pressure
B. Tone, colour, respiratory effort, heart rate and reflex irritability
C. Tone, colour, pulse, reflex irritability and blood pressure
D. Tone, colour, pulse, respiratory effort and blood pressure
E. Tone, colour, cry, blood pressure and heart rate

7. Post-partum haemorrhage

An 18-year-old woman has been successfully delivered of a healthy female infant by elective caesarean section for maternal request. Estimated blood loss was 1120 mL. Forty minutes after return to the recovery area, she has a brisk vaginal bleed of around a litre. Her pulse rate is 120 bpm and blood pressure is 95/55 mmHg. What should the immediate management process be?

- A. Rapid fluid resucitation, uterine massage, intravenous ergometrine
- B. Rapid fluid resuscitation, intravenous ergometrine and bimanual compression of the uterus
- C. Rapid fluid resuscitation, insertion of an intrauterine balloon catheter device
- D. Rapid fluid resuscitation, uterine massage, oxytocin infusion and vaginal assessment
- E. Rapid fluid resuscitation and administration of direct intramyometrial uterotonic agents

8. Post-partum problems

A 34-year-old woman develops a significant post-partum haemorrhage and hypotensive shock following vaginal delivery of a healthy infant at term. The labour was uncomplicated. She recovers well with volume replacement and oxytocin and returns to the post-natal ward. She is unable to breast feed on the ward and 2 months later has neither started breastfeeding nor resumed her periods and is increasingly fatigued. What is the most likely diagnosis?

- A. Addison's disease
- B. Syndrome of inappropriate antidiuretic hormone hypersecretion (SIADH)
- C. Sheehan's syndrome
- D. Panhyperpituitarism
- E. Post-partum depression

9. Infection in pregnancy

A 30-year-old French woman delivers a live female infant by spontaneous vaginal delivery at term. In the eleventh week of pregnancy she developed a flu-like illness which resolved spontaneously a week later. Her newborn child has severe hydrocephalus and chorioretinitis. Four days after birth, she develops severe convulsions and efforts to revive her are unsuccessful. Which pathogen is most likely to be responsible?

- A. Cytomegalovirus (CMV)
- B. Human immunodeficiency virus
- C. *Toxoplasma gondii*
- D. Group B *Streptococcus*
- E. *Listeria monocytogenes*

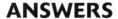

ANSWERS

Post-partum coagulopathies

1 C   Disseminated intravascular coagulation (DIC) is a consumptive coagulopathy in which both tissue factor (extrinsic) and contact activation (intrinsic) pathways are activated throughout the body causing the utilization of clotting factors, the build up of clotting degradation productions and a widespread increased tendency to bleed. In DIC, both PT and aPTT are prolonged, so only (C) and (D) remain possible answers. However, only (C) includes a decreased platelet count – owing to platelets being utilized in the clotting process – and the existence of active bleeding, both of which would likely exist in a profoundly unwell patient with DIC. Although this appears a tricky question, principally, because the candidate must assess five answers with five different data items each, the answer becomes obvious if you realize that in DIC, all measures of the speed of clotting increase while products of clotting go down (the 'consumptive' element of the coagulopathy). Options (A) and (B) do not make clinical sense as the bleeding time is increased despite a decreased PT time and normal aPTT. With these parameters, there would be an increased tendency to clotting and a decreased bleeding tendency, neither of which is supported by the other data. Option E, which also does not describe a consumptive coagulopathy, could describe von Willebrand's disease, a hereditary deficiency of von Willebrand factor, which is required for platelet adhesion.

Intraoperative complications

2 D   This woman is in extremis. Primary post-partum haemorrhage in this case has been due to the retained placenta accreta. Once the placenta is removed (often they are left *in situ*) the aim is to help the uterus contract and compress any remaining bleeding uterine vessels. Syntocinon (A) may well be part of the initial management. The crucial part of this question is how unwell she is. No obstetrician wants to perform a hysterectomy (D) on a 30-year-old but this may be necessary. She has already lost 5 L of blood so this has been a complicated operation so far. A B-Lynch suture (B) is an external uterine suture that helps uterine contraction. A balloon (E) would provide internal uterine tamponade against any bleeding vessels. Internal iliac artery ligation (C) would prevent blood flow down the uterine artery reducing the blood volume reaching the uterus. All of the above could be part of her management but in this case she is so unwell that performing a caesarean hysterectomy would be the correct course of management.

Post-partum complications (1)

3 C This woman appears to be unwell. Her tachycardia, tachypnoea, low grade pyrexia and cough would give weight to the diagnosis of a lower respiratory tract infection (A). She is hypoxic, raising the suspicion of a pulmonary embolus (B) but she has no chest pain, does not have a respiratory alkalosis on her ABG and there are chest x-ray findings that could otherwise explain her hypoxia. She does not meet the diagnostic criteria for SIRS (D) and there is no proof of infection yet. Her haemoglobin is low (E) but we would not expect to see this level of symptomatic anaemia at 8.9 g/dL. The diagnosis is to exclude is peripartum cardiomyopathy (C). Although it is rare it has a mortality rate of 9–15 per cent. It usually develops in the last month of pregnancy and up to 5 months post-partum. Risk factors include multiple pregnancies, hypertension in pregnancy and advanced maternal age. It presents as shortness of breath, tachycardia, tachypnoea and signs of congestive cardiac failure. In this case the x-ray findings of cardiomegaly and pulmonary oedema give weight to the diagnosis.

Post-partum complications (2)

4 C Puerperal psychosis (C) affects around one in 1000 mothers and normally presents within the first 2 weeks after delivery. Caesarean section, emergency delivery and a primiparity are independent risk factors for puerperal psychosis. It commonly presents with delusional ideation and hallucinations, with a religious aspect to the delusions often being noticeable. It is clinically similar to bipolar affective disorder (B), though depressive episodes are much less common in puerperal psychosis, and depression (A) is not evident here. Schizophrenia (D) would normally be associated with third person hallucinations which are not present here. An acute confusional state is a clinical syndrome normally caused by a non-psychiatric process such as infection. Although hallucination may be present, as in this case, acute confusional state classically fluctuates and its onset is much quicker, usually over the course of hours or a few days. In this case, her behaviour has become more odd over the course of a fortnight, and there are features of frank psychosis. The time from delivery within which acute-onset psychosis has occurred, coupled with the risk factors, makes puerperal psychosis the most sensible diagnosis.

Fetal physiology

5 D After birth the umbilical vessels are occluded. This subsequently reduces the venous return (B) back to the right side of the heart reducing the right atrial pressure and closing the patent foramen ovale (C). As the fetus starts to breath, the pressure in the pulmonary circulation lowers and right ventricular output increases (A). The pulmonary artery vasodilates, not constricts (D), to allow this new low-pressure system on the right side of the heart to develop. The increased flow through the pulmonary system leads to more venous return to the left side of the heart via the pulmonary veins, leading to an increase in the pressure on the left side. In turn, the ductus arteriosus (E) in response to the rising oxygen levels will close.

Assessment of the newborn

6 B Apgar scores were developed in the 1950s. They provide a unified way of assessing a newborn baby to determine the level of care they require and predict the risk of long-term morbidity. Apgars take account of the infant's tone, colour, breathing, heart rate and reflex irritability (B). The scores are measured at 1, 5 and 10 minutes. Infants' Apgar scores at 1 minute are often low but usually they improve with the simple resuscitative measures of stimulation and inflation breaths. Blood pressure (A, C, D, E) is not measured in newborn babies.

Post-partum haemorrhage

7 D Recognizing that this woman has a primary post-partum haemorrhage is of vital importance. All the options listed are recognized options in the management of post-partum haemorrhage, but of these, fluid resuscitation, oxytocin infusion and uterine massage (D) are the most commonly employed first line techniques to arrest haemorrhage. Intravenous ergometrine (A) and bimanual compression (B) of the uterus may be employed if initial measures have not controlled bleeding, while intrauterine balloons (C) and intramyometrial uterotonics (E) are employed if bleeding continues in spite of other measures.

Post-partum problems

8 C In a well-motivated mother, the inability to lactate so far after delivery is a cause for concern. This, coupled with an absence of periods requires ruling out hypopituitarism (C). This woman suffered a post-partum haemorrhage significant enough to cause hypovolaemia. Since the anterior pituitary is hyperplastic during pregnancy, it is acutely sensitive to acute falls in blood pressure. If hypotension is severe, necrosis or infarction of the anterior pituitary can occur, rendering it hypofunctional, i.e. Sheehan's syndrome (C). This can commonly result in absence of lactation and periods, fatigue and, less commonly, diabetes insipidus. This is the opposite of panhyperpituitarism, which is neither a recognized post-partum condition nor a complication of post-partum haemorrhage. Post-partum depression (E) can occur soon after pregnancy or up to a year after delivery. Younger and unsupported mothers, women with previous depression or drug use and those with a strong family history are most at risk of post-partum depression. It can cause fatigue and difficulty in breastfeeding, but is unlikely to stop periods or completely prevent any lactation. SIADH (B) would present with features of hyponatraemia, and although this can happen after Sheehan's syndrome has been long established, it does not account for this woman's symptoms at present. Adrenal insufficiency/Addison's disease (A) could account for this woman's fatigue but not the other symptoms and more often would present with symptoms associated with glucocorticoid insufficiency.

Infection in pregnancy

9 C   Cytomegalovirus (CMV) infection is very common, with about 60% of the population having had a prior infection. If it is contracted in pregnancy about 40–50% of fetuses will become infected. The manifestations of such an infection can be very broad. Complications include visual and hearing loss, microcephaly and long-term neurodevelopmental disability. Babies do not have hydrocephalus (so (A) is incorrect). HIV (B) infection is screened for routinely at booking, so with full antenatal care you should detect those mothers at risk. Admittedly, the flu-like illness here could represent seroconversion but you would not expect chorioretinitis or hydrocephalus. Group B *Streptococcus* (D) is a pathogen that is present in the genital tract of 25% of women. It has the ability to cause infection in the baby in the puerperium but not hydrocephalus. *Listeria monocytogenes* (E) is a bacterium that is present in unpasteurized cheeses and pâtés. It can lead to miscarriage, stillbirth or preterm delivery. The correct answer is (C) – toxoplasmosis. This is caused by the protozoon *Toxoplasma gondii* and can be contracted form undercooked meat and cat faeces. It can lead to chorioretinitis, macro- or microcephaly, convulsions and long-term neurodevelopmental delay. Initial infection in the mother is usually mild, and often she is not aware of it.

SECTION 7:
SEXUAL AND
REPRODUCTIVE HEALTH
AND UROGYNAECOLOGY

QUESTIONS

1. Gynaecological infections (1)

A 32-year-old woman has a routine cervical smear at her GP practice. The result returns as severe dyskaryosis. Following colposcopy and cervical biopsy, formal histological examination reveals cervical intraepithelial neoplasia 3 (CIN 3). Which of the following pathogens is the most likely to have caused this disease?

    A.   *Candida albicans*
    B.   Human immunodeficiency virus (HIV)
    C.   Human papilloma virus (HPV)
    D.   Herpes simplex
    E.   *Treponema pallidum*

2. Paediatric and adolescent gynaecology

A 15-year-old girl attends the paediatric gynaecology clinic with primary amenorrhoea and features of secondary breast development. She has intermittent abdominal bloating and is extremely worried that she is 'not like other girls'. On speculum examination of the vagina, which is normal externally, a bulging red disc is seen 3 cm proximal to the introitus. What is the most likely diagnosis?

    A.   Turner's syndrome
    B.   Congenital adrenal hyperplasia
    C.   Imperforate hymen
    D.   Anorexia nervosa
    E.   Delayed puberty

3. Management of miscarriage

A 19-year-old woman undergoes surgical evacuation of the retained products of conception (ERPC). Histological examination of the sample shows genetically abnormal placenta with a mixture of large and small villi with scalloped outlines, trophoblastic hyperplasia. What is the most likely diagnosis?

    A.   Choriocarcinoma
    B.   Degenerated uterine leimyoma
    C.   Uterine dysgerminoma
    D.   Hydatidiform mole
    E.   Complete miscarriage

4. Urogynaecology

An 89-year-old woman attends the gynaecology clinic with a long history of a dragging sensation in the vagina. Apart from severe aortic stenosis, she has no significant medical history. She leaks fluid when she sneezes or coughs. On examination with a Sims' speculum in the left lateral position, a grade 1 uterine prolapse is seen, with an additional cystocoele. What is the most appropriate management?

A. Vaginal hysterectomy with anterior colporrhapy (cystocoele repair)
B. Vaginal hysterectomy alone
C. Tension-free vaginal tape (TVT)
D. Weight loss and pelvic floor exercises
E. Twice weekly 0.1 per cent estriol cream and insertion of shelf pessary

5. Incontinence

A 46-year-old woman presents to your clinic with a 6-year history of Incontinence. She has had four children by vaginal deliveries, has a body mass index (BMI) of 35 kg/m^2 and suffers from hayfever. Initial examination reveals a very small cystocele. A mid-stream urine culture is negative and urodynamic studies show a weakened urethral sphincter. What is the most appropriate first line management?

A. Fesoterodine 4 mg daily
B. Weight loss and pelvic physiotherapy
C. Tension free vaginal tape
D. Solifenacin 5 mg daily and pelvic physiotherapy
E. Anterior repair and insertion of a transobturator tape

6. Gynaecological infections (2)

A 16-year-old girl attends the gynaecology clinic complaining of vaginal itching and lumpy labia. On examination the area is covered with vulval warts. Which is the causative pathogen for vulval warts?

A. Human papilloma virus type 16
B. Human papilloma virus type 18
C. Human papilloma virus type 6
D. Herpes simplex virus
E. *Epidermophyton floccosum*

7. Gynaecological infections (3)

A 25-year-old woman attends accident and emergency with an exquisitely sore, large swelling of her vagina which she noticed only a couple of days before. It has steadily got much bigger. On examination there is a soft fluctuant mass on the right labia minora which is very tender. What is the most appropriate management?

A. Marsupialization
B. Oral ofloxacin and metronidazole
C. Sebaceous cystectomy
D. Local 2 per cent clotrimazole (Canestan)
E. Referral to a vulval clinic

8. Contraceptive risks

An 18-year-old woman attends clinic seeking contraceptive advice. She is currently using condoms only and is keen to start taking the combined oral contraceptive pill (COCP). Her sister used to take it but told her there were lots of problems with it. Her aunt has bowel cancer and she has no other past medical history. Appropriate counselling should cover all of the following except:

    A.   There is an overall 12 per cent risk in reduction of cancers
    B.   There is a small increase in cervical cancer with prolonged use (>8 years)
    C.   There is a reduction in the risk of bowel cancer ✓
    D.   There is an increase in the risk of ovarian cancer ✗
    E.   There is no need for a cervical smear prior to starting the pill

9. Subfertility treatments

A 49-year-old woman presents to a private clinic expressing her desire to become pregnant. She has no past medical history. Initial investigations show that she still has ovarian function, is ovulating and is having regular periods. An ultrasound of her pelvis shows no structural abnormality and an hysterosalpingography demonstrates patent fallopian tubes. Analysis of her partner's semen is normal. Which would not be an appropriate first line management option?

    A.   *In vitro* fertilisation (IVF)
    B.   Intracytoplasmic sperm implantation
    C.   Intrauterine insemination
    D.   Clomiphene
    E.   Egg donation IVF

10. Urge incontinence

A 42-year-old woman presents to the urogynaecology clinic with a 3-year history of urge incontinence. She has features of an overactive bladder and is desperate to start treatment for her problem as it is affecting her quality of life. She opts for medical treatment. What is the most appropriate first line pharmacological therapeutic?

    A.   Darifenacin
    B.   Oxybutynin
    C.   Fesoterodine
    D.   Solifenacin
    E.   Oxybutynin dermal patch

11. Assisted reproductive technologies

A 41-year-old woman is about to undergo her first cycle of IVF. As part of the consultation, she is counselled about the maternal and fetal risks involved with IVF-conceived pregnancies. All of the following occur in such pregnancies except:

A. Increased risk of low birth weight infants
B. Increased risk of fetal congenital abnormalities
C. Decreased risk of ectopic pregnancies
D. Increased risk of small for gestational age (SGA) fetuses in singleton pregnancies
E. Increased risk of maternal pregnancy-induced hypertension (PIH)

12. Pre-termination assessment

A 16-year-old presents to the termination of pregnancy service 6 weeks into her second pregnancy requesting surgical termination (STOP). What is not required as part of her work-up for the procedure?

A. Antibiotic prophylaxis for *Chlamydia*
B. Gaining consent from her mother
C. Contraception discussion
D. Explaining the risks of STOP
E. Explaining that the risk of uterine perforation is one in 300

13. Subfertility (1)

A 35-year-old woman is seen in the assisted conception unit. She has been trying to conceive for 4 years. In this period she has been having regular intercourse. Her periods have been irregular and recently she has had no periods at all. Her BMI is 19.5 kg/m², she has had an appendectomy and is otherwise well. Her biochemistry comes back as follows: luteinizing hormone (LH) 0.5 IU/L, follicle-stimulating hormone (FSH) 1.0 IU/L, prolactin 490 mIU/L, thyroxine (T4) 12, thyroid stimulating hormone (TSH) 4.2 mIU/L, oestradiol 60 pmol/L. What is the most likely cause of her subfertility?

A. Polycystic ovarian syndrome (PCOS)
B. Hypothyroidism
C. Microprolactinoma
D. Hypothalamic hypogonadism
E. Anorexia

14. Pre-conception advice

A 19-year-old comes to you for some pre-conception advice. Some members of her family and her partner's family have a sickle cell anaemia. She reveals that her sister and his sister are both affected. Tests have shown that they are both carriers. What is the chance that if their child was a boy he would have sickle cell anaemia?

A. 50 per cent
B. 67 per cent
C. 100 per cent
D. 33 per cent
E. 25 per cent

15. Post-coital bleeding

An 18-year-old girl is seen in the colposcopy clinic after having had persistent post-coital bleeding. She has been sexually active since the age of 14 and has no past medical history. She is studying for her A-levels and has been doing a lot of reading. She is concerned that she might have cervical cancer. Which of the following is not a risk factor for cervical cancer?

A. Herpes simplex virus (HSV)
B. Smoking
C. HIV
D. Use of the oral contraceptive pill
E. Multiparity

16. Mixed urinary incontinence

A 49-year-old comes to the urogynaecology clinic with a history of leaking urine for the last year. There are associated stress symptoms and some urge symptoms. Interestingly she says that it seems to come from inside the vagina as well. She had a hysterectomy last year for endometrial cancer and had quite a prolonged recovery. She has a BMI of 30 kg/m², does not smoke and is otherwise fit and well. You are suspicious that she might have a vesico-vaginal fistula secondary to her operation. What is the most appropriate first line investigation?

A. Examination under anaesthesia (EUA) and cystoscopy
B. Pelvic MRI
C. Instillation of methylene blue into the urinary bladder and speculum examination
D. Pelvic computed tomography
E. Urodynamic study

17. Emergency contraception

A 16-year-old girl presents to your surgery with a history of unprotected sexual intercourse (UPSI) 70 hours ago. Her last menstrual period was 8 days ago. Her only past medical history of note is that of epilepsy which is well controlled by carbamazepine. She is worried about becoming pregnant, does not want her mother to find out and is in a hurry to get home before suspicions are raised. Which of the following options are available to her?

A. Take the combined oral contraceptive pill (COCP) continuously for the next month
B. A copper intrauterine device (IUD) should be inserted with prior screening for sexually transmitted infections (STIs)
C. Levonorgestrel 1.5 mg should be given as she is within 72 hours of UPSI

D. Reassure and tell her to come back when she has made her mind up as ulipristal can be taken up to 7 days after UPSI

E. Reassure her that she is in the safe part of her cycle and she should try and use condoms in the future

18. Contraception

A 40-year-old woman comes to your clinic alone wanting an effective form of contraception. She has two children from a previous marriage and has recently started a new relationship. She says that she does not want any further children. She has regular heavy periods, no menopausal symptoms and she is otherwise well with no past medical history. A recent ultrasound showed a normal sized uterus and pipelle biopsy revealed normal secretory endometrial tissue. What is the most appropriate form of contraception?

A. Combined oral contraceptive pill with <30 µg of oestrogen
B. Mirena coil
C. Laparoscopic sterilization
D. Vasectomy
E. Total abdominal hysterectomy

19. Secondary amenorrhoea

In a busy gynaecology clinic you are assessing a 22-year-old woman who has not had a period for 18 months. She is not pregnant and previously had regular periods. She has had two surgical terminations of pregnancies (STOP), an underactive thyroid gland and an appendectomy. Clinical examination is unremarkable with a BMI kg/m² of 20. Biochemical investigations reveal a T4 of 17 pmol/L, TSH 4.6 kg/m², prolactin of 570 mU/L, and testosterone of 42 ng/dL. LH and FSH are normal. Vaginal ultrasound shows a normal sized uterus and the left ovary contain four cysts. Which of the answers listed below is the most likely cause?

A. Polycystic ovarian syndrome (PCOS)
B. Prolactinoma
C. Sheehan's syndrome ×
D. Asherman's syndrome ×
E. Anorexia nervosa ×

20. Subfertility (2)

A 26-year-old woman is otherwise fit and well has been trying to conceive for over 2 years. On questioning she has regular periods and has been having regular intercourse. There are no abnormalities on clinical examination. What would be your first line investigations for her subfertility?

A. Day 14 FSH and LH, ultrasound and hysterosalpingogram (HSG), semen analysis
B. Day 1–3 FSH and LH, mid-luteal progesterone, semen analysis

C. Day 1–3 FSH and LH, mid-follicular progesterone, semen analysis
D. Random LH, FSH, HSG, semen analysis
E. Ultrasound, laparoscopy, semen analysis

21. Semen analysis

A 42-year-old man undergoes semen analysis as part of the investigation of subfertility with his wife. What result would most likely contribute to their subfertility?

A. Sperm count 30 million/mL
B. Volume 2.5 mL
C. 40 per cent have normal motility
D. 5 per cent normal morphology
E. pH 7.4

22. Assisted reproduction

A 46-year-old women in her fifth IVF cycle is admitted to the emergency department 4 days after egg collection. She is complaining of a swollen abdomen and shortness of breath. She is reviewed and a diagnosis of ovarian hyperstimulation syndrome (OHSS) is made. Which of the following is not a clinical feature/complication of OHSS?

A. Hydrothorax
B. Deep vein thrombosis
C. Haemodilution
D. Oliguria
E. Marked ascites

23. Primary amenorrhoea

A 17-year-old girl comes to clinic with her mother as she has not started having periods yet and they are worried. On examination she is of short stature, with a slightly widened neck and has no secondary sexual characteristics and there is no obvious abnormality of the external genitalia. What is the most likely diagnosis form this limited information?

A. Androgen insensitivity syndrome
B. Turner's syndrome
C. Congenital adrenal hyperplasia
D. Kallmann's syndrome
E. Rokitansky's syndrome

24. Vaginal discharge

A 22-year-old woman presents to the GUM clinic with an offensive smelling discharge. She is sexually active and is in a monogamous relationship. She describes no pain or soreness just an offensive smelling discharge. After examination and taking swabs for the second time she is diagnosed with bacterial vaginosis. Which of the following organisms is not likely to be the cause?

    A.   *Gardnerella* species
    B.   *Mobiluncus*
    C.   *Bacteroides*
    D.   *Trichomonas*
    E.   *Mycoplasma*

ANSWERS

Gynaecological infections

1 C HPV (C) is attributed to the development of cervical intraepithelial neoplasia and adenocarcinoma. Of the subtypes of HPV, 16 and 18 are among the most highly oncogenic. These are responsible for around 70 per cent of all cervical cancer cases. Routine vaccination against the virus is now offered to all girls at around 12 years of age. Herpes simplex (D) is responsible for oral cold sores and genital herpes, not cervical cancer. *Candida albicans* (A) is a yeast which causes vaginal candidiasis or 'thrush,' which can cause pain and embarrassing discharge. HIV (B) is a retrovirus which is now readily treatable but as yet incurable. Immune destruction gradually causes the onset of opportunistic infection, and, eventually, an AIDS-defining infection. HIV-positive women are at high risk of contracting human papilloma virus and therefore at an increased risk of intraepithelial neoplasias. *Treponema pallidum* (E) is a spirochaete bacterium which is responsible for clinical syphilis infection. Histological examination of the cervix would not demonstrate any bacterium. Although young women with syphilis infection would be more likely than those without to have a concurrent HPV infection, and therefore a higher risk of cervical intraepithelial neoplasia, there is no direct link between the two and the risk is raised due to the confounding effect of sexual behaviour.

Paediatric and adolescent gynaecology

2 C Primary amenorrhoea is a failure to start periods. To begin menstruating, the girl must be structurally normal and have a properly functioning hypothalamic-pituitary axis (HPA). The fact that this girl has normal external genitalia and has normal pubertal breast development suggests that secondary sexual development is occurring normally, and the HPA is functioning. The speculum examination reveals what is most likely to be haematocolpos – blood inside the vagina – the most common cause for which in the presence of amenorrhoea is an imperforate hymen (C). This is where the hymen does not separate at the time of the menarche and thereafter blood cannot escape with each period, but builds up behind the intact hymen. This would also explain her intermittent bloating. Patients with anorexia nervosa (D) would either have complete lack of secondary development, if the condition started early, or a secondary amenorrhoea. Turner's syndrome (A) – XO karyotype – is associated with short stature, wide carrying angles, a broad chest and a lack of sexual development. Congenital adrenal hyperplasia (B) results from inadequate cortisol production positively feeding back on adrenocorticotrophic hormone production, resulting in adrenal hyperplasia and excessive adrogenic cortisol precursors. Females normally have ambiguous or masculinized genitals, and suffer from hyponatraemia, hyperkalaemia and dehydration. This girl has shown signs of secondary development, so (E) is incorrect.

Management of miscarriage

3 D The pathological findings are consistent with a diagnosis of hydatidiform mole (D). Hydatidiform moles are part of a spectrum of pathological pregnancies and are essentially benign trophoblastic tumours. They occur in between 1:20 000 and 1:50 000 pregnancies. Risk factors include extremes of age, previous molar pregnancy and race; an increased rate of molar pregnancy is seen in people from South East Asia, although the reasons are unclear. Women usually present with unusual or heavy bleeding beyond the sixth week of pregnancy with a pregnancy which is larger than dates would suggest. Due to the size of theca lutein cysts, the ovaries are often enlarged. Pre-eclampsia, thyrotoxicosis and hyperemesis gravidarum are common in molar pregnancy. Diagnosis involves clinical assessment for the features above, coupled with serum beta hCG assessment (which is often significantly higher than would be expected in an early pregnancy) and ultrasonography which may demonstrate a classical 'snowstorm appearance'. Follow-up is of vital importance to ascertain whether the hCG level is falling: if it does not, further treatment may be necessary, including surgical evacuation of the uterus. One in 80 women will go on to have a further molar pregnancy. Choriocarcinoma (A) is also a form of gestational trophoblastic disease, but it is aggressive and malignant. It readily metastasizes to the lungs. Closely related syncytiotrophoblasts and cytotrophoblasts are typical, with syncytiotrophoblasts often displaying abnormal nuclei containing cytoplasm with abnormally high eosiniphil counts. Hydatidiform moles can rarely progress to choriocarcinoma, and around half of all cases of choriocarcinoma will have developed from a hydatidiform mole. Degenerated uterine leimyoma (B) is the result of 'red degeneration' of a fibroid and would not show any histological features of pregnancy (e.g. trophoblasts). A complete miscarriage (E) constitutes a failed pregnancy in which all products of conception have been expelled from the uterine cavity. As there is still tissue found at ERPC, this cannot be the diagnosis. Dysgerminomas (C) are germ cell tumours which would be histologically distinct from molar pregnancy by the presence of lobular cells with fibrous stromal cells with lymphocytic invasion.

Urogynaecology

4 E This woman has symptomatic uterine and bladder prolapse into the vagina. When it is significant and symptomatic, surgical treatment is most appropriate. Urodynamic studies should be performed to guide the choice of operation. This woman, however, has a significant medical co-morbidity (severe aortic stenosis) which in a patient of her age makes her a poor surgical candidate: (A)–(C) are therefore least appropriate. Vaginal hysterectomy (A, B) is a suitable surgical therapy for women who have completed their family, have a normal sized uterus (enabling vaginal extraction) and would benefit from it (indications include uterine prolapse and heavy menstrual bleeding among others). Vaginal repairs (A) may be performed concurrently with vaginal hysterectomy, either of the anterior wall (anterior colporrhapy) or posterior wall (posterior colporrhapy) for cystocoele and rectocoele, respectively. TVT is a procedure for urinary stress incontinence involving the insertion of a tape, not under tension, underneath the urethra to support failed native tissue. Of the two non-operative interventions available, estriol cream and a shelf pessary (E) are most likely to bring symptomatic relief from her prolapse. Weight loss and pelvic floor exercises (D) would be appropriate non-medical interventions, though in a woman of 89 years weight loss and effective pelvic floor exercises are probably as unachievable as they are inadvisable.

Incontinence

5 B   This woman has symptoms and urodynamic evidence of stress incontinence. She does not have any urge symptoms or frank urinary incontinence. Fesoterodine (A) and solifenacin (D) are used to treat urge incontinence. She has a high body mass index (BMI) which is an independent risk factor for developing stress incontinence. Conservative options should be attempted before more complex medical or surgical stratgies. A TVT (C) or a transobturator tape (TOT) (E) are both appropriate surgical options for persistent stress incontinence but simple measures should be undertaken first such as weight loss, smoking cessation and physiotherapy (B). The TOT procedure carries a lower risk of iatrogenic bladder damage as the tape is passed through the obturator foramen. The choice of procedure in practice often falls to the operator's preference and surgical experience. In the presence of a cystocoele, an anterior repair may be appropriate but not as a first line treatment for symptomatic stress incontinence. For this reason option (B) is the correct answer.

Gynaecological infections (2)

6 C   Human papilloma virus types 6 (C) and 11 are associated with vulval warts. Subtypes 16 (A) and 18 (B) are strongly associated with cervical cancer. Herpes simplex virus (D) causes cold sores on the lips or genital herpes, which are distinct from warts and have a papulovesicular morphology. *Epidermophyton floccosum* (E) is the fungus responsible for athlete's foot which can manifest in the groin as jock itch or tinea cruris.

Gynaecological infections (3)

7 A   The clinical history and examination findings make it clear that this is a Bartholin's abscess. The paired Bartholin's glands, about 0.5 cm in diameter, are commonly found at the 4- and 8-o'clock positions in the labia minora. They are normally non-palpable. Their role is to secrete vaginal lubricant into the vestibule via the Bartholin's ducts during sexual arousal. If the ducts become blocked, an abscess of the gland can develop. Treatment of this is normally with marsupialization (A): surgery involving opening the abscess and suturing its lining to the outside to create a permanent opening, thereby preventing recurrence. Oral antibiotics (B) may be useful after surgery, or before if the abscess is small, but not when it is large like in this case. Note however that ofloxacin and metronidazole are agents commonly used for pelvic inflammatory disease and not usually for abscesses. Sebaceous cystectomy (C), as the name implies, is a treatment for sebaceous cysts, and is only employed if the cyst is very symptomatic. Vaginal clotrimazole (D) is a treatment for thrush. Simple Bartholin's abscesses do not require specialist assessment in a vulval clinic (E) unless there are signs of Bartholin's gland malignancy which is very rare (<1:1 000 000).

Contraceptive risks

8 D   It is important that before starting any therapy the patient is informed of the potential risks and benefits. There is a decreased risk of bowel (C) and rectal cancer with use of the COCP. The risk of any cancer developing overall is reduced by 12 per cent for women on the COCP (A) while there is a small but statistically significant increase in the risk of cervical cancer with prolonged use (B). Option (D) is the appropriate option because there is no proven increased risk of ovarian cancer in women taking the combined oral contraceptive: in fact there is a protective effect. Before starting the pill, a full sexual history should be taken. There is no requirement to start cervical smears (E) until she is 25 unless there are specific patient-specific risks of developing cervical neoplasia. There is a small increase in cervical cancer with prolonged pill usage but this risk is mitigated through regular routine cervical screening.

Subfertility treatments

9 D   Most students, and indeed many postgraduate trainees, will have little experience with which to tackle this question since only in private practice would a 49-year-old woman normally be offered IVF. The important point is that in 2008 the average success rate of IVF with a patient's own eggs if she was over 44 years old was 2.5 per cent. (A), (B) and (C) would be appropriate measures to try and achieve a pregnancy. Option (E) may well provide a better success rate as the donor's eggs will be potentially of a better quality than the patient's. Clomiphene is the wrong answer. Clomiphene is a selective oestrogen receptor modulator which, by inhibiting negative feedback on the hypothalamus, increases the production of gonadotrophins. In this way, it is used to induce ovulation. Given that the woman in this case is ovulating, treatment with clomiphene would be inappropriate.

Urge incontinence

10 B A diagnosis of an overactive bladder can be based on history. Urodynamic studies will confirm the diagnosis but this is an invasive procedure. It is appropriate in most women to start a trial of therapy and assess the response. Conservative measures include keeping a bladder diary and bladder retraining. The first line treatment is immediate release oxybutynin (B). All of the other answers (A, C, D, E) are appropriate second line agents. It is important to counsel the patients about the side effects of antimuscarinics which include dry mouth, constipation and urinary retention. If there is no improvement following trials of alternative medical treatments, and if diagnosis of overactive bladder is confirmed with urodynamic studies, other treatment modalities such as sacral nerve stimulation may be appropriate.

Assisted reproductive technologies

11 C Since the birth of the first baby conceived through IVF in 1978, IVF has offered women the chance of successful healthy pregnancy which nature would have otherwise denied them. There is good evidence demonstrating various increased maternal and fetal risks of IVF-conceived pregnancies compared with natural conception. There is in fact an increased risk of ectopic pregnancies, not a reduced risk (C). There is an increased risk of fetal congenital abnormalities (B). IVF pregnancies are more likely than naturally conceived pregnancies to be multiple (twins, triplets etc.), which carry their own increased risks such as pre-eclampsia. There is an increase in SGA babies (D) and low birth weight deliveries (A). If the pregnancy is a result of egg donation there is an as yet unexplained a seven-fold increase in PIH (E).

Pre-termination assessment

12 B This patient is 16 years old and is therefore able to consent to an operation under the concept of 'Gillick competence'. If she shows that she has the capacity to consent to the procedure then parental request is unnecessary (B). Screening for *Chlamydia* or treating empirically should be offered (A). A very important part of a termination of pregnancy service is to offer women post-termination contraception (C). The risks of a termination (D), including bleeding, infection, failure of the procedure, the need for a repeat procedure and perforation of the uterus (E), must be explained clearly to the patient for consent to be valid. Perforation of the uterus occurs in approximately one in 300 surgical terminations of pregnancy.

Subfertility (1)

13 D From these results you can see that her pituitary is not producing FSH and LH in adequate quantities to cause the ovaries to produce oestradiol. In fact, the negative feedback loop is not activated – the pituitary is not responding to the low oestradiol levels by increasing the FSH as in the menopause. Therefore, this could be attributed to hypothalamic hypogonadism. Her BMI is at the low end of normal but is not pathological (E). Her prolactin (C) level is normal. A microprolactinoma can be diagnosed on MRI of the brain. Her TSH (B) is at the high end of normal but again is not pathological and could not explain her subfertility. The diagnosis of PCOS (A) needs two of oligo/anovulation, signs of hyperandrogenism or polycystic ovaries. Although we do not have any comment about the ovaries or clinical hyperandrogenism, the pituitary profile is not typical of PCOS.

Pre-conception advice

14 E Sickle cell anaemia is an autosomal recessive condition. The gender of the offspring is irrelevant as sickle cell is not an X-linked condition. If both parents are carriers of this autosomal recessive gene then the chance of having a child with sickle cell anaemia is 25 per cent, being a carrier 50 per cent and not being affected at all 25 per cent. Other autosomal recessive conditions include Tay–Sachs disease, phenylketonuria and cystic fibrosis.

Post-coital bleeding

15 A Cervical cancer typically affects women between the age of 45 and 55. The majority of cancers are squamous cell with 10 per cent being adenocarcinomas. There is a clear association with human papilloma virus (HPV) but there is no clear association with HSV (A). Smoking (B) is an independent risk factor and any condition that renders the patient immunocompromised, such as HIV (C), increases the risk of cervical carcinoma. There is an association with COCP use (D) and having children (E). Both of these are not causal factors for the development of cervical cancer but instead are relative risk factors conferred by the increased sexual activity associated with them.

Mixed urinary incontinence

16 C Vesico-vaginal fistulae are common around the world, mainly as a result of obstructed labour. The fetal head can sit adjacent to the bladder for days before medical help is sought. By this time the tissues become necrotic, break down and a fistula develops. In resource-rich countries the most common cause is pelvic surgery. This woman may have a connection from the bladder to the vagina. A simple test you could do in clinic is to pass a catheter and fill the bladder with some methylene blue dye (C). You can then perform a speculum examination to see if the dye is in the vagina. Second line investigation would involve an EUA and cystoscopy (A). Urodynamics (E) and imaging (B, D) are unlikely to aid in diagnosis as stress incontinence is the loss of native supporting tissue allowing incontinence and is likely to be undetectable on x-ray. Once a fistula has been identified, referral to a centre that has experience in repair is advised. They can be repaired abdominally or vaginally depending on their site and size.

Emergency contraception

17 This is a difficult conversation under time pressures. Ideally you would prefer to counsel the patient about all the options of emergency contraception and the ramifications of unprotected sexual intercourse. An important part of your counselling will involve future contraception advice. This patient has three options for emergency contraception. A copper IUD (B) inserted up to 5 days after the UPSI, the progesterone antagonist Ulipristal (D) up to 5 days after and the more common levonorgesterol 1.5 mg within 72 hours (C). She meets the timeline for all options. Importantly she is taking an enzyme inducer carbamazepine so you could not guarantee the success of levonorgesterol. The Diploma of the Faculty of Sexual and Reproductive Healthcare (DFSRH) recommends increasing the dose of levonorgesterol to 3 mg but this is off licence. A copper coil would be the most appropriate contraception under these circumstances, also allowing you to perform a full STI screen simultaneously. Option (A) would not be effective as an emergency contraception and she is on an enzyme-inducing drug. Option (E) is not appropriate as depending on her cycle length she may well ovulate in the next 5–6 days. Sperm can survive for a week so she may well fall pregnant if no action is taken.

Contraception

18 B Although there is much in the press about the cardiovascular/carcinogenic/venous thromboembolism (VTE) risks of the COCP there is no contraindication to prescribing them in a low risk woman (A). The DFRSH states that there is a small increase in the risk of breast cancer and a recent study suggested that VTE risk was lower if oestrogen was <30 μg. The Mirena coil (B) would be a good choice of contraception as she has a normal endometrium and heavy periods. She must be warned that she can expect up to 6 months of irregular bleeding post insertion but a third of women at 1 year have no periods and 70 per cent report significant reduction in bleeding 12 months after insertion. Laparoscopic sterilization (C) is appropriate if she really does not want more children. She is still only 40 and in a new relationship and may change her mind so this would not be first line. Similarly, a hysterectomy (E) would not be appropriate purely for contraceptive reasons in an otherwise well woman. Vasectomy (D) is an excellent form of contraception (one in 2000 failure rate) but you would need to speak to her partner about this. Most clinicians would recommend the Mirena coil for this woman as it will treat her heavy periods and provide an effective contraception for the next 5 years.

Secondary amenorrhoea

19 D PCOS (A) is a multisystem disorder classically diagnosed by two of the following three criteria: anovulation/oligo-ovulation, biochemical or physical evidence of hyperandrogenism and an ultrasound scan showing 12 or more follicles in the ovary. This woman has secondary amenorrhoea but has no evidence of PCOS physically, biochemically or on ultrasound. Her prolactin level (B) is at the high end of normal. With a prolactinoma one should be vigilant for visual field defects. If the adenoma compresses the optic chiasm you can develop visual field defects. Other symptoms of hyperprolactinaemia include galactorrhea. Sheehan's syndrome (C) is a post-partum complication, classically after a large haemorrhage causing hypoperfusion of the pituitary gland leading to ischaemia and necrosis. She has not carried a pregnancy past the first trimester so this is not possible. Her BMI is normal but further questioning would be needed to ascertain whether this was the cause. In light of a normal LH and FSH, anorexia (E) being the cause is unlikely as it leads to a hypothalamic hypogonadism. Asherman's syndrome (D) is intrauterine scar tissue and adhesion formation seen after instrumentation of the uterus. It is not common but should be considered with a history of two STOPs. To diagnose, a hysteroscopy would need to be performed.

Subfertility (2)

20 B The causes of subfertility can be viewed broadly as male and female. Semen analysis is vital in the assessment of the subfertile couple. Female causes include anovulation, tubal/uterine blockage and endometriosis. It would be advisable to check day 1–3 LH and FSH as well as a mid-luteal phase progesterone (B). This will give you the best indication as to whether the woman is ovulating. If she is not ovulating then pregnancy will not be possible. Further investigations can include an ultrasound to look at the size of the uterus and the presence of fibroids/polyps. An HSG is an assessment of tubal patency. A laparoscopy (E) would be considered after all the above to investigate endometriosis and direct vision of tubal patency by passing dye through the cervix and watching it exit via the fimbrial ends of the fallopian tubes. (A) would not be an appropriate first step as day 14 – around ovulation – would provide little information to help your diagnosis. You would expect an LH surge to be present at this time. A mid-follicular phase progesterone (C) would be low. Mid-luteal phase progesterone >30 nmol/L would lead you to believe that she is ovulating. Answer (D) has no place in the initial investigation as it is important to know whereabouts in the cycle this woman is.

Semen analysis

21 C Male factor subfertility is the cause for somewhere between 25 and 40 per cent of subfertile couples. The average ejaculate volume is 1.5–6 mL (B) and the pH should be between 7.2 and 8.0 (E). The sample is considered normal if 4 per cent or more have normal morphology (D). Sperm count should be over 15 million per millilitre (A). Fifty per cent of the sperm should have normal motility so (C) is the correct answer.

Assisted reproduction

22 C OHSS is diagnosed after ovarian stimulation in IVF cycles. Thirty-three per cent of all IVF cycles will lead to mild OHSS and 3–8 per cent into severe OHSS. It typically presents with abdominal pain and swelling and vomiting. It is important to consider differentials including an ectopic pregnancy, pelvic infection, ovarian cyst torsion or appendicitis. Classically the blood will become haemoconcentrated (C) with a hypoproteinaemia and ascites (E) will be present which may lead to a pleural effusion (A). The ovaries will be enlarged on ultrasound and in severe OHSS will be over 12 cm. Due to the haemoconcentration these patients are at particularly high risk of venous thromboembolism (B) so thromboembolic decompression stockings and enoxaparin while in hospital is appropriate. This is partly attributable to the hypoproteinaemia – low albumin – leading to decreased intravascular plasma and hypercoagulability. If the OHSS is severe there may be problems perfusing the kidneys well if much of the intravascular volume is being drawn into the third space by the decrease in oncotic pressure in the blood vessels. This may lead to oliguria. Fluid balance and management is key to these patients.

Primary amenorrhoea

23 B Androgen insensitivity syndrome (AIS) (A) is very unlikely in a female as carriers are not generally affected and the likelihood of a fertile male with AIS is very small. Turner's syndrome (B) is most likely because of the sexual development, short stature and the neck webbing. Turner's syndrome is 46×0 leading to gonadal dysgenesis and sterility. Congenital adrenal hyperplasia (C) is autosomal recessive and is a disruption of steroid production. There are various enzymes that lead to different versions but the most common is 21 hydroxylase deficiency. This leads to hyperandrogenism and virilization of the female genitalia. Kallmann's syndrome (D) would have been the next best answer as it is a result of decreased gonadotrophin-releasing hormone leading to hypogonadism, delayed puberty and lack of secondary sexual characteristics. Rokitansky's syndrome (E) is characterized by Müllerian agenesis. So a girl will be 46XX, will have ovaries that function and will develop secondary sexual characteristics. There will, however, be no development of fallopian tubes or uterus and she may have a shortened vagina.

Vaginal discharge

24 D Bacterial vaginosis (BV) is not felt to be a sexually transmitted disease but is seen in people who are sexually active. It is a result of an imbalance of the naturally occurring flora in the vagina. It presents as an off-white offensive discharge with a fishy odour. Diagnosis is made with swabs showing clue cells and a loss of vaginal acidity. *Trichomonas* (D) is a separate infection caused by a protozoon that leads to a greenish discharge. It is a sexually transmitted infection. All the other flora above are responsible for bacterial vaginosis. (A, B, C and E) can all cause BV secondary to the reduction in the normal levels of lactobacilli found in the vagina. This reduction may be due to a recent antibiotic course or a change in pH of the vagina allowing these other bacteria to multiply.

SECTION 8:
SURGICAL GYNAECOLOGY AND ONCOLOGY

QUESTIONS

1. Gynaecological oncology (1)

A 28-year-old woman attends her GP clinic for routine cervical screening. Liquid-based cytology (LBC) shows mild dyskaryosis. A repeat sample again shows mild dyskaryosis. What is the most appropriate management?

    A.   Repeat the LBC smear test in 6 months
    B.   Repeat the LBC smear test in 3 months
    C.   Arrange colposcopy at the gynaecology clinic
    D.   Knife cone biopsy of the cervix
    E.   Large loop excision of the transformation zone

2. Female pelvic anatomy (1)

When assessing the fetal presenting part in labour it is important to know the anatomy of the pelvis. What are the bony landmarks of the pelvic outlet?

    A.   Pubic arch, ischial tuberosities and the coccyx
    B.   Pectineal line, ischial spines, coccyx
    C.   Pubic symphysis, pubic rami, sacrum
    D.   Pectineal line, ischial tuberosities and the coccyx
    E.   Pubic arch, ischial spines, sacrum

3. Postoperative complications (1)

A 26 year old undergoes potassium-titanyl-phosphate (KTP) laser laparoscopic excision of endometriosis. Her postoperative haemoglobin is 8.1 g/dL. Six hours postoperatively she complains of increased umbilical swelling, abdominal pain and shortness of breath and she appears pale. A repeat full blood count now shows a haemoglobin count of 6.5 g/dL. What are the most appropriate steps you should take next?

    A.   Transfuse one unit of cross-matched packed red cells and await events
    B.   Volume replacement with colloids and reassessment of the haemoglobin level
    C.   D-dimer and computed tomography (CT) pulmonary angiogram (CTPA)
    D.   Insertion of a large-bore nasogastric tube on free drainage
    E.   Transfuse four units of cross-matched packed red cells and return to theatre for further laparoscopy

4. Abdominal cramps

A 54-year-old woman presents to her GP with a 1-year history of bloating, early satiety and occasional crampy pelvic pain. She was diagnosed a year ago with irritable bowel syndrome (IBS). A serum CA 125 is 62 IU/mL (normal range <36 IU/mL). What is the most appropriate management?

    A.   Pelvic examination and pipelle biopsy
    B.   Ultrasound of the abdomen and pelvis

C. Computed tomography of the abdomen and pelvis
   D. Urgent referral to the gynaecology clinic under the 2-week rule for
      suspected cancers
   E. Trial of mebeverine and lifestyle modification

5. Acid-base physiology

A 24-year-old woman is admitted to the gynaecology ward with a 4-day history
of severe hyperemesis gravidarum. She has been unable to tolerate food or fluid
orally for 2 days. On the second day of admission she develops signs of a severe
pneumonia. This is presumed to be a hospital-acquired infection. She deteriorates
rapidly. An arterial blood gas shows:

pH 7.68
PO_2 10.0 kPa
PCO_2 4.26 kPa
HCO_3 32 mmol/L
K^+ 1.9 mmol/L
Lactate 1.2 mmol/L

What is the most accurate description of the acid-base disorder?

   A. Metabolic alkalosis
   B. Respiratory alkalosis
   C. Mixed respiratory alkalosis and metabolic acidosis
   D. Respiratory alkalosis with inadequate respiratory compensation
   E. Mixed metabolic alkalosis and respiratory alkalosis

6. Oncology

A 61-year-old woman has recently been diagnosed with a stage 1a endometrial
carcinoma. She has had four children, she has mild utero-vaginal prolapse and she has
never been operated on. She needs to have surgery. You see her in clinic and talk about
the different operations available to her. Which is the most appropriate operation?

   A. Wertheim's hysterectomy
   B. Total abdominal hysterectomy
   C. Laparoscopic hysterectomy
   D. Subtotal hysterectomy
   E. Posterior exenteration

7. Endometrial cancer

A 58-year-old woman presents to the clinic with post-menopausal bleeding. A
pipelle biopsy confirms adenocarcinoma of the endometrium. Further imaging of
the pelvis shows that there is spread of the tumour outside of the uterus into the
left adnexa. There is no other spread. What is the most likely stage of the tumour?

   A. Stage 1A
   B. Stage II

    C.   Stage IIIA
    D.   Stage IVA
    E.   Stage IIIC2

8. Gynaecological oncology (2)

A 65-year-old woman is referred by her GP to the gynaecology clinic with increasing bloating and a raised CA 125 level. A CT scan shows an irregular, enlarged left ovary and several well-circumscribed nodular lesions in the liver and on the omentum which are highly suspicious for metastatic ovarian cancer. What is the most appropriate treatment regimen?

    A.   Total hysterectomy, bilateral salpingo-oophorectomy and omentectomy along with concomitant stereotactic radiotherapy of the liver lesions
    B.   Total hysterectomy, bilateral salpingo-oophorectomy, omentectomy, aortopelvic lymphadenectomy
    C.   Staging laparotomy and optimal cytoreduction
    D.   Palliative care
    E.   Total pelvic exenteration

9. Pleural effusion

A 62-year-old woman presents to accident and emergency with shortness of breath. Examination reveals reduced breath sounds and a swollen, distended abdomen. Chest x-ray demonstrates a left-sided pleural effusion. On further questioning the woman has had a poor appetite for the last 6 months and recently had some vaginal bleeding. An ultrasound revealed large quantities of ascites, which were drained. Analysis of the ascites shows a high protein content. What is the most likely diagnosis?

    A.   Congestive cardiac failure (CCF)
    B.   Carcinoma of the ovary
    C.   Meigs' syndrome
    D.   Cirrhosis of the liver
    E.   Carcinoma of the cervix

10. Emergency gynaecology

A 28-year-old woman attends accident and emergency unable to walk because she is so faint. She has had heavy vaginal bleeding for 4 hours since she engaged in sexual intercourse with a new partner, which she described as 'rough and very painful'. She is still bleeding and cannot tolerate vaginal examination due to the pain. A point-of-care haemoglobin estimation is 6.4 g/dL and she is haemodynamically unstable. What is the most appropriate management?

    A.   Discharge with oral iron supplementation and follow up in the gynaecology clinic in 2 days
    B.   Discharge with oral iron supplementation and follow up on the ward in 24 hours

C. Admit, resuscitate and prepare her for immediate transfer to theatre
D. Admit to the gynaecology ward, cross-match four units of packed red cells and send a formal full blood count
E. Admit to the gynaecology ward having packed the vagina

11. Peri-operative management

A 64-year-old woman with asthma is admitted to the ward prior to an elective vaginal hysterectomy for symptomatic uterine prolapse. Her medications include Seretide (fluticasone/salmeterol 500/50) four times daily and oral prednisolone 20 mg twice daily. What is the most important peri-operative consideration?

A. Steroid cover with 50 mg hydrocortisone intravenously at induction of anaesthesia
B. Steroid cover with 100 mg hydrocortisone intravenously at induction of anaesthesia
C. Steroid cover with 50 mg hydrocortisone intravenously at induction of anaesthesia and 50 mg 8-hourly for 3 days
D. Bronchodilator cover with intravenous salbutamol infusion postoperatively
E. Continue regular medications and postoperative review by respiratory physician

12. Female pelvic anatomy (2)

A woman is undergoing surgery to enhance the cosmetic appearance of her labia. A bleeding vessel is encountered at the labia majora which cannot be controlled through pressure alone. The surgeon believes it to be a branch of the posterior labial artery. The posterior labial artery is a branch of which artery?

A. Internal pudendal artery
B. Inferior gluteal artery
C. Uterine artery
D. Obturator artery
E. Inferior vesical artery

13. Female pelvic anatomy (3)

Following surgery to place a tension-free transobturator tape for stress incontinence, a 54-year-old woman loses some sensation in part of her labia anterior to the anus. Damage has most likely been caused to which nerve?

A. Perineal nerve
B. Peroneal nerve
C. Pudendal nerve
D. Dorsal nerve of clitoris
E. Inferior anal nerve

14. Postoperative complications (2)

A 54-year-old woman with a history of significant ischaemic heart disease undergoes vaginal hysterectomy for symptomatic uterine prolapse. She develops significant surgical site bleeding which is repaired at reoperation the same day. Her postoperative haemoglobin is 6.4 g/dL. Later the same day she develops chest pain. Her observations, blood gas and cardiac enzymes are within normal limits. An electrocardiogram (ECG) shows sinus rhythm without ST changes. She is charted for thromboprophylaxis. What is the most likely cause of the chest pain?

    A. Non ST-elevation myocardial infarction
    B. Anaemia
    C. Pulmonary embolism
    D. Atelectasis
    E. Postoperative sepsis

15. Postoperative complications (3)

A 46-year-old woman is returned to the ward from the recovery room following a routine vaginal hysterectomy for heavy periods and prolapse. The estimated blood loss at operation was 200 mL. Two hours later the ward sister becomes concerned that her urine output is low and calls the doctor. Her observations show: pulse 115 bpm, BP 90/62 mmHg, temperature 37.1°C. What are the most appropriate next steps in her management?

    A. Aggressive fluid resuscitation, alert the operating surgeon and prepare for a return to theatre
    B. Fluid challenge, haemoglobin estimation and arterial blood gas
    C. Vaginal examination, haemoglobin estimation and arterial blood gas
    D. Establish large-bore intravenous access, alert the operating surgeon and perform arterial blood gas
    E. Establish large-bore intravenous access, alert the operating surgeon and perform a fluid challenge

16. Female pelvic anatomy (4)

The peritoneal lining drapes over the pelvic viscera and forms the part of the peritoneal cavity. Which is the most inferior extent of the peritoneal cavity?

    A. Vesicouterine pouch
    B. Paravesical fossa
    C. Rectouterine pouch (Pouch of Douglas)
    D. Pararectal fossa
    E. Rectovesical pouch

17. Cancer risk

A 74-year-old woman has an annual health check up with her private insurer. They arrange an ultrasound scan that shows a cyst on her right ovary. It is multiloculated and has solid components. She is post-menopausal and otherwise well. A doctor has sent for a CA 125 which comes back as 120 U/mL. What is her risk of malignancy index score (RMI)?

    A.   120
    B.   240
    C.   60
    D.   720
    E.   480

18. Irregular vaginal bleeding

A 21 year old comes to the clinic with a history of intermenstrual bleeding for the last 6 weeks. She has regular periods and does not experience post-coital bleeding. She is not on the oral contraceptive pill and has no other past medical history. What is the most appropriate first line investigation?

    A.   Hysteroscopy and biopsy
    B.   Cervical smear test
    C.   Triple swabs for pelvic infection
    D.   Ultrasound scan of the pelvis
    E.   Pipelle biopsy

19. Postoperative complications (4)

Two days after undergoing posterior exenteration for recurrence of cervical adenocarcinoma a 53-year-old woman develops a tachypnoea, tachycardia of 125 bpm and a fever of 39°C. Blood cultures have grown methicillin-resistant *Staphylococcus* aureus (MRSA). She requires intravenous vasopressors. What is the most appropriate diagnosis?

    A.   Sepsis
    B.   Systemic inflammatory response syndrome
    C.   Septic shock
    D.   Septicaemia
    E.   Adult respiratory distress syndrome

20. Female pelvic anatomy (5)

A 60-year-old woman is undergoing abdominal hysterectomy for a fibroid uterus. During suture ligation of the right uterine pedicle, iatrogenic injury to the ureter is confirmed. Which of the following statements is correct?

    A.   The ureter passes through the mesometrium and posterior to the uterine artery on its course to the urinary bladder
    B.   The ureter passes outside of the mesometrium and anterior to the uterine artery on its course to the urinary bladder

C. The ureter lies posterior to the internal iliac artery and lateral to the obturator nerve opposite the lower part of the greater sciatic notch
D. The ureter passes inferior to the cardinal ligament before coursing anteriorally to enter the urinary bladder
E. The ureter is not closely related to the uterine arteries

21. Vaginal bleeding

A 57-year-old woman has been referred by her GP under the 2-week suspected cancer referral approach with vaginal bleeding. She has been post-menopausal for the last 4 years and she has been taking Elleste Duet to treat her vasomotor symptoms. Two weeks ago, after reading about the risks associated with hormone replacement therapy (HRT) she stopped taking any medication. This is the first unscheduled bleeding she has ever had. She had a normal smear 2 years ago and is otherwise well. What would be your first line investigation?

A. Pipelle biopsy
B. Hysteroscopy
C. Smear test
D. Ultrasound of the pelvis
E. CT abdomen and pelvis

22. Gynaecological pathology

A 39-year-old woman attends the gynaecology clinic complaining of long-standing pelvic pain. Routine bimanual examination and abdominal ultrasonography do not detect any abnormality. At diagnostic laparoscopy, multiple tiny dark brown nodular lesions are noted covering the surface of the uterus, tubes and left ovary, as well as in the Pouch of Douglas. Which finding is most likely from histological examination of the excised lesions?

A. Krukenberg tumour
B. Vacuolated clear cells
C. Endometrial glands with stromal cells
D. Multiple leiomyomata
E. Enucleolated hyperplastic smooth muscle cells

23. Operative laparoscopy

A 21-year-old woman with dysmenorrhorea, dyspareunia and dyschezia has been scheduled for a laparoscopy to investigate possible endometriosis. You are asking for her consent and you describe the risks of laparoscopy, which include bleeding and damage to blood vessels, viscera and nerves. Which of the following is not at risk when inserting a lateral port?

A. Superficial epigastric artery
B. External iliac vein
C. Iliohypogastric nerve
D. Superior epigastric artery
E. Ilioinguinal nerve

ANSWERS

Gynaecological oncology (1)

1 C Cervical screening is an important public health strategy introduced to reduce the morbidity and mortality of cervical cancers. It is based on the premise that abnormal cells can be detected early, well before they undergo malignant change and appropriate treatment can be instituted to prevent progression to invasive disease. Women in the UK are first invited for cervical screening at 25 years of age and then every 3 years until 50, whereafter they are screened every 5 years. The programme ends when they are 65 years of age unless abnormal results have been shown. Mild dyskaryosis detected on one sample should prompt a repeat smear within 3 months. A second sample reported as mild dyskaryosis warrants referral for colposcopy (C). Knife cone biopsy (D) and loop excision (E) are normally performed only after a histological rather than cytological diagnosis of dyskaryosis. Referral for colposcopy should also be made after three consecutive borderline results at LBC, after two results of mild dyskaryosis, or when there is any moderate or severe dyskaryosis.

Female pelvic anatomy (1)

2 A The pelvic outlet is delineated by the inferior margin of the pubic symphysis (pubic arch), the ischial tuberosities (left and right, sometimes called the ischial spines) and the tip of the coccyx. Answer (A) is correct. The pectineal line is part of the pubic bone forming the pelvic inlet so (B) and (D) are wrong. (C) and (E) are wrong because the sacrum forms the posterior aspect of the pelvic inlet.

Postoperative complications (1)

3 E In a postoperative patient, a low haemoglobin count which is continuing to fall must always be treated as due to ongoing haemorrhage until proven otherwise. In this patient, the combination of the haemoglobin drop and increasing abdominal distension, alongside the umbilical pain, points towards an umbilical port site bleed. Where there is evidence of continuing blood loss, as in this case, resuscitation followed by reoperation (E) is the most appropriate management. Her paleness and shortness of breath are probably due to blood loss. Volume replacement (B) and blood transfusion (A) are appropriate management methods but they are 'holding options' and by no means definitive in correcting continuing surgical bleeding. Although abdominal distension may point to obstruction, requiring a nasogastric tube (D), in this situation and in the absence of vomiting it is an unlikely diagnosis. CTPA (C) to exclude pulmonary embolism is not indicated in the absence of other more specific signs pointing towards this diagnosis, and D-dimer would be raised after surgery anyway.

Abdominal cramps

4 B A history of progressive bloating, fullness, early satiety and abdominal or pelvic pain should raise suspicions, particularly in a woman of this age, of ovarian cancer. Although she has been diagnosed with irritable bowel syndrome (IBS), which could account for her symptoms, a new diagnosis of IBS at this age is rare and treating these symptoms (E) without further investigation is inadvisable. The GP has rightly arranged a CA 125 test, which is high. In this case, ultrasound of the abdomen and pelvis (B) should be organized as a matter of urgency. The results of this, coupled with the raised CA 125, will then determine the degree of urgency in relation to the potential diagnosis (D). CT of the abdomen and pelvis (C) is more appropriately used as part of a work-up for suspected ovarian cancer in a specialist setting where there is a need for staging the disease. Pipelle biopsy (A) is used when there is suspicion of endometrial abnormality, not ovarian cancer.

Acid-base physiology

5 E This woman is clearly very unwell with a profound alkalosis. As there is a low PCO_2 as well as a raised bicarbonate, there is a mixed acid-base disturbance (E). In a purely metabolic alkalosis (A) the PCO_2 should be higher, whereas with a pure respiratory alkalosis (B) one would expect a much lower compensatory bicarbonate, given that the respiratory alkalosis is likely to have been chronic. This is therefore a mixed respiratory and metabolic alkalosis (E). In this case, the respiratory alkalosis is most probably due to a high respiratory rate due to the significant acute pneumonia while the metabolic alkalosis is most probably due to the hypokalaemia (potassium 1.9 mmol/L), in turn caused by her repeated vomiting of potassium-rich gastric contents secondary to hyperemesis gravidarum. Answer (D) is a distractor which most candidates can easily dismiss: respiratory alkalosis is marked by low PCO_2 due to an increased respiratory effort 'blowing off' the carbon dioxide, and a respiratory compensation would mean the patient had reduced but not normalized their respiratory rate. All respiratory alkaloses therefore have 'inadequate respiratory compensation'!

Oncology

6 C A Wertheim's hysterectomy (A) is an operation for cervical cancer. It involves removing the uterus, upper third of the vagina and all the parametrium. A total abdominal hysterectomy (B) would be an appropriate choice as it is important that the ovaries are removed as well. This woman may well be an ideal candidate for a laparoscopic hysterectomy as she is multiparous, has mild prolapse, has an early stage endometrial cancer and has had no operations. The recovery time is much quicker compared to a laparotomy. For this reason answer (C) would be most appropriate. Subtotal hysterectomy (D) is inappropriate since not removing the cervix may inadvertently leave some malignant endometrial tissue. A pelvic exenteration (E) usually involves a Wertheim's hysterectomy as well as a bowel resection of sorts (either abdominoperineal or anterior resection). This is employed for significant recurrent cervical and upper vaginal cancers.

Endometrial cancer

7 C   Endometrial cancer is the most common genital tract cancer. It usually presents between the ages of 50 and 60 with post-menopausal bleeding. FIGO (the International Federation of Obstetrics and Gynaecology) changed the staging of endometrial cancers in 2010 to the following:

- IA tumour confined to the uterus, no or $<\frac{1}{2}$ myometrial invasion (A)
- IB tumour confined to the uterus, $>\frac{1}{2}$ myometrial invasion
- II cervical stromal the invasion, but not beyond the uterus (B)
- IIIA tumour invades the serosa or adnexa
- IIIB vaginal and/or parametrial involvement
- IIIC1 pelvic lymph node involvement
- IIIC2 para-aortic lymph node involvement, with or without pelvic node involvement
- IVA tumour invasion bladder and/or bowel mucosa (D)
- IVB distant metastases including abdominal metastases and/or inguinal lymph nodes

This tumour is a IIIA tumour – answer (C).

Gynaecological oncology (2)

8 C   The diagnosis and management of ovarian cancers is principally surgical. A full work-up for women undergoing evaluation for ovarian cancer includes CT of the abdomen. This may, as in the case here, reveal extra-abdominopelvic disease which is classified as stage IV (metastatic) ovarian cancer. However, imaging does not replace the need for histological diagnosis at operation. A staging laparotomy establishes the type and extent of the primary cancer and allows optimal cytoreduction (or 'debulking surgery') (C) where as much of the disease as possible is removed at operation. Even in advanced cancers, the preferred treatment for all women who are fit for operation is optimal cytoreductive surgery. Chemotherapy may also be indicated since ovarian cancers are highly sensitive to platinum based agents and the vinca alkaloids. Indeed, many centres now pre-empt debulking surgery with chemotherapy (so-called interval debulking procedures). In an otherwise fit woman of 65 years, offering no active treatment for a disease (D) which can be effectively managed is inappropriate, unless the patient expressly wishes it. Total hysterectomy, bilateral salpingo-oophorectomy and omentectomy are often employed during surgery for early ovarian cancers. However, performing radiotherapy of another organ system (A) at the same time as radical surgery has significant risk attached. Aortopelvic lymphadenopathy (B) is not widely used given that it does not increase 5-year survival and is associated with operative risk.

Pleural effusion

9 B   This woman is unwell as a result of the pleural effusion and ascites. All of the options can cause ascites and pleural effusions. The high protein content of the ascitic fluid suggests an inflammatory or malignant cause rather than CCF (A) or cirrhosis of the liver (D). CCF involves both left and right ventricular failure. Left ventricular failure will lead to pulmonary oedema while right-sided failure leads to hepatomegaly, ascites and peripheral oedema. Cirrhosis of the liver is characterised by ascites and hepatomegaly. Other complications may include oesophageal varices and hepatic encephalopathy. The history of decreased appetite and vaginal bleeding raises the possibility of an advanced gynaecological cancer with metastatic spread outside the abdomen – (B) or (E). CCF (A) and hepatic cirrhosis (D) do not cause vaginal bleeding. Once an ovarian tumour (B) has spread to the pleural cavity it is by definition a stage IV tumour. Ovarian cancers usually present late because symptoms are often non-specific. This woman needs investigation to rule out ovarian cancer as a matter of urgency. Cancer of the cervix (E) tends to present earlier than ovarian cancer so distant spread is not as common. This patient is most likely to have an ovarian tumour. Meigs' syndrome (C) is a pleural effusion associated with an ovarian fibroma which is rare. It is benign and classically causes a right-sided pleural effusion.

Emergency gynaecology

10 C   This woman must have bled a significant amount to cause such a marked degree of anaemia and faintness. Furthermore, she is still actively bleeding. Since it is not possible to examine her, packing the vagina (E) would be impossible. Discharging a woman (A, B) in this condition would be negligent. Both of the two remaining options – theatre (C) and cross-matching blood (D) – would be appropriate but this woman requires examination under anaesthesia and primary treatment of any vaginal trauma to prevent further blood loss. It is likely that she will require transfusion, so requesting cross-matched blood and a formal blood count would also be appropriate, but only in tandem with definitive management of her genital tract trauma.

Peri-operative management

11 C Patients on long-term steroids prior to surgery are at risk of postoperative shock as a result of secondary corticosteroid insufficiency. Most studies have shown that patients taking less than 10 mg of prednisolone/day (or the equivalent) have a normal hypothalamic-pituitary axis (HPA) response to major surgery and do not need additional steroid cover. However, evidence suggests that those on more than 10 mg/day for 3 months or more prior to surgery require adequate steroid supplementation. For major gynaecological surgery, such as vaginal hysterectomy, 50 mg of hydrocortisone 8-hourly from induction (C) is the standard practice, and may be stopped after 2 or 3 days, or when normal gut function returns and the patient can resume oral steroids. Giving a single dose of steroids and anaesthesia induction (A, B) is unlikely to cover the patient for the increased postoperative demand on the HPA, and cover is necessary until such time as the patient can resume oral steroids. Peri-operative cover for asthma (D) is not routinely employed in surgery. Patients whose asthma is uncontrolled, or who are having a mild asthma attack, would normally have their elective procedure cancelled. Patients should continue to take regular asthma inhalers before and after surgery. Postoperative exacerbations should be managed as for any other non-surgical patient. Respiratory physiotherapy may be useful postoperatively to encourage the use of accessory muscles and full inflation of the lungs and reduce the risk of atelectasis or postoperative respiratory tract infection. Inpatient review by a respiratory physician (E) is not warranted in an otherwise well and well-controlled asthmatic.

Female pelvic anatomy (2)

12 A The labia majora are supplied by branches of the posterior labial artery, which is supplied by the internal pudendal artery (A), itself originating from the internal iliac artery. The inferior gluteal (B), uterine (C) and obturator (D) arteries are similarly all supplied by the internal iliac artery, and supply, respectively, the buttock and posterior thigh, the uterus, and the medial compartment of the thigh. The inferior vesical artery (E) is a branch of the internal iliac artery and often arises in common with the middle rectal artery. It supplies the lower part of the bladder.

Female pelvic anatomy (3)

13 A Damage to the perineal nerve (A), which is a branch of the pudendal nerve, can cause localized loss of sensation of parts of the labia (usually anterior) and perineum. Damage to the pudendal nerve (C) itself would likely cause much more extensive sensory loss over the entire perineum, perianal skin and some of the labia. The dorsal nerve of the clitoris

(D) and inferior anal nerves (E) are similarly branches of the pudendal nerve and supply part of the clitoris and the anal skin and external anal sphincter, respectively. The peroneal nerve (B) is a distractor which should be easily dismissed. Also referred to as the common fibular nerve, it originates from the sacral plexus (L4–S3) and innervates the anterior and lateral compartments of the lower leg.

Postoperative complications (2)

14 B This woman has a history of significant ischaemic heart disease. In the presence of such a profound anaemia, the myocardium will be sufficiently deprived of oxygen that chest pain can develop, even if this is not significant enough to cause frank infarction (A). Myocardial infarction is very unlikely in the presence of normal troponin-I and a normal ECG. Pulmonary embolism (C) is a possible differential diagnosis, although this woman is on thromboprophylaxis. Atelectasis (D) would typically occur some time later, after surgery, usually after 48 hours. Similarly, this would be a very rapid onset for sepsis (E) and an unusual presentation in the absence of fever.

Postoperative complications (3)

15 A In a postoperative patient, signs of shock must be assumed to be due to haemorrhage until proven otherwise. In a fit 46 year old, significant blood loss is required to invoke a response of tachycardia, hypotension and reduced urine output. The concerns of a senior nurse should always be treated seriously. Although a fluid challenge (B, E) may help to stabilize the patient, it is not definitive management. Similarly, arterial blood sampling (C) and haemoglobin measurement (which may be estimated on an arterial blood gas machine) may assist diagnosis but in this case they should be performed concurrently with definitive, life-saving actions. The only response which combines these two is (A). This woman needs returning to the operating theatre, where even if surgery does not take place, invasive monitoring and aggressive resuscitation facilities, as well as anaesthetists, are more readily on hand. Always alert the operating surgeon (D) when a patient on whom they have just performed surgery develops signs of significant postoperative haemorrhage.

Female pelvic anatomy (4)

16 C The rectouterine pouch, or Pouch of Douglas (C), is formed by the draping of the peritoneum over the pelvic organs. It is the extension of the peritoneal cavity between the rectum and the posterior aspect of the uterus. A second pouch, the vesicouterine pouch (A), lies between the anterior surface of the lower uterine body and the posterior surface of the bladder.

The vesicouterine fold is dissected off the anterior wall of the uterus at caesarean section to deflect the bladder inferiorly and reduce the likelihood of iatrogenic bladder damage when incising the uterus. The pararectal fossa (D) is formed by lateral reflections of the peritoneum over the superior third of the rectum. The rectovesical fossa (E) does not exist in the normal female pelvis as the bladder and rectum are separated anatomically by the uterus. The paravesical fossa (B) is formed by the anterior pelvic wall peritoneum covering the superior surface of the bladder; either side of this is a depression that is termed the paravesical fossa.

Cancer risk

17 D Ovarian cysts in post-menopausal women may be managed conservatively if they meet certain criteria. A risk of malignancy can be calculated using the CA 125 value, the characteristics of the cyst on ultrasound and the menopause status. The concerning ultrasound features include the presence of bilateral cysts, multiloculated cysts, cysts with solid components, ascites and metastases. The score is calculated as one point for every ultrasound feature (0 to 5) multiplied by the CA 125. This is then multiplied by three if they are post-menopausal. Thus, with two features on ultrasound, RMI = $2 \times 120 \times 3$, which is 720. RMI <50 has a 3 per cent chance of cancer. RMI between 50 and 250 has a 20 per cent chance of cancer and an RMI >250 has a 75 per cent chance of cancer. This woman should be referred to a specialist cancer unit for work-up and surgery.

Irregular vaginal bleeding

18 C When assessing intermenstrual bleeding, a full history and examination need to be performed. Pelvic swabs (C) are essential as pelvic infection is a very common cause of new-onset intermenstrual bleeding. If the woman does have an infection such as chlamydia, early treatment can prevent the long-term sequelae of pelvic inflammatory disease, including subfertility. As she is only 21, it is unlikely this woman will have had a cervical smear test (B). However, as she is sexually active it would be prudent to perform a cervical smear as well. There is no need to perform biopsy of the endometrium (A) yet, given the short duration of her symptoms. If she has no cause identified on these first line investigations and the bleeding continues, then an ultrasound (D) estimating endometrial thickness should be undertaken. Only if this were abnormal, in someone so young, would you consider obtaining an endometrial biopsy (E).

Postoperative complications (4)

19 C Systemic inflammatory response syndrome (SIRS) (B) is evidence of the body's continuing inflammatory mechanism against a pathological insult and is present when two of the following are present: temperature <36°C or >38°C, pulse >90 bpm, tachypnoea >20 min or white cells <4 or >12 × 10^9/L. This patient meets the requirement for a diagnosis of SIRS, but in addition there is microbiological evidence of infection with MRSA: this meets the definition of sepsis (A) (SIRS in the presence of a demonstrated pathogen). The fact that she requires intravenous vasopressor support to maintain a cardiac output is evidence of haemodynamic shock, and coupled with sepsis means that the patient is in septic shock (C). Septicaemia (D) is simply the presence of a proven pathogen in the bloodstream. Adult (or acute) respiratory distress syndrome is caused by insult to the lung parenchyma causing impaired gas exchange. There are also systemic effects resulting from associated massive release of inflammatory mediators.

Female pelvic anatomy (5)

20 A Understanding of pelvic anatomy and the course of the ureters is of vital importance if ureteric injury is to be avoided during hysterectomy. The ureters run down the lateral pelvic side walls, along the anterior border of the greater sciatic notch and under the peritoneum. Medial to the obturator nerve, the ureter lies anterior to the internal iliac artery. It enters the pelvis crossing over the iliac vessels at the level of the bifurcation. The ureter passes underneath the uterine artery about 15 mm lateral to the supravaginal cervix (remember 'water under the bridge') before coursing towards the urinary bladder. Iatrogenic injury is most common during hysterectomy during ligation of the uterine artery pedicle.

Vaginal bleeding

21 D Post-menopausal bleeding can be a symptom of ovarian, endometrial and cervical cancer. It is likely that this woman's post-menopausal bleed is secondary to her stopping HRT. However, it is important that these symptoms are investigated. A pipelle biopsy (A) is invasive and sometimes technically difficult to perform in a post-menopausal woman. A hysteroscopy (B) will be necessary if there is a thickened endometrium on ultrasound. Her smear tests (C) are up to date, so repeating this test is unnecessary unless abnormality is seen at speculum examination. Ultrasound (D) would be the investigation of choice. If the endometrium is smooth in outline with a thickness less than 4 mm the woman's vaginal bleeding is most likely due to withdrawing the HRT. There is no indication for a CT (E) though one would be performed as a staging tool if endometrial cancer were discovered.

Gynaecological pathology

22 C It should be fairly obvious that the findings described during the operation are those of endometriosis. Pelvic pain is a prominent feature.

Once you understand that endometriosis is simply the deposition of endometrium-like tissue outside of the uterine cavity then it follows that the histology of any excised samples of endometriosis will be similar to that of normal endometrium: that is, containing endometrial glands, stroma and/or epithelium (C). Krukenberg tumours (A) are metastatic neoplasms of the ovary from a gastric primary. Smooth muscle cells (E) would have suggested a diagnosis of fibroids, also called leiomyomata (D), while vacuolated clear cells (B) are seen in clear cell adenocarcinoma.

Operative laparoscopy

23 D Laparoscopies are not without risk. Risks include damage to bowel, bladder and blood vessels. Blood vessels can be damaged deep in the pelvis or superficially. When inserting a transverse port the skin should be transilluminated to avoid the superficial epigastric artery (A) that arises from the femoral artery and ascends to the umbilicus. In addition, care is needed to avoid the inferior epigastric artery that runs medial to the obliterated umbilical artery. It begins at the external iliac artery and anastamoses with the superior epigastric artery around the umbilicus. The superior epigastric artery (D) can therefore not be damaged by lateral port insertion. The ilioinguinal (E) and iliohypogastric (C) nerves both originate from L1 and are at risk of damage with lateral port insertion. The ilioinguinal nerve passes through the superficial inguinal ring and provides sensation over the thigh and the labia majora. The external iliac vein (B) originates at the inferior margin of the inguinal ligament and is nowhere near where a lateral port could be placed.

PART II
PAEDIATRICS

SECTION 9:
GROWTH, DEVELOPMENT AND PUBERTY

QUESTIONS

1. Menstrual cycle delay

A 14-year-old girl comes to see you as she has not had her periods yet. You note that her breasts are stage II and her nipples are set lateral to the mid-clavicular line. She has no pubic hair. Her weight is on the 50th centile but height is on the 9th centile. Her parents are both of average height. What is the most likely diagnosis?

A. Turner's syndrome
B. Polycystic ovary syndrome
C. Anorexia
D. Constitutional delay
E. Underlying undiagnosed chronic illness

2. Development milestones (1)

A 2-year-old child is referred to you by the GP because he has not started walking. His mother says that he can stand but cries to be picked up or sits down shortly. His older sister was walking by 14 months. You note that he is talking well with short two to three word phrases. He is able to build a tower of six blocks. What is your management plan?

A. Advise mum to work harder at giving him independence and follow up in 4 months.
B. Request blood tests including a creatinine kinase
C. Refer for physiotherapy
D. Reassure and discharge as his development is normal
E. Refer to orthopaedics

3. Developmental milestones (2)

You see a boy in outpatients whose parents are concerned he is not talking yet. You do a developmental assessment and find he is walking well and able to build a tower of three blocks. He will scribble but does not copy your circle. He is able to identify his nose, mouth, eyes and ears as well as point to mummy and daddy. You do not hear him say anything but his parents say he will say a few single words at home such as mummy, daddy, cup and cat. He is a happy, alert child. Parents report him to be starting to feed himself with a spoon and they have just started potty training but he is still in nappies. What is the child's most likely age?

A. 12 months
B. 15 months
C. 18 months
D. 2 years
E. 2.5 years

4. Failure to thrive

A one-and-a-half-year-old Caucasian child is referred to paediatrics for failure to thrive. On examination he is a clean, well-dressed child who is quite quiet and withdrawn. He is pale and looks thin with wasted buttocks. His examination is otherwise unremarkable. What is the most likely cause of this child's growth failure?

His growth chart shows good growth along the 50th centile until 6 months followed by weight down to the 9th, height down to 25th and head circumference now starting to falter at 1.5 years.

    A.   Coeliac disease
    B.   Neglect
    C.   Constitutional delay
    D.   Normal child
    E.   Beta thalassaemia

5. Puberty

A 12-year-old boy presents to his GP with left-sided unilateral breast development stage III. He is very upset as he is being bullied at school. His mother is worried as her friend's sister has just been diagnosed with breast cancer and wants to know if he could have breast cancer? What is the management?

    A.   Refer for a breast ultrasound
    B.   Test sex hormone levels
    C.   Test alpha fetoprotein
    D.   Reassure and explain this is a normal part of puberty; it will resolve but the other breast may enlarge transiently as well
    E.   Do a fine needle aspirate on his left breast

6. Neonatal examination

You see a baby for the first baby check at 6 weeks. Mum reports no problems and he is feeding well. On examination you are unable to palpate the testicles on ether side and do not feel any lumps in the groin area. He has a normal penis with no hypospadias and the anus is patent. He is otherwise a normal baby on examination. What is the most important diagnosis to rule out?

    A.   Klienfelter's syndrome
    B.   Congenital adrenal hyperplasia
    C.   Undescended testicles
    D.   Virilized female infant
    E.   Testicular cancer

7. Growth (1)

You see an 8-year-old boy in accident and emergency who fell off his bike 3 days ago and scraped his left calf. The cuts are now angry, red and painful. You note he is a big boy and plot his growth: his weight is on the 99th centile and height is on the 75th centile. You note mild gynaecomastia and stretch marks on his abdomen which are normal skin colour. His past medical history is unremarkable except for mild asthma. What is the most likely cause of his large size?

    A.   Cushing's syndrome secondary to a pituitary adenoma

    B.   Cushing's syndrome secondary to becotide inhaler use

    C.   Obesity

    D.   His size is within the normal range and is a variant of normal

    E.   Liver failure

8. Growth (2)

A 16-year-old boy is brought to the GP by his parents. They are concerned he is the shortest boy in his class. He is otherwise well. His height and weight are on the 9th centile. His father plots on the 75th centile and his mother on the 50th centile for adult height. On examination, his testicular volume is 8 mL, he has some fine pubic and axillary hair. The rest of the physical examination is normal. On further questioning you elicit from his father that he was a late bloomer and did not reach his full height until he was at university. What is the most likely cause of the boy's short stature?

    A.   The 9th centile is a normal height and weight so there is nothing wrong with him

    B.   Growth hormone deficiency

    C.   Constitutional delay of growth and puberty

    D.   Underlying chronic illness should be sought

    E.   Anorexia

9. Child development

A mother comes to see you with her 2-year-old daughter, Stacey, out of frustration that her daughter is so ill behaved. She does not know how to make her listen and is worried that she is going to get hurt. Yesterday she ran ahead and did not stop when her mother called to her. She ran into the street and was hit by a cyclist, but fortunately he was OK and Stacey had only had a few cuts and scrapes and seems alright! On questioning you hear other stories of a naughty child. She is active and eats well, feeding herself a lot now, but her mother does say she gets frequent coughs and colds. Her mother says that Stacey only says about 5–10 words and only she can understand what Stacey says. What is the best next management?

    A.   Ask the health visitor to visit mum for parenting advice and support

    B.   Order blood tests for full blood count to check for leukaemia as she has recurrent coughs and colds

    C.   Give Stacey a tetanus shot to cover her after her fall the day before

D. Refer for a hearing test
E. Tell Stacey that she needs to listen to her mother and not have any
    more accidents

10. Down's syndrome

An older mother books in to see you after attending the health visitor for a weight check at 2 months for her first child. She and her husband have had a hard time coming to terms with their daughter's diagnosis of Down's syndrome. She is relieved that the appointment with the cardiologists went well and the heart is normal. However they have a lot of trouble getting her to take the whole bottle, she was slow to regain her birth weight and looking at the plotted weight yesterday she is not growing along her birth centile and the mother is worried she is not doing a good enough job. She is not vomiting except for small possets after feeds, is passing urine and opening her bowels. The red book growth chart shows the weight to be falling off centiles. What is the most appropriate management?

A. Contact the cardiologists in light of the poor feeding and slow weight
    gain for a second opinion as baby's with Down's syndrome are at high
    risk of heart problems and they may have missed it
B. Refer to the dietician for nutritional support
C. Replace the growth chart in their red book with a Down's syndrome
    growth chart, reassure mum by re-plotting her growth and explain she
    is normal but arrange to review again
D. Tell the mother to try a different milk and come back in 2 weeks
E. Advise the mother to change to a faster flow teat for their bottles so
    that she takes her feed faster

ANSWERS

Menstrual cycle delay

1 A The answer is Turner syndrome (A) (45,X), which may go undiagnosed in many women until they try to start a family. It is associated with lymphoedema of the hands and feet as a neonate, webbing of the neck, short stature, wide spaced nipples, congenital heart defects (coarctation of the aorta) delayed or absent puberty and infertility. Polycystic ovarian syndrome (B) would be unlikely in a girl who has not started puberty yet. She is of average weight so this is not anorexia (C). Constitutional delay (D) is much more common in males and is the isolated finding of delay in skeletal growth, i.e. height. A chronic illness (E) significant enough to delay puberty would also be associated with failure to thrive.

Development milestones (1)

2 B The best answer here is requesting blood tests including a creatinine kinase (CK) (B). His development is not normal (D). He has delayed gross motor skills but seems otherwise normal. Therefore, an important diagnosis to make would be muscular dystrophy and the mother should not be told to try harder (A). This presentation is more severe than is often seen; typically children are a bit clumsy and walk with a waddling gait. If the blood test shows a raised CK then he will need a muscle biopsy to confirm the diagnosis. Until you have established the diagnosis, it would be inappropriate to refer to physiotherapy (C). Developmental hip dysplasia could present with failure to walk and would require orthopaedic referral (E) but a hip ultrasound to confirm the diagnosis would be the appropriate first step in management.

Developmental milestones (2)

3 C Developmental assessment should involve assessing the child in all four areas: gross motor; fine motor and vision; speech, language and hearing; and social, emotional and behaviour. This child is scoring 18 months old (C) in all four areas. He is walking steadily (gross motor), scribbling (fine motor), identifies four body parts (speech and language) and reportedly has several single words – he should have at least 10 words and you have not elicited this from him, but he is not worryingly delayed. This would warrant some follow-up. Likely, his older sister is saying everything for him so he does not have to talk yet. He is feeding himself with a spoon and starting to potty train (social and behavioural). At 12 months (A) he would be walking unsteadily and have 2–3 words; he does more than this. At 15 months (B) he would be scribbling and likely walking well but not managing to feed himself with a spoon. At 2 years (D) you would expect him to build a tower of six blocks and be putting words together. He may also be getting close to potty trained, although modern nappies keep children dry so they are not learning to potty train as early. At 2.5 years (E) he should build a tower of eight blocks.

Failure to thrive

4 A   The answer here is coeliac disease (A). The clue to this is that his growth was normal until the age of weaning, 6 months. With the introduction of gluten into the diet his growth began to falter. You also note he is pale, likely anaemic, suggestive of malnutrition. One of the classic signs of coeliac disease is the wasted buttocks. Neglect (B) should always be considered in any case of failure to thrive, especially in a child who seems withdrawn, but it is important to remember that chronic illness may make children listless and withdrawn and it is always important to rule out physical illness. You would need multidisciplinary input prior to making the diagnosis of neglect. Constitutional delay (C) is the isolated finding of delay in skeletal growth, i.e. height, and is typically seen around the time of puberty; as his growth failure started with weight this answer is incorrect. He is not a normal child (D) as he was born on the 50th centile and his weight is now on the 2nd centile with other parameters following in the traditional pattern of growth failure: weight followed by height, followed by head circumference. Beta thalassaemia (E) is highly unlikely in a Caucasian child. You would expect them to be pale and develop symptoms including growth failure around 6 months of age, but without transfusions he would be unlikely to survive to a year-and-a-half old.

Puberty

5 D   This is a common presentation for adolescent males and the correct answer is to reassure (D). Normal puberty for boys starts between 9 and 13 years old with increasing testicular volume above 4 mL. This is followed by penis enlargement, pubic hair growth and lastly the growth spurt. It is not uncommon for boys to develop transient gynaecomastia during puberty. He does not need investigation (A, B, C or E) or intervention, unless the problem does not resolve.

Neonatal examination

6 B   The correct answer is congenital adrenal hyperplasia (CAH) (B), which is most commonly due to 21-hydroxylase deficiency. These infants may present with ambiguous genitalia or bilateral undescended testicles and are at risk of a salt-losing adrenal crisis (vomiting, weight loss, floppy unwell infant), typically around 1–3 weeks of age. It is therefore important to measure urea and electrolytes in addition to chromosomal analysis and a pelvic ultrasound to look for the location of the sex organs. This baby could be a virilized female (D) infant secondary to CAH but the important diagnosis is the underlying cause for the virilization. Undescended testicles (C) are important to identify as they should be followed up to ensure they do descend by 2 years of age. If they remain out of the scrotum they are at increased risk of developing testicular cancer (E) but this would not be a diagnosis found at this stage. Klinefelter's syndrome (A) has a karyotype 47XXY and typically presents as tall stature, delayed puberty and possibly mild learning difficulties but not undescended testicles.

Growth (1)

7 C This child is obese (C). He should be advised to continue exercise, such as bike riding, and make healthy choices for his diet, such as eating fruit rather than potato chips for snacks. Children should not be put on diets under normal circumstances as a normal healthy diet with regular exercise will improve his weight as he grows. In the context of a wound infection and abdominal striae, many worry that obesity may be Cushing's syndrome but this would typically present with growth failure and his height is above average (A), which is typical of obesity (C). Cushing syndrome is not caused by steroid inhalers (B) but may be seen in children with severe asthma on oral steroids. While both his height and weight plot on the lines of the centile chart, only 1 per cent of the population of 8 year olds have his weight normally and his height does not match his weight centile, suggesting that he is overweight (D). The mild gynaecomastia is unlikely to be made of breast tissue and is more likely to be fat pads as he is active riding bikes. It is unlikely that he is unwell enough to be in liver failure despite possibly having gynaecomastia (E).

Growth (2)

8 C This is constitutional delay of growth and puberty (C). It classically runs in families in the male line and presents with delayed puberty and growth spurt. He has started puberty and it seems to be progressing in the normal pattern so he should be reassured that he will get his growth spurt as he finishes puberty. While 9 per cent of the population will have his height and weight (A) and be normal, the mid-parental height suggests he should be taller than he is (the mean parental height plus 7 cm for boys or minus 7 cm for girls predicts the adult height of the child ± two standard deviations). As he has started puberty and is otherwise well this is unlikely to be growth hormone deficiency (B) or underlying chronic illness (D). In anorexia (E) you would expect the weight to be less than the height centile and to be more extremely low.

Child development

9 D Stacey seems to have some speech delay. She is feeding herself and running which is appropriate for a 2 year old but she is only talking at about a year-and-a-half's age level and she is difficult to understand. This, along with a story of poor attentiveness in a child, raises concerns of hearing problems. The most common cause would be glue ear associated with recurrent coughs and colds and she should have a hearing test (D). She does not need any blood tests (B) as all children at this age have recurrent coughs and colds, the average being eight illnesses a year. Only recurrent severe infections warrant investigation for immune deficiency. The routine childhood vaccinations cover her for tetanus (C); unless her records say she has not had them she does not need a booster, and she will have the pre-school booster and one when she is a teenager. Answer (E) will not change Stacey's behaviour; young children respond to positive and negative reinforcement techniques to modify behaviour.

Down's syndrome

10 C Children with Down's syndrome do have different growth patterns to other children and should be given special growth charts in their red books, so the correct answer is (C). If the cardiologist has carried out an echocardiogram (A) and discharged the patient, unless there are clinical signs and symptoms to warrant re-referral, this would be a waste of resources and needless worry for the parents. A dietician referral (B) will be needed if she is failing to thrive and continues to have difficulty feeding, but this should be done with investigations for a cause. Parents do shop around to find a milk their child prefers but in the absence of an intolerance the over the counter milks (D) are all equally good and this is unlikely to help. A faster teat (E) may make things worse as Down's syndrome is associated with low tone and swallowing difficulties, so she may choke if the flow is too fast.

SECTION 10:
PAEDIATRIC EMERGENCIES

QUESTIONS

1. Identifying the unwell child

Which child should be moved to the resuscitation area for urgent management in accident and emergency?

A. A miserable 2 year old with a fever and vomiting temperature of 38.5°C, heart rate of 150, respiratory rate 42, capillary refill time 2–3 seconds who is alert and clinging on to his father and has just been given paracetamol and started on a fluid challenge with oral rehydration salts 5 minutes ago by the triage nurse

B. A quiet 4 year old brought in with an asthma attack who is sitting upright with a respiratory rate of 50, heart rate of 162, capillary refill time of 3 seconds, subcostal recessions and poor air entry on chest auscultation following a salbutamol nebulizer

C. An 8 year old, known diabetic, brought in vomiting with her glucose reader saying HI. She is able to tell you her history and has a heart rate of 120, respiratory rate of 25, capillary refill time of <2 seconds

D. An alert 3 year old who has had a cough and cold for the past 3 days which is keeping him up at night and mum noticed a rash on his neck and face which did not disappear when she pressed a glass tumbler against it. His temperature is 37.8°C, heart rate is 110, respiratory rate is 30, capillary refill time is <2 seconds

E. A 15 year old, known to social services for a family history of domestic abuse, brought in to accident and emergency by her best friend after she admitted to taking 20 paracetamol tablets 4 hours ago. She is alert but does not make eye contact, her heart rate is 98, respiratory rate is 20, capillary refill <2 seconds

2. Management of the unwell child (1)

A 4-year-old child has been losing weight recently and has been vomiting for the past 24 hours, unable to eat anything. His mother has brought him into accident and emergency out of concern as he seems confused. The triage nurse has taken him to the resuscitation room and asked for your help. On examination he is drowsy, has a heart rate of 150, respiratory rate of 60 and a central capillary refill of 5 seconds. He has subcostal recessions and good air entry bilaterally with no added sounds. He moans when you examine his abdomen but there are no masses. You put in a canula and take bloods. The venous blood gas shows:

pH 7.12
PCO_2 2.3 kPa
PO_2 6.7 kPa
HCO_3^- 15.3 mmol/L
BE −8.6
Glucose 32.4 mmol/L

What is the most likely diagnosis and what is the first management step?

A.   Diabetic ketoacidosis, start an insulin infusion
B.   Diabetic ketoacidosis, give a fluid bolus
C.   Pneumonia, start IV co-amoxiclav
D.   Ruptured appendix, give a fluid bolus and book the emergency operating theatre
E.   Gastroenteritis with severe dehydration, give a fluid bolus

3. Asthma

An 8 year old known asthmatic is brought into accident and emergency by ambulance as a 'blue call'. He has been unwell with an upper respiratory tract infection for the past 2 days. For the past 24 hours his parents have given him 10 puffs of salbutamol every 4 hours, his last dose being 90 minutes ago. The ambulance staff have given him a nebulizer but he remains agitated with a heart rate of 155, respiratory rate of 44 and sub/intercostal recessions and on auscultation there is little air movement heard bilaterally. Saturations in air are 85 per cent. He is started on 'back to back' nebulizers with high flow oxygen. How severe is his asthma exacerbation and what other bedside test would support this?

A.   Moderate, venous blood pH 4.4, gas PCO_2 = 3.1 kPa
B.   Severe, peak flow <33 per cent expected
C.   Severe, venous blood pH 4.4, gas PCO_2 = 3.1 kPa
D.   Life-threatening, peak flow <33 per cent expected
E.   Life-threatening, venous blood pH 4.4, gas PCO_2 = 3.1 kPa

4. Management of the unwell child (2)

The accident and emergency triage nurse asks you to look at a 3-year-old child with a short history of waking up this morning unwell with a cough and fever. She looks unwell, heart rate is 165, respiratory rate 56, saturations of 96 per cent in air, temperature of 39.3°C and central capillary refill of 4 seconds. She has a mild headache but no photophobia or neck stiffness and you notice a faint macular rash on her torso and wonder if one spot is non-blanching. You ask the triage nurse to move her to the resuscitation area and call your senior to review her. Fifteen minutes later your senior arrives and the spot you saw on the abdomen is now non-blanching and there is another spot on her knee. What are the three most important things to give her immediately?

A.   High flow oxygen, IV fluid bolus, IV ceftriaxone
B.   IV fluid bolus, IV ceftriaxone, IV methylprednisolone
C.   High flow oxygen, IV ceftriaxone, IV fresh frozen plasma
D.   IV fluid bolus, IV ceftriaxone, IV fresh frozen plasma
E.   High flow oxygen, IV ceftriaxone, IV methylprednisolone

5. Examination

A 9-year-old boy is brought in by ambulance having been hit by a car while playing football in the street. You have been assigned to do the primary survey in resus when the ambulance arrives. The patient is receiving oxygen, crying for his mummy and holding his right arm, but able to move over from the stretcher to the bed when asked. Which is the correct examination procedure?

A. The trachea is deviated to the right. On auscultation you hear decreased air entry on the left. Percussion note is hyper-resonant on the left. He is tachycardic and his heart sounds are muffled, heard loudest at the right lower sternal edge. You ask for a left-sided thoracocentesis.

B. You introduce yourself and tell him that you will be gentle but need to check that he is okay. You see his left wrist is deformed and swollen and check the fingers which are cool and note the capillary refill is 4 seconds. He is able to feel you touching him and moans when you examine the wrist. You call for an x-ray to assess the probable fracture in the wrist.

C. You introduce yourself and tell him that you will be gentle but need to check that he is okay. You listen for equal air entry and think there is decreased air entry on the left but there is air entry on the right. He is tachypnoeic and has a pulse which is tachycardic. His capillary refill is 4 seconds. You expose his abdomen and notice bruising and grazes to the left side. He moans as you palpate in the left upper quandrant and has guarding. You ask for an IV canula or intraosseous needle and a 20 mL/kg fluid bolus while organizing an urgent CT chest and abdomen.

D. You introduce yourself and tell him that you will be gentle but need to check that he is okay. He is tachypnoeic. The trachea is deviated to the right. On auscultation you hear decreased air entry on the left. Percussion note is hyper-resonant on the left. He is tachycardic and his heart sounds are muffled, heard loudest at the right lower sternal edge. You ask for a left-sided thoracocentesis.

E. You listen for equal air entry and think there is decreased air entry on the left but there is air entry on the right. He is tachypnoeic and has a pulse which is tachycardic. His capillary refill is 4 seconds. You expose his abdomen and notice bruising and grazes to the left side. He moans as you palpate in the left upper quandrant and has guarding. You ask for an IV canula or intraosseous needle and a 20 mL/kg fluid bolus while organizing an urgent CT chest and abdomen.

6. Shock

A 6-year-old boy with a history of anaphylaxis to peanuts is brought in by ambulance unconscious. He was attending a children's birthday party. His mother says there was a bowl full of candy and he may have eaten a Snickers bar but she is not sure and she did not have his EpiPen with her. His face and lips are swollen and erythematous, he is still breathing but weakly and there is wheeze. His pulse is tachycardic and thready. Which type of shock is this?

A. Hypovolaemic
B. Distributive
C. Septic
D. Cardiac
E. Obstructive

7. Cardiopulmonary resuscitation (CPR)

A 13 month old is brought in having had a blue floppy episode at home lasting 1 minute. While you are taking a history from the mother, you notice the baby has gone blue again and seems to be unconscious in her arms. You call for help and place the baby on the examination table. There is no obvious work of breathing. The nurses bring the crash trolley and give you a bag valve mask, which they are connecting to the oxygen. You give two inflation breaths but do not see the chest rise. You reposition the air way and this time the breaths go in. You feel for a pulse and there is none. When asked to do CPR the nurse asks for direction on how many breaths and compressions you both need to do.

A. Two inflation breaths per 30 compressions
B. Two inflation breaths per 15 compressions
C. Continuous inflation breaths about 10–12 per minute and compressions 100–120 per minute
D. One inflation breath per five compressions
E. Two inflation breaths per five compressions

8. Status epilepticus

A 10-year-old child is brought in by ambulance with seizure activity. His mother reports it starting 30 minutes ago in his right arm and quickly became generalized tonic clonic jerking. She gave him his buccal midazolam after the first 5 minutes and called an ambulance when he did not respond after another 5 minutes. The ambulance crew gave him rectal diazepam on arrival at 15 minutes into the seizure. He is receiving high flow oxygen via a face mask and continues to convulse. The mother tells you that he was weaned from his long-term seizure medication, phenytoin, 2 weeks ago and that he has had a cold for the past 2 days. What is the next step in management?

A. Gain intravenous or intraosseous access and administer lorazepam
B. Gain intravenous or intraosseous access and administer ceftriaxone
C. Repeat the rectal diazepam
D. Gain intravenous or intraosseous access and start a phenytoin infusion
E. Gain intravenous or intraosseous access and start a phenobarbital infusion

9. Overdose

A 3-year-old boy is brought in by ambulance fitting. You are assigned to get the history from the father. Harry is normally fit and well with no significant past medical history or allergies. He is up to date with his immunizations and has been growing and developing normally. His behaviour has been difficult for the past 2 weeks since the birth of his little sister. Mum has been unwell as she developed HELLP syndrome and was in hospital for a week following the delivery. Yesterday, he was quite unwell with a tummy bug, vomiting and had black diarrhoea. That evening they found a mess he had made in the bathroom with all of his mum's things strewn over the floor including her tablets from the hospital. By that time, Harry was getting better so they did not think anything of it. Today he has been acting strangely and has been difficult to understand, he then became lethargic at about 4 pm and started fitting 15 minutes ago. What is the most likely diagnosis?

A. Paracetamol overdose
B. Aspirin overdose
C. Tricyclic antidepressant overdose
D. Bleach intoxication
E. Iron overdose

10. Management of the unwell child (3)

A 6-year-old boy with a history of asthma and eczema is brought in to accident and emergency from a local restaurant. He is on high flow facial oxygen with significant facial oedema and generalized erythema. On auscultation there is widespread wheeze for which the ambulance crew gave a salbutamol nebulizer. What is the next step in management?

A. Insert an IV line and give 10 mg slow intravenous antihistamine
B. Insert an IV line and give 100 mg slow intravenous hydrocortisone
C. Insert an IV line and give 200 μg of 1:10 000 intravenous adrenaline
D. Give intramuscular 1:1000 adrenaline, 250 μg
E. Repeat the salbutamol nebulizer and call for an anaesthetist for intubation

ANSWERS

Identifying the unwell child

1 B   Child (B) is the sickest here and should be moved to the resuscitation area with a dedicated nurse and doctor to manage her. She is having a severe asthma attack: she is tachycardic and tachypnoeic with circulatory compromise, a prolonged capillary refill time and she has not responded to initial management. Child (A) is unwell with tachycardia, tachypnoea and a slightly prolonged capillary refill time but is pyrexic and has just been given treatment. He should be reviewed in 30 minutes to see that his parameters are improved. Child (C) is at risk of diabetic ketoacidosis and should be assessed quickly with a blood gas but she remains alert and orientated with no evidence of circulatory compromise so she is stable enough to remain in general paediatric accident and emergency, but it important to be aware that these patients can get very sick. Patient (D) has a non-blanching rash in the superior vena caval distribution and has normal observations. This is unlikely to be meningococcal sepsis and more likely to be a petechial rash related to the pressure of coughing; however any non-blanching rash should be reviewed by a senior clinician and should be isolated in a side room in accident and emergency. Patient (E) also has the potential to become quite sick but she is currently stable and may need privacy for talks with the mental health team once she is medically cleared; she would benefit from a side room if it is free.

Management of the unwell child (1)

2 B   This child has new-onset, type 1 diabetes; he has been losing weight and the blood gas shows a very high glucose and a metabolic acidosis (remember that in paediatrics, arterial gases are rarely used, and that a venous PO_2 will be low; this gas does not show respiratory failure.) The chest is clear on examination and the gas does not show a respiratory acidosis; therefore this is not pneumonia (C). The first management for him is rehydration (B). Only after an hour of rehydration should he be started on intravenous insulin. It is important to correct his dehydration and hyperglycaemia slowly over 2 days due to the risk of brainstem demylination with rapid shifts in salts in the cerebrospinal fluid; therefore (A) is incorrect. Appendicitis (D) or gastroenteritis (E) would be reasonable if the glucose were normal. In the context of a tachycardia with prolonged capillary refill, a patient should be given a fluid bolus and reassessed. Patients should be stabilized before going to the operating theatre.

Asthma

3 D   This child has signs of a life-threatening asthma exacerbation: agitation, cyanosis, silent chest. Other signs would be fatigue, drowsiness or poor respiratory effort and a peak flow of less than 33 per cent expected (D). Therefore, (B) is incorrect as severe would be a peak flow between 33 and 55 per cent expected. In addition, signs of severe exacerbation include being too breathless to talk or feed, tachycardia and tachypnoea. A blood gas is not part of the guidelines for assessing asthma severity but in this child a worrying gas reading would show a respiratory acidosis, i.e. a rising CO_2 suggests that he is unable to maintain the respiratory effort and is therefore failing to clear CO_2 leading to a rise in the pH. For this reason (A), (C) and (E) are all incorrect as they are signs of a moderate exacerbation showing hypocapnia associated with hyperventilation, which is typical of asthma.

Management of the unwell child (2)

4 A   The correct answer is (A): she has presented with a classic presentation of meningococcal sepsis. Do not forget to always give sick children oxygen; if the mask makes them more distressed a minimum of wafted high flow O_2 may suffice. The child has a prolonged capillary refill and is tachycardic; she should have a fluid bolus (20 mL/kg) and be reassessed. As soon as intravenous or intraosseous access is obtained she should be given IV ceftriaxone, but only after the blood culture has been taken. (B) and (E) are incorrect as there is no mention of the child having meningitis. Currently there is no formal consensus as to whether steroids should be routinely used but administration before or with the first dose of antibiotics has been shown to be beneficial for some types of bacterial meningitis. (C) and (D) are incorrect as you do not yet have clotting results. She will likely need fresh frozen plasma to correct her disseminated intravascular coagulation which is evidenced by the forming non-blanching rash.

Examination

5 D   Answer (D) is correct, you introduce yourself to the patient and follow the ABCD approach: A is for Airway, he is crying therefore it is patent. B is for Breathing; you find evidence of a pneumothorax therefore you do not proceed further in your assessment until B is addressed with a needle thoracocentesis decompression. (A) is incorrect as you have not introduced yourself which is very important in gaining patient trust and examination cooperation. (B) is examination of D = disability, you have skipped the ABC and missed several life-threatening conditions. (C) is incorrect as you failed to respond to a problem in (B) despite noticing signs of a tension pneumothorax. (E) is incorrect as you failed to introduce yourself and to address the pneumothorax noted in assessing breathing.

Shock

6 B   Shock is inadequate perfusion of tissues which is insufficient to meet cellular metabolic needs. This child presents with anaphylaxis, but did not have early intramuscular adrenaline to prevent the capillary leak of fluid into his airway tissues. Due to oedema his airway is closing off. The rapid shifts in fluid to the interstitium results in intravascular hypovolaemia and shock. This is distributive shock (B). Hypovolaemic shock (A) is due to haemorrhage or dehydration, and the patient would be pale, cool and poorly perfused. In septic shock (C) you would expect a fever and history suggesting infection. In cardiac shock (D) the heart is unable to meet the circulatory demands of the body, resulting in shock. There is chest pain or other cardiac symptoms and this is rare in childhood outside of congenital heart or Kawasaki's disease. Lastly, obstructive shock (E) is due to blockage of blood flow from the heart, either due to cardiac tamponade, fluid in the pericardial sac compressing the heart or tension pneumothorax.

Cardiopulmonary resuscitation (CPR)

7 B   As of November 2010 the paediatric advanced life support guidelines for CPR recommend two inflation breaths per 15 chest compressions (B). This is different from the adult guidelines of two breaths to 30 compressions (A). Answer (C) is correct once the child is intubated but in this scenario, the child is not. Answer (D) is the old neonatal guidelines and is no longer used. Answer (E) is not used at all.

Status epilepticus

8 D   The child has now had two doses of barbiturate and management should proceed to the next step in management of status epilepticus (seizure lasting greater than 30 minutes): IV phenytoin (D). Due to the risk of respiratory depression further doses of barbituates ((A) or (C)) should be avoided. It should be noted that many text books still recommend the use of per rectum peraldehyde if two doses of barbituates fail; however this is now not routinely used in management of status epilepticus due to significant rates of drug errors such as IV rather than rectal administration. If his epilepsy was currently managed by phenytoin he should be given intravenous phenobarbital (E) but he was recently taken off of it. Intravenous ceftriaxone (B) may be indicated in a situation of status epilepticus associated with fever as encephalitis may present with seizures, but it is not the next step in management.

Overdose

9 E   The answer is iron overdose (E) which classically is a two phase illness with early vomiting and diarrhoea due to gastric irritation and may present with haematemesis or malaena (the black diarrhoea). There is a period up to 24 hours of improvement and then deterioration with liver failure, drowsiness and coma. The liver failure can produce hypoglycaemia and seizures. The mother has recently had HELLP syndrome, liver failure, thrombocytopenia and hypertension in pregnancy. These patients often have significant haemorrhage and go home on iron supplements. Paracetamol overdose (A) in young children is often not in large doses due to the tablets being difficult to swallow; it may present with gastric irritation or a history that the child took some tablets, liver failure develops on day 3–5, our case presented on day 2 and you would not expect malaena from paracetamol intoxication. Tricyclic antidepressant (C) overdose would present much earlier than 2 days, with tachycardia, anticholinergic symptoms (dry mouth, blurred vision, agitation). Patients become shocked with seizures or coma and develop severe metabolic acidosis and this is one of the few indications for giving intravenous bicarbonate. Bleach intoxication (D) should be thought of as he was in the bathroom playing on his own; however problems are rare as the bleach does not taste nice and typically there will only be localized lesions where the bleach contacted the mucous membranes.

Management of the unwell child (3)

10 D All of the answers are correct except for (C) which is the dose of adrenaline for cardiac arrest. (D) is the best answer as it is the most important life-saving treatment; IM adrenaline will work to reduce the capillary leak which is producing airway oedema. Once the fluid has shifted out of the vascular space, there is no way to rapidly move it out of the tissues; therefore the key first management of anaphylaxis is to administer IM adrenaline. In reality you would put out an emergency call for an anaesthetist (E) to manage the rapidly closing airway, give further salbutamol nebulizers and gain intravenous access to give hydrocortisone and antihistamine. Give (A) to block the histamine release which is driving the capillary leak and (B) to reduce general inflammation and aim to prevent the late type IV hypersensitivity. It is important not to forget about delayed type IV hypersensitivity; these children should be observed and sent home with two further doses of prednisolone for the next 2 days to cover this.

SECTION 11:
GENETIC AND METABOLIC DISORDERS

QUESTIONS

1. Turner's syndrome

A newborn baby is born to non-consanguineous parents. She is noted to have puffy feet on her 1st day check. She weighs 2.0 kg with widely spaced nipples and absent femoral pulses. You have asked your registrar to review her as you think she may have Turner's syndrome. She agrees and asks you to send blood tests for karyotyping. Which is the chromosomal diagnosis of Turner's syndrome?

    A. 47XXY
    B. 45YO
    C. 46XY
    D. 46XX
    E. 45XO

2. Down's syndrome

A 15-year-old boy was diagnosed with Down's syndrome at birth. He is short for his age, had cardiac surgery as a baby, has treatment for hypothyroidism and now attends mainstream school with some support. His parents are enquiring now about what complications he faces. Which of these is not a recognized complication of Down's syndrome?

    A. Retinoblastoma
    B. Atrioventricular septal defect (AVSD)
    C. Type 1 diabetes
    D. Leukaemia
    E. Alzheimer's disease

3. Prader–Willi syndrome

A baby is born and you are asked to do the baby check at 6 hours post-natal age. You go to see the baby and mum states that he has not yet had a feed. You advise they stay in hospital until the feeding is established. This is the first child of non-consanguineous parents. On day 4 when you review the baby he has still not had an adequate intake, has lost over 10 per cent in birth weight and is markedly hypotonic. Your consultant asks you to request genetic testing for Prader–Will syndrome. What is the inheritance of Prader–Willi syndrome?

    A. X-linked
    B. Imprinting
    C. Monosomy
    D. Microdeletion
    E. Trisomy

4. Septic neonate

A 5-day-old baby who is formula fed is on the neonatal unit being treated for sepsis secondary to an *Escherichia coli* urinary tract infection. He has been on antibiotics for 5 days. He is still unwell and vomiting. The parents are consanguineous and this is their first child. He has had repeat blood and urine cultures taken. Urine reducing substances are positive. What is the most likely underlying diagnosis?

    A.   Fructose intolerance
    B.   Galactosaemia
    C.   Phenylketonuria
    D.   Lactose intolerance
    E.   Glycogen storage disease

5. Marfan's syndrome

A 10-year-old boy is brought to the GP with tall stature. He is taller than his peers at school. His arm span is greater than his height, he has long, thin fingers, scoliosis and pectus excavatum. He is also concerned that he gets short of breath at school during PE lessons. You refer him for an echocardiogram and chest x-ray. You make a clinical diagnosis of Marfan's syndrome. What is the inheritance of Marfan's syndrome?

    A.   X-linked recessive
    B.   Autosomal recessive
    C.   Sporadic
    D.   X-linked dominant
    E.   Autosomal dominant

6. Phenylketonuria

A pregnant woman seeks advice from you regarding her condition and its impact on the pregnancy and risk to the baby. She has phenylketonuria (PKU) and has been on a phenylalanine-free diet for life. She was told that it was very important during her pregnancy to be compliant with this diet. She would like to know how the baby will be tested for the condition as she is aware that is an inherited condition. What is the initial investigation you will advise?

    A.   Serum tyrosine levels
    B.   Genetic screening
    C.   Serum phenylalanine levels
    D.   Urine phenylketones
    E.   Newborn blood spot screening

7. Oculocutaneous albinism

You see an 18-year-old boy who is the first child of his African parents and was born in Kenya before moving to the UK 1 year ago. He has white skin and pink irises. He was diagnosed with oculocutaneous albinism at birth. He has difficulty with his sight but has recently developed a skin lesion on his face. His mother has brought him to his GP as it has recently started to increase in size. On examination you note is an elevated, 3 cm diameter lump on the left of his nose. It has irregular edges, is firm and immobile and pigmented in areas. What is the likely diagnosis?

    A. Benign naevus
    B. Scar from a healing wound
    C. Malignant tumour
    D. Abscess
    E. Wart

8. Delayed walking

A 20-month-old boy has been referred due to delayed walking. On further questioning you establish he has no difficulty feeding, had head control at 3 months of age, and sat up by 8 months. He has been crawling for the last 8 months, but he does not pull to stand or walk with support. He has no dysmorphic features. There is no known family history of muscle problems. His mother has no myotonia. His mother is very concerned and asks you what is wrong. What is the most likely diagnosis?

    A. Myotonic dystrophy
    B. Duchenne's muscular dystrophy
    C. Down's syndrome
    D. Myasthenia gravis
    E. Becker's muscular dystrophy

9. Congenital adrenal hyperplasia

You are asked to see a 3-day-old baby on the post-natal ward. The baby was born at term and is the first child of consanguineous parents. The baby is drowsy and vomiting, with no fever, rash or diarrhoea. On examination, the baby is noted to have ambiguous genitalia. You do some blood tests: white cell count 5×10^9/L, C-reactive protein 2 mg/L, Na$^+$ 125 mmol/L, K$^+$ 8 mmol/L, glucose 1.7 mmol/L. 17-OH level progesterone is low. You make a diagnosis of congenital adrenal hyperplasia. What is the best initial management plan?

    A. IV hydrocortisone
    B. IV dextrose
    C. IV dextrose and IV hydrocortisone
    D. IV 0.9 per cent saline
    E. IV 3 per cent saline and IV hydrocortisone

10. A syndromic diagnosis

A 10-year-old boy is brought to the paediatric outpatient department for a review of his height. He was found to be on the 0.4th centile and his mid-parental height is the 98th centile. He also has widely spaced nipples, wide carrying angle, hypogonadism, pulmonary stenosis and developmental delay. What is the most likely diagnosis?

    A.   Angelman's syndrome
    B.   Williams's syndrome
    C.   Turner's syndrome
    D.   Prader–Willi syndrome
    E.   Noonan's syndrome

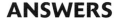

ANSWERS

Turner's syndrome

1 E Turner's syndrome is due to the absence of two sex chromosomes (pair number 23). Therefore the child is a girl (due to the absence of the Y chromosome) and has only 45 chromosomes. The physical characteristics may be noted at birth, particularly lymphoedema and cardiac anomalies, or noted later in life, such as short stature, delayed puberty, thyroid disorders, coarcation of aorta, aortic stenosis, horseshoe kidney and coeliac disease. (C) and (D) are normal gentoypes for males and females respectively. (A) is the karyotype of Klinefelter's syndrome which presents in boys with tall stature, delayed puberty and gynaecomastia.

Down's syndrome

2 A Down's syndrome affects many systems. Cardiac: ventricular septal defect, AVSD (B) and Tetralogy of Fallot. Endocrine: hypothyroidism, Addisons disease, type 1 diabetes (C). Ocular: cataracts, but not retinoblastoma (A). Malignancy: leukaemia (D). Gastrointestinal: duodenal atresia, Hirschprung's disease. Musculoskeletal: atlanto-axial instability. They are also at risk of Alzheimer's dementia (E) in later life.

Prader–Willi syndrome

3 B Prader–Willi syndrome is inherited by the phenomenon of genetic imprinting (B). It is due to the fact that for some chromosomes, you need the paternal or maternal chromosome to be present for normal functioning. To inherit Prader–Willi syndrome, there is loss of part of the paternal chromosome 15. X-linked conditions include Duchenne's muscular dystrophy, Fragile X syndrome (A) monosomy is seen in Turner's syndrome with only one X chromosome in girls (C), microdeletions cause DiGeorge's syndrome and Williams' syndrome (D) and trisomy 21, 13 and 18 are seen in Down's, Patau's and Edwards' syndromes, respectively (E).

Septic neonate

4 B Galactosaemia (B) is due to a deficiency in galactose-1-phosphate uridyl transferase. It results in illness with lactose-containing milks, with vomiting, cataracts and recurrent episodes of *Escherichia coli* sepsis. Fructose intolerance (A) can also produce a metabolic acidosis and vomiting, but is distinguished from galactosaemia by the *E. coli* sepsis. Phenylketonuria (C) presents with developmental delay when the child is older and a musty smelling urine, not acute illness and sepsis. Lactose intolerance (D) is unlikely as lactase levels are usually high at birth and may present with diarrhoea and poor weight gain. Glycogen storage diseases (E) are a heterogeneous group of disorders that present with liver, muscle and cardiac defects.

Marfan's syndrome

5 E Marfan's syndrome is an autosomal dominant (E) condition affecting the fibrillin gene. It is a connective tissue disorder that affects the musculoskeletal, ocular and cardiac systems. X-linked conditions affecting the musculoskeletal system include Duchenne's and Becker's muscular dystrophy, which can present with muscle weakness or delayed motor milestones (A). Autosomal recessive conditions affecting the musculoskeletal system include homocysteinuria, which has similar skeletal characteristics but also thromboembolic tendency (B). Klinefelter's syndrome is sporadic and can present with tall stature (C). Hypophosphataemic rickets is an X-linked dominant condition, which can present with genu varum and short stature (D).

Phenylketonuria

6 E PKU is an autosomal recessive metabolic condition resulting in a defect in enzyme phenylalanine hydroxylase, which converts phenylalanine to tyrosine. Due to the accumulation of phenylalanine and conversion to phenylketones, unrecognized and untreated PKU can result in seizures and musty smelling urine and eventually microcephaly and learning difficulties. PKU is screened on the newborn blood spot screening test (E). It is a rare but treatable condition with a good prognosis if management is started from birth (phenylalanine-free diet for life). (A), (C) and (D) can be measured but not usually as the diagnostic test, but they can be useful for monitoring of treatment. (B) is not performed routinely for PKU.

Oculocutaneous albinism

7 C This boy has oculocutaneous albinism, a metabolic condition affecting the production of skin pigment melanin. He is therefore at higher risk of skin malignancy (C) due to the lack of melanin. There is no history of trauma (B) or infection or fever (D) so both are less likely. Benign naevus or mole (A) would be static in size, smooth and regular edged in comparison to a malignant tumour. Warts caused by human papilloma virus (E) may be in the differential diagnosis but are rarely located on the face. With the medical background of albinism, (C) is more likely.

Delayed walking

8 B Delayed walking is a common paediatric presentation. Of the causes listed, Duchenne's muscular dystrophy (B) is the most common, with Becker's muscular dystrophy (E) being less severe but a similar presentation. Both are due to defects in the dystrophin gene and are inherited in an X-linked manner. Myotonic dystrophy (autosomal dominant) (A) and Down's syndrome (C) may present with hypotonia from birth, both centrally and peripherally, though children with Down's syndrome may have other features including dysmorphic facies (low set ears, epicanthic folds, protruding tongue, flattened nasal bridge), single palmar crease, sandal gap toes. Myasthenia gravis (D) can present with delayed walking, but fatigability is a key sign that differentiates it from the others.

Genetic and metabolic disorders

9 C Congenital adrenal hyperplasia is due to a deficiency of the enzymes that metabolize sex hormones (testosterones) to cortisol. Hence the accumulation of sex hormones can result in masculinized female genitalia or abnormal male genitalia. The lack of cortisol presents as a salt-losing crisis, as in this child, with low glucose and vomiting. Replacement of glucose and steroids is required in the first instance (C); they are both of high priority, so not (A) or (B). This will help to correct the electrolyte imbalances. Sodium disturbance should generally not be corrected too quickly; therefore (E) is incorrect. Normal saline (0.9 per cent) alone will not help, although may be required if there is hypotension.

A syndromic diagnosis

10 E Noonan's syndrome has a similar phenotype to Turner's syndrome but can present in both girls and boys (unlike Turner's syndrome which only occurs in girls (C)). These features are not typical of the other syndromes: (A) developmental delay and happy demeanour, (B) typical facial features, aortic stenosis, developmental delay, (D) poor feeding and weight gain in the neonatal period, followed by overeating in later life and obesity.

SECTION 12:
NEONATAL MEDICINE

QUESTIONS

1. Jaundiced baby

A 2-week-old baby was referred to the prolonged jaundice clinic by the community midwife. The pregnancy was unremarkable, and she was born at term with no antenatal abnormalities on ultrasound (US) scans or blood serology. She is now 17 days old and has been jaundiced since day 5 of life and never required phototherapy. She is breastfed and feeds 3-hourly for 20–25 minutes. She is afebrile and not lethargic. Her mother reports that the stools are pale and she has dark coloured urine. The bilirubin is 300 μmol/L, and conjugated bilirubin 100 μmol/L. What is the most important diagnosis to exclude?

A. Breast milk jaundice
B. ABO incompatibility
C. Biliary atresia
D. Neonatal hepatitis
E. Hypothyroidism

2. Neonatal sepsis

A 1-day-old baby is on the post-natal ward. You are asked to review her as she is febrile and lethargic. On examination she is tachycardic, has a capillary refill time of 3 seconds centrally and reduced urine output. Her blood culture 24 hours later grows Gram-positive cocci. Which is the most likely causative organism?

A. *Streptococcus pneumoniae*
B. *Staphylococcus aureus*
C. Group B *Streptococcus*
D. *Streptococcus viridans*
E. Group A *Streptococcus*

3. Preterm baby with breathing difficulty

A preterm baby is born at 25 + 6 weeks gestation. He is delivered by caesarean section due to maternal pre-eclampsia. He is intubated at birth and given surfactant via the endotracheal tube. He is ventilated and commenced on IV dextrose. After 4 hours of age he has increased work of breathing, with intercostal and subcostal recession and a respiratory rate of 60/min. A chest x-ray shows a ground glass pattern in both lung fields. He has no audible murmur. He is afebrile. You diagnose respiratory distress syndrome. What is the aetiological factor responsible for respiratory distress syndrome?

A. Pneumonitis
B. Lung hypoplasia
C. Surfactant deficiency
D. Immature lung parenchyma
E. Infection with group B *Streptococcus*

4. Preterm with bowel problems

A preterm baby is now 25 + 7 weeks corrected gestation. He is on the neonatal unit being cared for while his mother recovers on ITU after he was born secondary to an eclamptic seizure. He has been receiving formula milk as the parents have not consented to donor breast milk. He has been having bilious aspirates from his nasogastric tube and today his abdomen in very distended and tense. He has had one episode of bloody stools. You are going to treat him for nectrotizing enterocolitis (NEC). What is the best initial management plan?

    A.   Conservative management, observe and reassess
    B.   Nil by mouth (NBM), IV antibiotics and emergency exploratory laparotomy
    C.   IV fluids, emergency laparotomy and bowel resection
    D.   IV fluids and IV antibiotics
    E.   NBM, IV fluids, abdominal X-ray and surgical review

5. Hypotonic baby

A 3-day-old baby is seen by the midwife for a routine post-natal review. She notices that he is very floppy and his mother has raised concerns about his poor feeding. He has a protruding tongue, epicanthic folds, low set ears and sandal gap toes. She explains to the parents she thinks he may have Down's syndrome and refers him to the paediatrician. What is the diagnostic test for Down's syndrome?

    A.   Serum alpha fetoprotein, beta human chorionic gonadotrophin, oestriol, inhibin
    B.   Gene mutation analysis
    C.   Clinical diagnosis
    D.   Karyotype
    E.   FISH

6. Coughing baby

A baby is born by emergency caesarean section due to fetal tachycardia. His delivery was uneventful and you are asked to see him 5 hours later on the post-natal ward. He has just taken his first feed and has been coughing and spluttering since. He had an episode with blue lips transiently and this has now improved; his oxygen saturations are 97 per cent in air and he is apyrexial. On examination, you note other features including vertebral and limb abnormalities, imperforate anus, pansystolic murmur at the lower left sternal edge and renal anomalies noted on antenatal scans. What is the most likely cause for his coughing episode?

    A.   Cleft palate
    B.   Tracheoesophageal fistula
    C.   Choanal atresia
    D.   Incoordinated swallowing reflex
    E.   Pneumonia

7. Cyanotic baby

A term baby is awaiting his discharge check when you are called to see him at 10 hours of age. His mother reports that he has turned a dusky colour and is not as alert as he has been. On examination he has central cyanosis, pulse 150 bpm regular, and both brachial and femoral pulses are palpable. He has normal heart sounds with no murmur. His oxygen saturations are 65 per cent in air. What is the most likely underlying diagnosis?

    A.   Transposition of the great vessels
    B.   Ventricular septal defect (VSD)
    C.   Tetralogy of Fallot
    D.   Aortic stenosis
    E.   Coartation of the aorta

8. Fitting baby

A 12-hour-old baby on the post-natal ward has just had a seizure lasting 2 minutes. It resolved spontaneously and was generalized in nature. Her mother had gestational diabetes and poor glucose control in pregnancy. The baby's birth weight was 5 kg. There were no abnormalities noted on antenatal US scans or maternal serology. On examination she has no dysmorphic features and handles well. What initial blood tests would you do for the baby?

    A.   Liver function tests
    B.   Boehringer Mannheim (BM) glucose
    C.   Full blood count, C-reactive protein
    D.   Electrolytes
    E.   Calcium, magnesium

9. Gastroschisis

A pregnant woman is admitted to the labour ward for an elective caesarean section at 38 weeks for her baby who had an antenatal diagnosis of gastroschisis. The paediatric team are called to attend the delivery. The baby is born in good condition with no resuscitation required. He is taken to the neonatal unit for further care. Which of these is a complication of gastroschisis?

    A.   Dehydration
    B.   Hyperthermia
    C.   Necrotizing enterocolitis (NEC)
    D.   Fluid overload
    E.   Hypernatraemia

10. A baby with intrauterine growth restriction (IUGR)

You are called to see a baby who has just been born at 39 weeks' gestation, as the midwife thinks he is small and should be admitted to the neonatal unit for his care. You review the baby. His weight is 1.8 kg, below the 0.4th centile and his head circumference is 35 cm – 50th centile. He has no dysmorphic features. Which is the most likely cause of this IUGR?

  A. Chromosomal anomaly
  B. Maternal smoking
  C. Congenital infection
  D. Maternal alcohol use
  E. Placental insufficiency

ANSWERS

Jaundiced baby

1 C Jaundice is important in neonates, particularly the timing of onset and duration. Jaundice in the first 24 hours may be due to haemolysis either immune (ABO incompatibility or rhesus disease) or non-immune (G6PD, spherocytosis) and is unconjugated; therefore (B) is incorrect. Jaundice between 24 hours and 2 weeks can be physiological as the phenomenon of breast milk jaundice (A) but should not persist. Hypothyroidism is very important to exclude in the neonate due to the potential learning difficulties that can ensue, but it is unlikely to present with acholic stools. Neonatal hepatitis (D) can be secondary to infection (congenital) or metabolic diseases (alpha-1-santitrypsin, cystic fibrosis), but with the history of pale stools and dark urine a diagnosis of biliary atresia (C) must be fully investigated due to the risk of liver cirrhosis.

Neonatal sepsis

2 C Group B *Streptococcus* (GBS) (C) can colonize the reproductive tract of women. When babies are delivered through this tract, they can become infected with GBS. This may manifest as sepsis, pneumonia, meningitis, urinary tract infection and septic arthritis among others. All others are possible but in this demographic, the three most common pathogens are group B *Streptococcus*, *E. coli* and *Listeria monocytogenes*.

Preterm baby with breathing difficulty

3 C Respiratory distress syndrome (C) is secondary to surfactant deficiency due to immaturity of type 2 pneumocytes in the alveoli of the developing lung. Preterm babies are at risk by virtue of their gestational age. They have respiratory distress, and require artificial surfactant and ventilatory support as their lungs are prone to atelectasis. The lung parenchyma is structurally immature but functional (D). Congenital pneumonia (E) may present with increased work of breathing and focal signs on chest x-ray. Lung hypoplasia (B) occurs due to renal problems or diaphragmatic hernia, where the underlying lung is unable to develop and therefore is impaired functionally. (A) occurs as a part of meconium aspiration syndrome, and is due to the irritation to the lung caused by the chemicals in meconium.

Preterm with bowel problems

4 E NEC is a complicated disease occurring in preterm and also term babies. It has many risk factors, in this case formula feeding, prematurity and potential ischaemia at birth. The suspicion for NEC must remain high and therefore in this child where there are clear signs of bowel pathology, must be treated as such. He should therefore be managed actively, not conservatively (A). As with any suspected surgical problem, patients should be made NBM and given IV fluids, hence (D) is incorrect. He needs to be reviewed by a surgeon and imaging may assist this assessment (E). He cannot be operated on unless he is first seen by a surgeon and initial investigations are carried out; therefore (B) and (C) are incorrect. However he may require laparotomy and bowel resection.

Hypotonic baby

5 D Down's syndrome is due to trisomy 21 (three copies of chromosome 21) and therefore karyotyping will identify this extra chromosome (D). Women can be screened in pregnancy for the condition using various serum markers in combination with US scan (A). There is no gene mutation to identify (B); this would be more suitable in the diagnosis of cystic fibrosis. Although identification of a syndrome does involve elucidating clinical features, this needs to be confirmed with a diagnostic test if there is one available and karyoptying is the most definitive investigation in confirming a suspected diagnosis of Down's syndrome (C). Fluorescence *in situ* hybridization (FISH) (E) is used for the identification of microdeletion syndromes such as DiGeorge's or cri du chat syndrome.

Coughing baby

6 B All the above may result in coughing in this baby. With the constellation of other signs suggestive of VACTERL (vertebral, anal imperforation, cardiac, tracheo-oesophageal fistula, renal and limb anomalies) it makes (B) the correct answer. Babies with a cleft palate (A) also have a similar history but you should expect to see or feel the cleft palate and other dysmorphic features perhaps consistent with DiGeorge's or Down's syndrome. Choanal atresia (C) is associated with CHARGE (coloboma, heart defects, atresia choanae, retardation of growth and development, genitourinary abnormalities and ear anomalies) syndrome. An incoordinated swallowing reflex (D) may exist if there was concern about the neurological or neuromuscular status, but there is no evidence of this from the history. Pneumonia (E) is likely as a consequence of tracheo-oesophageal fistula (B) and may exist independently but the child's afebrile state makes this less likely.

Cyanotic baby

7 A This child has a cyanotic defect affecting the oxygenation of the blood. Transposition of the great vessels (whereby the aorta is attached to the right ventricle and the pulmonary artery attached to the left ventricle) (A) and the Tetralogy of Fallot (multiple defects including VSD, right ventricular outflow tract obstruction, right ventricular hypertrophy and overriding aorta) (C) are both cyanotic presentations but the Tetralogy of

Fallot more commonly presents at around 6 months of age with cyanotic spells. Transposition of the great vessels is more likely to present at birth and is only compatible with life if there is a mixing defect in addition (VSD, atrial septal defect, persistent ductus arteriorus). In this child the ductus arteriosus helps to shunt blood to the lungs until it starts to close physiologically. He then is at risk of worsening cyanosis. He needs a prostaglandin infusion to keep the duct open and surgical intervention. The other answer options (B) (VSD is a communication between the left and right ventricles allowing left-to-right shunting), (D) (narrowing of the outflow tract of the left ventricle) and (E) (narrowing of a section of the aorta) are acyanotic and therefore do not account for this presentation.

Fitting baby

8 B Infants of diabetic mothers are at risk of congenital malformations (if glucose control was poor around conception) and hypoglycaemia and macrosomia in the post-natal period. They become used to having high levels of circulating glucose from their mother and therefore increase their baseline insulin production. At delivery, this supply of glucose is removed and the residual insulin will decrease their glucose, predisposing to hypoglycaemia, so (B) is correct. Fits can occur in babies secondary to infection (C), or electrolyte disturbances (A), (D) and (E) but in this case (B) is more likely given the mother's history, though all should be considered after.

Gastroschisis

9 A Gastroschisis refers to herniation of the bowel through a defect in the anterior abdominal wall of the developing fetus. It is not covered with a membrane as in exomphalos and is rarely associated with other anomalies. Gastroschisis can lead to fluid, electrolyte and heat losses. The baby will require fluid replacement and strict fluid balance assessment, placing in a heated incubator and regular electrolyte monitoring. Dehydration (A) is a serious complication, not overload (D), along with hypothermia and not hyperthermia (B). Hyponatraemia is more likely than hypernatraemia (E). NEC (C) is not more likely in children with gastroschisis.

A baby with intrauterine growth restriction (IUGR)

10 E Placental insufficiency is the most likely cause of IUGR. This child has asymmetrical IUGR, suggesting that the insult occurred late in pregnancy with head growth sparing. Causes include maternal diabetes or pre-eclampsia, both resulting in placental insufficiency due to their effects on placental microvasculature. Chromosomal anomaly (A), maternal smoking (B), congenital infection (C) and maternal alcohol use (D) would more likely cause low birth weight and head circumference changes, i.e. symmetrical IUGR is present from the first trimester.

SECTION 13:
GASTROENTEROLOGY

QUESTIONS

1. Vomiting

A mother brings her 4-week-old baby to see you for the third time. He was born at term by normal vaginal delivery with no complications. You started him on anti-reflux medicine last week but it has not helped. He is now vomiting his whole feeds and is becoming lethargic and passing less urine and stool. His mother says he is hungry even after he vomits. The practice nurse has weighed him and he has lost 200 g since last week. His mother was breastfeeding him while waiting to be seen and as you go to examine him, the baby has a large milky vomit, which cascades over the clinic floor. What is the most likely diagnosis?

A. Gastroenteritis
B. Volvulus
C. Necrotizing enterocolitis (NEC)
D. Intussusception
E. Pyloric stenosis

2. Failure to thrive

A 15-month-old girl has come to see you with her father. The family are worried that she has had diarrhoea for more than a month, occasional vomiting and is losing weight. She used to be a happy interactive baby but now seems lethargic and miserable most of the time. She has no significant past medical history, the rest of the family are well and there is no history of travel. Her mother has well-controlled type 1 diabetes. The child's weight at 6 months in the personal child health record ('red book') was on the 50th centile but she is now just below the 9th. What is the most likely diagnosis?

A. Crohn's disease
B. Ulcerative colitis
C. Coeliac disease
D. Irritable bowel syndrome
E. Giardiasis

3. Abdominal examination

A 13-year-boy is brought to see you as he has recently been complaining of abdominal pain and is increasingly tired. On examination you note some early clubbing and erythematous palms. His conjunctivae look pale. He has one or two spider naevi on his chest. His abdomen is soft with mild tenderness in the epigastrium and right upper quadrant. The liver is palpable at 1 cm and you feel the splenic tip. He has normal bowel sounds and no bruits. On slit lamp examination of his eyes, an amber ring is noted around the cornea. What is the most likely diagnosis?

    A.   Abdominal tuberculosis
    B.   Cystic fibrosis
    C.   Wilson's disease
    D.   Acute hepatitis A
    E.   Glandular fever

4. Chronic constipation

An 8-year-old girl is brought to see you, having not opened her bowels in 8 days. She complains of hard painful stools and recurrent abdominal pain for the past 6 months but no vomiting. Her mother thinks that she is avoiding going to the toilet and reports that she has always been a bit irregular opening her bowels, averaging about twice a week. In her past medical history, she passed meconium on day 1 of life and has had no significant medical problems. On examination she is a well-looking, normally grown child. Her abdomen is soft with a palpable indentable mass in the left iliac fossa. The anus is normal, as are her lower limbs. What is the first step in management?

    A.   Encourage her to increase her fluid intake, dietary fibre and exercise
    B.   Introduce scheduled toileting with a positive reward scheme such as a star chart
    C.   Refer for bowel disimpaction under anaesthesia
    D.   Start polyethylene glycol with electrolytes such as Movicol
    E.   Start a stimulant laxative such as senna

5. Infant abdominal pain

A 2-week-old baby is brought to accident and emergency by his parents because he has been intermittently inconsolable for the past 12 hours. He does not want to breastfeed and has vomited. The parents think his tummy is upset as he keeps drawing up his legs. He was born at term by normal vaginal delivery with no problems. On examination the abdomen is distended and tense. He is crying and there is a firm swelling in the right groin area. You can hear active bowel sounds. What is the most likely diagnosis?

    A.   Appendicitis
    B.   Right inguinal hernia
    C.   Gastroenteritis
    D.   NEC
    E.   Sepsis

6. Jaundice

A 5-year-old girl is brought to accident and emergency with a 24-hour history of vomiting and diarrhoea and now her eyes and skin have gone very yellow. She has been taking oral rehydration salts and is still passing urine. She is normally healthy and there is no family history of jaundice. On examination her heart rate is 130 and respiratory rate is 26. She is alert, warm and well perfused. The chest is clear, heart sounds are normal and the abdomen is soft with a 2 cm liver edge. What should the management be?

A. Reassure and discharge home, to return if not keeping fluids down
B. Take bloods to test for liver function, hepatitis, and urea and electrolytes; inform the Health Protection Agency and discharge home with follow-up to review results
C. Take bloods to test for liver function, hepatitis screen and urea and electrolytes and admit for IV fluids
D. Take bloods to test for liver function, hepatitis screen and urea and electrolytes and admit for observation with continued oral rehydration salts
E. Take bloods to check liver function and urea and electrolytes. If they are normal, discharge home with reassurance but to return if not keeping fluids down

7. Haematemesis

A 15 year old with well-controlled type 1 diabetes presents with frank haematemesis. Her blood tests in accident and emergency show: pH 7.37, glucose 18.3 mmol/L, haemoglobin 12.3 g/dL, white cell count 5.3×10^9/L, neutrophils 2.1×10^9/L, platelets 165×10^9/L, Na$^+$ 135 mmol/L, K$^+$ 3.5 mmol/L, urea 5.0 mmol/L, creatinine 83 µmol/L, alanine transaminase 740 IU/l, bilisubin 96 µmol/L, alkaline phosphatase 102 IU/l, and albumin 25 g/L. Further investigations once she is stable on the ward show hepatitis B surface antigen negative, anti-hepatitis C virus negative, anti-nuclear antibody (ANA) 1:320 and anti-smooth muscle antibodies are positive. What is the most likely diagnosis?

A. Autoimmune hepatitis with varices
B. Metabolic ketoacidosis
C. Gastroenteritis with a Mallory–Weiss tear
D. Pregnancy with hyperemesis and a Mallory–Weiss tear
E. Systemic lupus erythematosus (SLE)

8. Abdominal pain

An 18-month-old child is brought into accident and emergency with a 2-day history of vomiting, abdominal pain and fever. Which of the following is an unlikely cause of this clinical picture?

A. Lower lobe pneumonia with pain referred to the abdomen
B. Mesenteric adenitis
C. Diabetic ketoacidosis
D. Pyelonephritis
E. NEC

9. Acute abdomen management – intussusception

A 13 month old is referred up to her local district general accident and emergency by a GP who is concerned she has intussusception following an 18-hour history of fever, vomiting and intermittent colicky screaming. A kind radiologist agreed to do an urgent ultrasound which shows an area of invaginated bowel in the right side of the colon. What is the most appropriate management?

   A. Ask the radiologist to attempt a reduction by rectal air insufflation and if this fails make nil by mouth (NBM) and transfer to a local paediatric surgical unit

   B. Make NBM and start intravenous fluids while waiting for transfer to a paediatric surgical unit

   C. Move to theatre for an attempt of rectal air insufflation reduction and if this fails move to surgery in the local hospital as the patient will be too unstable for transfer

   D. Make NBM, start IV fluids and admit for observation

   E. Make NBM and start intravenous fluids, and book him onto the emergency theatre list as he is too unstable for transfer to a local paediatric surgical unit

10. Per rectum (PR) bleeding

Which of the following is not a cause of PR bleeding?

   A. Constipation with an anal fissure
   B. Intussusception
   C. Meckel's diverticulum
   D. Bacterial gastroenteritis
   E. Abdominal migraine

11. Diarrhoea

A mother brings her 2 year old to see you. She is very worried that he always has diarrhoea or loose stools. He eats a normal diet, and no particular foods seem to upset him but he often still has bits of vegetables or food he has eaten visible in the stool. She thinks he is losing weight and he is starting to potty train, so she is concerned this will affect his ability to anticipate needing the toilet. On examination he is an alert and well-looking child with a normal capillary refill, heart and respiratory rate. His abdomen is soft with no masses, there is no evidence of wasting and his weight and height are following the 50th centile. What is the most appropriate management?

   A. Reassure the mother, explaining this is toddler's diarrhoea and he will grow out of it

   B. Start loperamide as toddler's diarrhoea is affecting his toilet training
   C. Refer for endoscopy and biopsy to rule out coeliac disease
   D. Refer for a colonoscopy and biopsy for inflammatory bowel disease
   E. Order a blood test for thyroid function to rule out hyperthyroidism

12. Failure to thrive diagnosis

A 10-year-old boy presents with recurrent mouth ulcers, abdominal pain, distension and frequent episodes of diarrhoea with mucus. He has been losing weight. On examination he is slim and plotting his growth shows a fall in weight from the 50th centile to below the 9th. His abdomen is soft with generalized discomfort on deep palpation but no masses are present. What is the most likely diagnosis?

    A. Ulcerative colitis
    B. Crohn's disease
    C. Coeliac disease
    D. Gastroenteritis
    E. NEC

13. Bloody diarrhoea diagnosis

A 15-year-old boy comes to see you, complaining of recurrent abdominal and back passage pain relieved by passage of diarrhoea. He is also complaining of low back and knee pain and last week there was blood mixed into his stool. He has been losing weight recently. On examination he is slim and looks pale. His abdomen is soft but tender in the left iliac fossa with no masses. What is the most likely diagnosis?

    A. Ulcerative colitis
    B. Crohn's disease
    C. Coeliac disease
    D. Gastroenteritis
    E. NEC

14. Delayed passage of meconium

Ninety-nine per cent of healthy term infants will pass meconium within the first 24 hours of life and all should do so within 48 hours. Which of the following is not a cause of delayed meconium passage?

    A. Hirschsprung's disease
    B. Cystic fibrosis with a meconium ileus
    C. Choanal atresia
    D. Imperforate anus
    E. Meconium plug syndrome

15. Chronic vomiting and diarrhoea

A 3-month-old baby is brought to accident and emergency because he has been vomiting and having diarrhoea for the past month. His mother breastfed him until he was 8 weeks old and he is now taking formula milk, 4–5 oz every 4 hours. On examination he is alert but fussy and looks thin. He has eczema on his face, neck and torso and the mother says this is new. The abdomen is soft, the genitalia are normal with a significant nappy rash and the anal margin is erythematous. You plot his growth in his red book and find that he was born on the 50th centile and was following that but now he is on the 25th centile for weight. What is the most likely diagnosis?

A. Cow's milk protein intolerance
B. Lactose intolerance
C. Gastroenteritis
D. Hyper IgE syndrome
E. Wiskott–Aldrich syndrome

ANSWERS

Vomiting

1 E The most likely explanation is pyloric stenosis (E), which classically presents at 1 month with projectile vomiting and is more common in males. This is caused by hypertrophy of the pyloric muscle at the gastric outlet leading to delayed stomach emptying and gradually increased vomiting. These children are often hungry after the vomit. A volvulus (B) and intussusception (D) would have significant irritability, abdominal distension and tenderness associated with them, in addition to vomiting. NEC (C) is predominately an illness of the premature infant presenting with abdominal distension and bile stained gastric aspirates. When it occurs in term infants there is usually a history of birth asphyxia or severe growth restriction. Gastroenteritis (A) can occur in young infants especially if parents are not using sterilized (boiled and cooled) water to make up formula. It normally presents with a short history of vomiting and diarrhoea in an unwell infant.

Failure to thrive

2 C The most likely diagnosis is coeliac disease (C), an autoimmune sensitivity to dietary gluten which results in villous atrophy of the small intestine and corresponding malabsorption and malnutrition. Children usually present after weaning and exposure to wheat, with diarrhoea, abdominal distension, failure to thrive and wasting, especially of the buttocks. There is often a family history of autoimmune disease such as thyroid disease or diabetes. Crohn's disease (A) and ulcerative colitis (B) are rare in paediatrics outside of teenagers. Irritable bowel syndrome (D) would be unusual in such a young child but is associated with abdominal pain and bloating with altered bowel habit, including diarrhoea or constipation. It is primarily a diagnosis of exclusion and while weight loss can be seen if the child eats less to avoid symptoms, it is a less prominent presenting feature. Lastly, giardiasis (E) could easily present like this in a young child; however you would expect a travel history to an endemic area or other family members to be unwell having drunk contaminated water. It would be worthwhile sending a stool sample for cysts and parasites.

Abdominal examination

3 C He is presenting with signs of chronic liver failure, clubbing and palmar erythema. While he does have spider naevi you need at least five to be significant. Slit lamp examination of his eyes revealed Kayser–Fleischer rings which are a sign of Wilson's disease (C). This is an autosomal recessive defect in copper metabolism that results in copper deposition in the tissues and leads to liver failure with cirrhosis, neurological sequelae, renal involvement and cardiac complications. In addition patients develop haemolytic anaemia due to copper deposits in the red cell membrane. Thus, as he has a palpable liver and spleen, he is anaemic and complaining of upper abdominal pain with stigmata of liver failure, the most likely diagnosis is Wilson's disease (C). Abdominal tuberculosis (A) is part of the differential diagnosis, but is unlikely to cause such significant signs of hepatic dysfunction, and would not explain the eye findings. Cystic fibrosis (B) may cause clubbing, but you have been given no pulmonary information, making this diagnosis unlikely. Acute hepatitis A (D) would not produce signs of chronic liver failure and normally presents with vomiting and possible jaundice. There is often a palpable liver but splenic enlargement would be unusual. Similarly, glandular fever (usually caused by infection with the Epstein–Barr virus (EBV)), would not produce signs of chronic liver failure on examination, but the child may give a history of lethargy and have a palpable liver and spleen. Again, the eye findings would not be explained by EBV infection.

Chronic constipation

4 A   This is a common presentation of constipation and on examination she has faecal impaction. There are no red flags present in the history such as growth failure, a history of delayed passage of meconium, distended abdomen with vomiting, anal pathology or neurological complications affecting the lower limbs. The correct first line management would be advice on increased fluid/fibre intake and exercise (A). Once her stools are softer, behavioural change management around toileting using star charts will help her overcome the toilet avoidance (B). If lifestyle changes do not produce softer stools or she develops vomiting, she may need medical bowel disimpaction with non-stimulant laxatives (D) but this would not be first line management. Stimulant laxatives (E) should not be used as they may produce more abdominal pain, dependence and have an associated risk of bowel perforation. Referral to the surgeons for bowel disimpaction under anaesthesia would be a last resort after failed medical management and underlying causes of constipation have been ruled out or treated. It is worth reviewing the NICE guidelines on paediatric constipation (www.nice.org.uk/nicemedia/live/12993/48754/48754.pdf).

Infant abdominal pain

5 B   On examination you can feel a swelling in the groin which is associated with a tense abdomen. In a vomiting baby this is an incarcerated inguinal hernia (B) and needs to be seen urgently by the surgeons to go to theatre. Appendicitis (A) is common in childhood, most commonly seen between the ages of 11 and 20 years old. However, it is very unusual in the infant as the neck of the appendix is wide and unlikely to obstruct at this age. Gastroenteritis (C) can occur in young infants, especially if parents are not using sterilized (boiled and cooled) water to make up formula. It normally presents with a short history of vomiting and diarrhoea in an unwell infant, and there may be a contact history such as another family member with diarrhea or vomiting. NEC (D) is predominately an illness of the premature infant presenting with abdominal distension and bile stained nasogastric aspirates. When it occurs in term infants there is usually a history of birth asphyxia or severe growth restriction. In the absence of localizing signs to the abdomen in a child this young you would treat with IV antibiotics to cover neonatal sepsis (E) but this does not explain the swelling in the groin. It is worth noting that inguinal hernias all require surgical review whereas umbilical hernias will self-resolve and need no surgical intervention.

Jaundice

6 B   The mostly likely cause of this child's illness is hepatitis A, which should be reported to the Health Protection Agency (B). If at all possible she should not be admitted to reduce the spread to other patients (D). She is drinking and well hydrated. She does not need IV fluids (C). (A) would be reasonable as she is clinically well but the jaundice and palpable liver should be investigated. (E) is wrong as it does not have a hepatitis screen or health protection reporting.

Haematemesis

7 A   It is important to know some of the associated autoimmune diseases that type 1 diabetics may suffer from. The most common are coeliac and Graves' disease which are screened for yearly. Autoimmune hepatitis (A) is more common in females and typically presents between the ages of 10 and 30 with either chronic liver failure or acute hepatitis. The ANA will be positive in approximately 80 per cent and the anti-smooth muscle antibody with be positive in approximately 70 per cent of cases. Her pH is normal, so she is not in ketoacidosis (B), and her glucose is raised as a stress response. While she would be isolated in a cubicle on admission in case of gastroenteritis (C), there is no history of diarrhoea and the investigations do not support an infectious cause with a normal white cell count and autoantibodies positive. There is nothing in the history to suggest she is pregnant (D); however it would be good practice to test the urine of any woman of child-bearing age with vomiting or abdominal pain. ANA would normally be positive in SLE (E) but anti-smooth muscle antibodies are associated with autoimmune hepatitis.

Abdominal pain

8 E   The answer is NEC (E) which classically affects preterm babies in the neonatal period and would not be a cause of abdominal pathology in an 18-month-old child. Pneumonia in the lower lobes (A) may present as pain in the upper abdomen and fever. Any upper or lower respiratory tract infection in young children can be associated with vomiting, mostly because of inflamed upper airways triggering the gag reflex and increased work of breathing putting pressure on the stomach just below the diaphragm. Mesenteric adenitis (B) is the most likely answer as this is classically how mesenteric adenitis presents, although it is a diagnosis of exclusion, having ruled out other pathology. There is often a preceding viral illness (typically either upper respiratory or gastroenteritis). Enlarged mesenteric glands can be seen on abdominal ultrasound examination. Mesenteric adenitis may be mistaken for appendicitis. While it is unusual for such a young child to develop diabetes (C), even babies can. Infection is often a trigger for new onset or an episode of ketoacidosis in a known diabetic, and this may present with vomiting. Pyelonephritis (D) should always be ruled out in a child with fever and vomiting unless a clear alternative source of infection is identified.

Acute abdomen management – intussuception

9   B   Up to 75 per cent of cases may be reduced by air insufflation rectally, but if this fails the child will need to be taken directly to theatre as there is a risk of perforation with the procedure. As it is unlikely that a district general hospital will be able to take such a young child to theatre, all procedures should be carried out in a paediatric surgical centre; therefore (A), (C), (D) and (E) are all incorrect and the only option is to transfer (B).

Per rectum (PR) bleeding

10   E   Often the first presentation of migraine in children is abdominal pain, in the context of a family history of migraine. This diagnosis would not be supported if the child has per rectum bleeding (E). The most common cause of PR bleeding in children is constipation with an anal fissure and this would produce bright red blood on the toilet tissue or streaked on the surface of the stool (A). Intussusception has a late and uncommon sign of 'redcurrant jelly' stool (B) which is due to blood and mucus from the distal end of the invaginated segment of bowel becoming necrotic. At this stage there is a risk of perforation, especially if insufflation is attempted. The diagnosis should ideally be made long before these signs evolve. Two per cent of the population have a Meckel's diverticulum, an ileal remnant of the vitellointestinal duct which contains ectopic gastric mucosa and can lead to ulceration, perforation and a presentation with severe rectal haemorrhage of dark red blood (C). Bacterial gastroenteritis with *Shigella* or *Salmonella* may produce blood and/or pus mixed into the stool (D).

Diarrhoea

11   A   This is toddler's diarrhoea which is a common cause of loose stool in pre-school aged children and almost always requires no treatment (A).

It is likely to be related to immature development of intestinal motility and it resolves in most children by the age of 5. Rarely, if the diarrhoea is socially disruptive to the child, it can be treated with loperamide (B), but he is only just starting to potty train and should be given a chance to do so. 'Significant social disruption' would be considered if he has failed to potty train and was unable to start school. He is a well-grown child with no evidence of wasting, so coeliac disease (C) is unlikely and the first investigation for this would be a blood test for anti-endomesial antibodies, not endoscopy. Inflammatory bowel disease (D) would be rare in a child this young, and there is no mention of abdominal pain, passage of blood and mucus or any suggestion of growth failure. While diarrhoea is a common symptom of hyperthyroidism (E), it is more commonly seen in female teenagers or in the neonatal period in infants born to mothers with Graves' disease. He is growing normally and has no other features of hyperthyroidism such as restlessness, increased appetite, sweating or tachycardia.

Failure to thrive diagnosis

12 B Inflammatory bowel disease (IBD) can be difficult to separate clinically into Crohn's and ulcerative colitis. A younger child with IBD is more likely to have Crohn's disease (B), although its incidence increases with age. He has mouth ulcers which would not go with ulcerative colitis (A). Ulcerative colitis is a rectal disorder with proximal spread. Coeliac disease (C) would normally present in young children as it is associated with the weaning process and ingestion of wheat, although the diagnosis should be considered in all children with growth failure. This is a more chronic story than would be expected for gastroenteritis (D) which should not produce failure to thrive. NEC (E) is predominately an illness of the premature infant presenting with abdominal distension and bile stained aspirates.

Bloody diarrhoea diagnosis

13 A Ulcerative colitis (A) can affect any age but is rare in early childhood and increases in incidence with age. It is a recurrent inflammatory ulcerating disease of the mucous membrane layer of the rectum which spreads proximally to involve the colon. It classically presents with abdominal pain with blood or mucus mixed into diarrhoea. It is associated with erythema nodosum, pyoderma gangrenosum, arthritis and spondylitis, which may explain his back and knee pain. Crohn's disease (B) can be difficult to distinguish from ulcerative colitis but it is not commonly associated with spondylitis suggested by the back pain. The main distinction is on histology with Crohn's disease showing non-caseating granuloma and full thickness lesions. Coeliac disease (C) usually presents with malnutrition and abdominal bloating. Diarrhoea may be a presenting feature but blood would be unusual and would be digested, i.e. dark stools. This is a more chronic story than you would expect for gastroenteritis (D) and the arthritis does not tie in. NEC (E) is predominately an illness of the premature infant presenting with abdominal distension and bile stained aspirates.

Delayed passage of meconium

14 C Choanal atresia (C) is a congenital blockage of the nasal airway which presents with newborn cyanosis and respiratory distress, as infants are obligate nose breathers. The most common cause of delayed meconium passage is (E), which is a transient immaturity of the gut resulting in failure to move a plug of meconium along. The management is with anal stimulation with a glycerine chip. Approximately 20 per cent of cystic fibrosis cases will present with a meconium ileus (B) due to inspissated meconium. Approximately one in 4000 babies will have Hirschprung's disease (A) which is caused by the absence of ganglion cells from the myenteric and submucosal plexi in part of the rectum or colon which results in narrowed bowel in the denervated region. The lack of bowel wall movement fails to move the meconium along. The management is surgical resection of the denervated portion of bowel. An imperforate anus (D) is slightly less common than Hirschprung's disease, and will require surgical intervention.

Chronic vomiting and diarrhoea

15 A In light of the eczema that has developed since breastfeeding cessation, plus the nappy rash and anal inflammation, the most likely explanation is cow's milk protein intolerance (A), an allergic reaction to the cow's milk proteins, which is different from lactose intolerance (B). Cow's milk protein intolerance typically presents with exposure to cow's milk in infancy, although in severe cases maternal ingestion of dairy products may affect a breastfeeding infant. The infant has worsening skin inflammation (eczema), vomiting, diarrhoea (which may be bloody), failure to thrive, irritability and colic. Lactose intolerance (B) is typically acquired following acute gastroenteritis. It is unusual in infancy, although rarely it can be congenital. It is a deficiency in the enzyme, lactose dehydrogenase, which breaks down lactose (the disaccharide sugar in milk). The build up of sugars in the gut results in an osmotic diarrhoea and dehydration. This history is too long for gastroenteritis (C) which could be associated with the introduction of bottle feeds if the equipment and water has not been sterilized. Hyper IgE syndrome (D), sometimes referred to as Job's syndrome, is an autosomal dominant immunodeficiency which is associated with severe eczema and skin boils but does not have significant gastrointestinal presentations. Wiskott–Aldrich syndrome (E) is also associated with eczema. This is an X-linked recessive disorder associated with thrombocytopenia, eczema and lymphopenia, but no significant gastrointestinal symptoms.

SECTION 14:
INFECTIOUS DISEASES

Questions

QUESTIONS

1. Unusual cause of meningitis

A 15-year-old Asian girl with Down's syndrome came to accident and emergency with a prolonged fever. She has severe learning difficulties and was difficult to assess. Her parents think she is more unsettled than usual and not eating and drinking properly for the last 3 weeks. She is admitted as you cannot confidently find the source of the infection, but she has no cough, rash, vomiting, diarrhoea or meningism. The next day she complains of a headache and starts to vomit. She has a CT scan which is normal and then a lumbar puncture (LP). White cell count (WCC) 150×10⁹/L (20 per cent neutrophils), red blood count 0, protein 2 g/L, glucose 1.2 mmol/L (serum glucose 6.0 mmol/L). What is the most likely cause of this meningitis?

- A. *Mycobacterium tuberculosis*
- B. Herpes simplex virus (HSV)
- C. *Streptococcus pneumoniae*
- D. *Cryptococcus neoformans*
- E. *Neisseria meningitidis*

2. Malaria

You are on elective in Uganda and spending the day on the paediatric ward. You are told that it is the rainy season and malaria is now becoming increasingly problematic. Almost all the children on the ward are suffering with the effects of malaria. The first child is a 5-year-old boy with a cyclical fever, abdominal pain and a 4 cm splenomegaly. He has 2 per cent parasitaemia on blood film. You are asked how you would treat this child. What is the best initial management step?

- A. IM quinine
- B. IV fluids and IV quinine
- C. IV fluids and prophylactic splenectomy
- D. Emergency splenectomy
- E. Oral atovaquone

3. Febrile child

A 3-year-old girl presents to accident and emergency with a 6-day history of fever and she is over 38°C when measured by her mother with a tympanic thermometer. She has become very miserable for the last few days. She has developed a rash on her trunk, which is blanching, erythematous and confluent. On examination, you also note bilateral non-purulent conjunctivitis, cervical lymphadenopathy, and a red tongue with lip cracking. Her extremities are also erythematous but not peeling. WCC 14×10⁹/L, C-reactive protein 200 mg/L, and erythrocyte sedimentation rate 60 mm/hour. Blood culture is pending. What is the diagnosis?

A. Staphylococcal scalded skin
B. Toxic shock syndrome
C. Scarlet fever
D. Kawasaki's disease
E. Measles

4. Periorbital cellulitis

A 3-year-old boy presents with a right swollen eyelid. He has had a cold for the last week but his eyelid started swelling yesterday. He has had no injury or broken skin around the eye. On examination, his right eye is swollen and red, there is no discharge, he is now unable to open his right eye and he has proptosis. You are concerned about the complications of this infection. Within the last hour he has become more drowsy and started to vomit. His observations are all normal. What is the concerning complication in this case?

A. Visual loss
B. Abscess
C. Septicaemia
D. Orbital cellulitis
E. Meningitis

5. Pyrexia of unknown origin

A 14-year-old girl presented to the GP with an enlarged lymph node in her neck. She first noticed it 3 weeks ago and it is increasing in size. She has also had a dry cough, fevers, night sweats and weight loss. She has had a poor appetite over the last 2 weeks, which her mother blames for her weight loss. There is no history of foreign travel or tuberculosis (TB) contacts. A chest x-ray shows a mediastinal mass. What is the most likely diagnosis?

A. Lymphoma
B. Pneumonia
C. TB
D. Lung tumour
E. Leukaemia

6. Petechial spots

A 6-year-old girl presents to accident and emergency with a fever. She has no history of cough, cold, vomiting, diarrhoea, rash, headache or joint pain. On examination, she is tachycardic at 150 bpm and there are two petechial spots on her right ankle. Her capillary refill time is 4 seconds and she has cold feet. All her other observations are normal. What is the most appropriate course of action?

A. Inform the consultant about child protection concerns
B. IV ceftriaxone
C. IV fluid bolus and IV ceftriaxone
D. Admit to the ward for observation
E. Discharge home and advise to return if the rash spreads

7. Limping child

A 3-year-old boy was brought to accident and emergency with his mother. She says he has been limping for a day now and refusing to walk for the last 2 hours. He has had a fever to 39°C which can be brought down with paracetamol. He has had no vomiting, diarrhoea, rash, cough, coryza or injury. He lives with his mother and is her only child. She is currently unemployed and has a background of depression. On examination of the right leg he has a swollen thigh and cries inconsolably when it is touched. It is red and tender. He refuses to allow movement of the hip either passive or active. The left leg is unremarkable on examination. What is the most likely diagnosis?

A. Perthes' disease
B. Septic arthritis
C. Fractured femur due to accidental injury
D. Juvenile idiopathic arthritis
E. Fractured femur due to non-accidental injury

8. Intrauterine infection

A pregnant woman attends her booking appointment at the antenatal clinic and has her routine blood tests done. She is now 13 weeks pregnant with her first child and you have a positive result for cytomegalovirus (CMV) IgM. You need to discuss the implications of CMV infection on her unborn child. Which of the following are not features of congenital CMV infection?

A. Deafness
B. Intrauterine growth retardation
C. Hydrocephalus
D. Thrombocytopenia
E. Congenital cardiac defects

9. Returned traveller

A 5-year-old girl was admitted to the ward after she presented to her local accident and emergency with diarrhoea. She was passing 7–8 loose, watery stools per day for the last 4 days and had been vomiting for 1 day prior to this. There was blood in the stools and this had worried her mother. You ask about foreign travel and her mother reveals they had been in India until 2 weeks ago, staying with family and drinking tap water. She had no vaccines prior to travelling. On examination, she now has abdominal pain, swinging pyrexias, right upper quadrant tenderness but no rebound or guarding. You notice a pale pink (rose) spot on her trunk. What is the most likely infecting organism?

A. Rotavirus
B. *Shigella* spp.
C. *Vibrio cholerae*
D. *Salmonella typhi*
E. *Escherichia coli* 0157

10. Febrile fits

A 10-month-old baby is brought to accident and emergency by ambulance having had a seizure. His mother reports that he went floppy suddenly and then his right arm and leg started shaking and he was not crying. It lasted less than 5 minutes and he was sleepy afterwards. He has had a fever and runny nose for the last 2 days and is off his food. Why is this not a febrile seizure?

A. He is too young
B. He has had a focal seizure
C. He has recently had a viral illness
D. The seizure lasted too long
E. The fever was not high enough

ANSWERS

Unusual cause of meningitis

1 A The insidious onset of this case must raise the possibility of tuberculous meningitis (A). Although (C) and (E) are the most common causes of meningitis in the UK, the LP result and insidious nature make them less likely. An LP in these causes of meningitis may show raised white cells, normal protein and a glucose less than two-thirds of the serum glucose. *Cryptococcus neoformans* (D) is more likely in immunosuppressed patients, for example with coexisting HIV infection, which is not noted in this case. HSV results in encephalitis, which clinically is difficult to distinguish from bacterial meningitis so should be treated until you have confirmation that HSV is not present in the cerebrospinal fluid, which can now be done by laboratory test HSV polymerase chain reaction.

Malaria

2 B This child has moderate parasitaemia. This child requires antimalarial treatment, IV in the first instance (B) and when he is improving this could be changed to oral (E). With splenomegaly secondary to acute haemolysis he should not have a splenectomy (C) or (D) unless there is evidence of a ruptured spleen; signs include hypovolaemic shock and peritonism. The first choice of antimalarial depends on the local resistance of the mosquitoes. This can be checked on national websites if the patient has just returned from travelling in endemic areas. It is also important to know what prophylaxis, if any, was taken and duration of the course.

Febrile child

3 D This girl has all the features of Kawasaki's disease (D). This is an inflammatory disease of unknown aetiology. It shares many features with all the other diagnoses listed, but may also have cardiac involvement in the form of coronary artery aneurysms. (A) causes a peeling of skin with a fever. (B) presents with a red macular rash, fever and usually an additional diarrhoeal illness. (C) presents with a sandpaper rash and erythematous mucous membranes. (E) is now an uncommon disease due to vaccination, though with reducing uptake of the MMR vaccine, cases are increasing, causing a febrile child with an erythematous, macular rash.

Periorbital cellulitis

4 E All of these can be complications of periorbital cellulitis. This child, with reduced conscious level and vomiting, would raise concern about meningitis (E) as the infection spreads to the cerebrospinal fluid around the optic nerve. All of these complications are worrying and require further investigation. Septicaemia (C) may also cause these symptoms if the child is in shock with poor perfusion of the brain. (A), (B) and (D) need to be excluded with CT head and ophthalmology review.

Pyrexia of unknown origin

5 A There is a history of prolonged fever, which must raise the possibility of diagnoses other than infectious causes. There are no TB contacts and the x-ray does not show a focal collection, hence (C) and (B) are unlikely. The presence of a rapidly enlarging lymph node should prompt investigation for infection and malignancy. Primary lung cancer is rare in children, hence (D) is unlikely. Both (A) and (E) can present with lymphadenopathy and should be excluded with a lymph node biopsy and blood film/bone marrow aspirate. However, with the history of dry cough caused by a mediastinal mass and 'B' symptoms of fevers and night sweats, this should point towards (A) as the most likely diagnosis.

Petechial spots

6 C This girl is tachycardic and therefore should be investigated to find the cause. With the petechial spots in the presence of a fever and clinical signs of shock, one must consider meningococcal sepsis and commence antibiotics immediately. Since she has features of early shock, namely tachycardia and prolonged capillary refill time, she therefore requires a fluid bolus so (C) is correct, not (B). Although bruising must always raise suspicion and appropriate measures taken, in this case an alternative diagnosis is more likely; therefore (A) is not applicable on this occasion. She should not be sent home (E) as she is tachycardic. She needs prompt treatment after assessment to avoid progression to septic shock and therefore (D) is not appropriate.

Limping child

7 B This child has a fever and a limp, with limited movement and signs of acute inflammation in his right lower limb. The most likely diagnosis is septic arthritis of the right hip (B). He is too young for (A) which is due to avascular necrosis of the femoral head which usually occurs in children over 5 years of age. There is no history of trauma and therefore this makes (C) unlikely. (E) must remain a consideration, in particular in view of the social background. This history does not fit the definition of juvenile idiopathic arthritis (D), which is 6 weeks of joint pain and swelling which persists after other diagnoses have been excluded.

Intrauterine infection

8 E   CMV is the most common congenital infection acquired in pregnancy. It
results in all the features in (A), (B), (C) and (D) after infection in the first
trimester, but not (E). Cardiac defects are associated with other congenital
infections such as rubella. Mothers are routinely screened for rubella,
hepatitis B, HIV and syphilis in early pregnancy to ascertain risk to the
fetus and treatment is given during pregnancy and may be required for
the baby after birth.

Returned traveller

9 D   Although the most common cause of infective gastroenteritis worldwide
is rotavirus, causing over 50 per cent of all cases, this case has some
unusual features, excluding (A). Cholera (C) presents with dysentery not
just diarrhoea. Blood in the stool (although possible with severe rotavirus)
is more commonly caused by bacteria. With the history of travel to India
and the added risk factors of staying in the local community, a more
tropical cause should be considered. The presence of rose spots indicates
this is (D), excluding (B) and (E), though stool microscopy and culture will
provide the definitive diagnosis with sensitivities for effective treatment.

Febrile fits

10 B   Febrile seizures are common in children aged 6 months to 6 years, hence
(A) is incorrect. The aetiology is unknown, but it is thought to occur
with the rapid rise in temperature at the start of an infective illness,
most commonly a viral illness in children, (C) is incorrect. There is no
recognized range of temperatures, though there must be a documented
fever, i.e. >37.5°C; therefore (E) is incorrect. A febrile convulsion by
definition must be a generalized seizure that occurs in association with
a fever, in a child with no neurological abnormality, hence (B) is the
correct answer. Focal seizures are not categorized as febrile fits and this
child requires imaging of the brain and to commence antibiotics (to cover
Streptococcus pneumoniae and Neisseria meningitidis) and antivirals (to
cover HSV) as this seizure may be secondary to meningoencephalitis.
Seizures are categorized into simple (<5 minutes, self-resolving) or
complex (prolonged >15 minutes, requiring medical treatment) but must
fulfil the other criteria above; therefore (D) is incorrect.

SECTION 15:
ALLERGY AND
IMMUNOLOGY

QUESTIONS

1. Anaphylaxis

A 4-year-old boy has been brought into accident and emergency with breathing problems. He is assessed by the paediatric team and found to have inspiratory and expiratory stridor, audible wheeze, lip and tongue swelling, and an urticarial rash on his trunk and abdomen. His heart rate is 167 bpm and his respiratory rate is 40, BP 90/45 mmHg. What is the single most important management step?

    A. Do not examine his throat as this may distress him
    B. Give a normal saline fluid bolus
    C. Give IV adrenaline 0.1 mg/kg of 1:10 000
    D. Give IM adrenaline 0.01 mg/kg of 1:1000
    E. Mobilize the paediatric anaesthetist as his airway is compromised

2. Drug reaction

A 12-year-old girl with a history of discitis in her lumbar spine was admitted following investigation at her tertiary centre. She was started on IV benzylpenicillin and clindamycin. She received 24 hours of medication and a rash appeared on her trunk and arms. There were discrete red lesions which outlined a central target lesion. They were non-blanching and itchy. What is the most likely diagnosis?

    A. Erythema migrans
    B. Erythema toxicum
    C. Erythema marginatum
    D. Erythema nodosum
    E. Erythema multiforme

3. Severe combined immunodeficiency (SCID)

A 3-year-old boy is admitted to the children's ward. He has been isolated in a cubicle as he is at risk of infections. He is awaiting a bone marrow transplant and has a brother with the same condition. His mother tells you they both have SCID. What are the likely immune function test results in SCID?

    A. Normal B cells, normal T cells, normal immunoglobulins
    B. Low B cells, low T cells, low immunoglobulins
    C. Normal B cells, normal T cells, high immunoglobulin M subsets
    D. Low B cells, normal T cells, low immunoglobulins
    E. Normal B cells, low T cells, normal immunoglobulins

4. Diarrhoea

A 3-week-old baby attends accident and emergency with bloody diarrhoea. Mum says he has been having diarrhoea for the past 2 days since she started using formula milk. He was previously breastfed and mum was not having any dairy products due to lactose intolerance. He also has eczema on his cheeks and a strong family history or asthma and eczema. Mum is concerned that he may be allergic to milk too. What is the most likely diagnosis?

    A. Lactose intolerance
    B. Gastroenteritis
    C. Cow's milk protein intolerance
    D. Fructose intolerance
    E. Galactosaemia

5. DiGeorge's syndrome

A 2-year-old child is brought to cardiology clinic due to a heart murmur heard by the GP after an examination when she was recently unwell. She was born at 40 weeks by normal vaginal delivery but was noted to have a cleft palate at birth. She was kept in hospital for establishment of feeding but during this time she had a seizure, noted later to be because her calcium was low. You hear a harsh, grade 3/6 pansystolic murmur, loudest at the left lower sternal edge, consistent with a ventral septal defect (VSD) as seen on echocardiogram. With this history and current examination finding, you wish to exclude DiGeorge's syndrome. What is the best diagnostic test?

    A. Karyotype
    B. FISH (fluorescence *in situ* hybridization)
    C. ELISA (enzyme-linked immunosorbent assay)
    D. Geneticist review and diagnosis
    E. Identification of specific mutation

6. Transfusion reaction

A 13-year-old girl is on the ward having a bone marrow transplant for acute leukaemia. She is noted to be profoundly anaemic with haemoglobin 5.9 g/dL and she is due to receive a transfusion of one unit of red blood cells. You are called to see her 5 minutes after starting the transfusion. She has come out in a rash, is looking frightened, with a heart rate of 120 bpm and respiratory rate of 30. As you arrive, you can see she has swollen lips and tongue and her blood pressure is measured as 90/45 mmHg. What is the best initial management step?

A. Repeat a full set of observations as it is likely to be anxiety resulting in the abnormal heart rate, respiratory rate and blood pressure. If still abnormal, stop transfusion
B. Stop the transfusion and return the unit of blood to blood bank
C. Stop the transfusion, take down the giving set, give IM adrenaline immediately
D. Give IM adrenaline, stop the transfusion, take down the giving set
E. Stop the transfusion, give IM adrenaline immediately and restart if the reaction settles

7. Recurrence risk

A couple are referred to a geneticist as they are planning on having their first child. There is a history of Wiskott–Aldrich syndrome on the woman's side. The woman's father and great grandfather have the condition (eczema, thrombocytopenia, recurrent infection) but she is unaffected. There is no history of the condition in the man's family. What is the risk of having the condition if the child is a boy or a girl respectively?

A. Boy: 1/4; Girl: 1/4
B. Boy: 1/2; Girl: 0
C. Boy: 0; Girl: 0
D. Boy: 0; Girl: 1/2
E. Boy: 1; Girl: 0

8. Superinfection

A 4-year-old boy with severe ezcema is brought to accident and emergency by his mother. His skin has been worse recently since the weather has become colder. He is scratching a lot more and now is very miserable and has a temperature of 38.6°C today. On examination of his skin he has multiple areas of erythematous, excoriated lesions on his elbow and knee flexures as well as his trunk and back. In addition they are hot, tender and slightly swollen with areas of broken skin. There are also some yellow fluid-filled vesicles on some of these lesions. You send some blood tests and commence him on IV flucloxacillin and aciclovir. Which are the two most likely organisms that can complicate eczema?

A. Gram-positive cocci and herpes simplex virus
B. Gram-negative cocci and herpes simplex virus
C. Gram-positive cocci and varicella zoster
D. Gram-negative bacilli and herpes zoster
E. Gram-positive bacilli and herpes simplex

9. Immunodeficiency

A 3-year-old boy has been admitted to hospital with a right-sided pneumonia and pleural effusion. The pleural fluid grew Gram-positive cocci. He is on IV ceftriaxone, oral azithromycin and has a chest drain *in situ*. On further questioning of Richard's mother, you establish that he has had multiple chest infections since he was born (in the UK). He has been admitted three times before and also had a sinus wash out following an episode of sinusitis. He has no cardiac anomalies or dysmorphism. His mother also tells you about his older brother, who sadly died of meningitis aged 6 years old. He too had 'more than his fair share of infections'. The two brothers had different fathers but his mother is HIV negative. What is the most likely underlying immunodeficiency in this family?

    A.   DiGeorge's syndrome
    B.   Complement deficiency
    C.   X-linked agammaglobulinaemia
    D.   Subacute combined immunodeficiency disorder (SCID)
    E.   HIV

10. Complement deficiency

You are in immunology clinic and the first patient is a 2-year-old boy who has a complement deficiency. You know this involves a cascade of proteins involved with innate immunity but are unsure about the manifestations in children. The professor of immunology asks you which organism is this child at risk of being infected with. He gives you a clue by telling you the child has a late complement deficiency, meaning C5-C9. What is the most likely causative organism that infects these children?

    A.   *Streptococcus pneumoniae*
    B.   *Neisseria meningitidis*
    C.   *Haemophilus influenzae*
    D.   *Mycobacterium tuberculosis*
    E.   *Pneumocystis jiroveci*

ANSWERS

Anaphylaxis

1 D   He has clear signs of anaphylaxis, with involvement of cardiovascular and respiratory systems. He is hypotensive and tachycardic and although a fluid bolus is required (B), adrenaline IM (D) is the most important initial step. Adrenaline is a catecholamine which in anaphylaxis should be given IM and not IV (C) (this is in contrast to a cardiac arrest protocol where it is given IV or through an endotracheal tube). IM adrenaline will cause vasoconstriction, bronchodilation and temporarily slow the anaphylactic process, which is histamine driven. A paediatric anaesthetist will also be required to assess and manage airway obstruction due to the enlarged tongue and upper airway soft tissues (E); however adrenaline must be given first to buy time for them to arrive. The effects of adrenaline are short lived and continued assessment is necessary. Once the reaction has settled there is a biphasic response, meaning the child may have a second reaction despite no contact with the allergen 6–12 hours later. Not examining the throat (A) refers to upper airway obstruction caused by epiglottitis or bacterial tracheitis and is not appropriate here.

Drug reaction

2 E   Erythema multiforme (E) is the rash described with target lesions with a surrounding red ring. The causes are numerous including: drugs (e.g. penicillin), infection (e.g. atypical pneumonia) or idiopathic. Erythema nodosum (D) can have similar categories of causes including drugs (e.g. sulphonamides), infection (e.g. streptococcal spp.), autoimmune and malignancy, but inflammatory bowel disease is also a well-known cause. Erythema migrans (A) is a rash due to Lyme's disease. Erythema toxicum (B) is a benign rash (characteristically seen as small pustules or vescicles surrounded by an erythematous area) seen in newborns in the first 2 weeks of life. Erythema marginatum (C) in seen in rheumatic fever along with the other cardinal signs which include carditis, arthralgia, subcutaneous nodules and Sydenham's chorea.

Severe combined immunodeficiency (SCID)

3 B   SCID is a group of disorders caused by B and T cell dysfunction. SCID affects both B and T lymphocyte cell lines; therefore only (B) can be correct. Low B cell numbers result in reduced immunoglobulin production. (A) would be the result in an immunocompetent host. (C) may be due to hyper IgM syndrome, which is due to a defect in the CD40 ligand, resulting in defective class switching and T cell function and recurrent infections. (D) may be suggestive of Bruton's agammaglobulinaemia, where lack of B cells results in low immunoglobulins and predisposition to respiratory and central nervous system (CNS) infections. (E) may result from thymic hypoplasia or absence as the T cells alone are affected with normal B cells and immunoglobulins; this may be associated with DiGeorge's syndrome.

Diarrhoea

4 C Cow's milk protein intolerance (C) is an allergic reaction secondary to allergens in cow's milk. Babies may present with diarrhoea on introduction of cow's milk based formula or breast milk if the mother takes dairy products. Cow's milk protein intolerance may also be associated with eczema, commonly on the face. Lactose intolerance (A) can present similarly, but the congenital form is extremely rare (due to absolute lactase deficiency at the brush border) though lactase expression starts to reduce from 2 years of age in most people. Fructose intolerance (D) is a rare metabolic condition presenting with vomiting, hypoglycaemia, failure to thrive, hepatomegaly, jaundice, renal complications and severe metabolic acidosis. Gastroenteritis (B) should be considered, but in the presence of vomiting and fever which are absent here. Galactosaemia (E) is due to galactose-1-phosphate uridyl transferase deficiency, which can present with metabolic disturbances, sepsis, vomiting and collapse.

DiGeorge's syndrome

5 B DiGeorge syndrome is due to a microdeletion on chromosome 22q11.2. It manifests as a collection of features including cleft palate, aortic arch and other cardiac abnormalities, thymic hypoplasia, typical facial features and hypocalcaemia. Microdeletions are best detected with FISH (B). Abnormalities in chromosome number or translocations can be seen with karyotyping (A) and known mutations can be identified (E), but since DiGeorge's syndrome is not due to a specific mutation this is not appropriate. ELISA (C) is used for the identification of known proteins, e.g. autoantibodies, bacterial/viral detection. A geneticist review (D) may be helpful, particularly for planning of further pregnancies.

Transfusion reaction

6 C There are clear transfusion guidelines which you should be familiar with – see Handbook of Transfusion Medicine from the UK Blood Transfusion Services. There are multiple transfusion reactions, but this is an allergic/anaphylactic reaction. The blood should be stopped and taken down first (removal of the allergen); therefore (A) and (D) are incorrect. The patient is in anaphylactic shock and therefore should be given IM adrenaline (C), not (B). This unit of blood should most certainly not be restarted (E) and should be returned to the blood bank for further analysis.

Recurrence risk

7 B   Wiskott–Aldrich syndrome is an X-linked condition due to defects in the *WASp* gene, affecting cell cytosketeton protein actin and associated with the above features. It presents with this triad in approximately one-third of cases, with the other having predominantly haematological complications such as petechiae and bruising. The woman's father has the condition and therefore she is a carrier. The risk of her having a son with the condition is 1/2 and a daughter is 0 (she can only be a carrier) (B). (A) is based on an autosomal recessive condition, with both parents as carriers, and (C) occurs if the mother is a carrier and the father is not affected. (E) is based on the condition being X-linked dominant, but then the mother should have been affected.

Superinfection

8 A   Cellulitis (bacterial superinfection) and eczema herpeticum (herpes simplex virus infection) are the two important complications of eczema. Gram-positive cocci (*Staphylococcus* spp. and *Streptococcus* spp.) are responsible for cellulitis. These occur due to breakage of the skin barrier in the eczematous areas allowing entry of bacterial into an already inflamed epidermis and dermis. These require aggressive treatment to prevent spread of the organisms into the blood. (B) is not correct as Gram-negative cocci (*Neisseria meningitidis* and *N.gonorrhoeae*) do not produce skin infections. Varicella zoster is the causative organism for chicken pox, and reactivation of the virus which lays dormant in the dorsal root ganglion is known as herpes zoster (shingles). They do not specifically cause infection of eczematous skin; therefore (C) and (D) are incorrect. (E) is incorrect as Gram-positive bacilli such as *Clostridium* spp., *Bacillus* spp. or *Listeria* spp. do not typically cause primary skin infections.

Immunodeficiency

9 C   This boy presents with recurrent respiratory tract infections and although these are common in childhood, the frequency, severity and causative organisms are important to consider. It is difficult to clearly differentiate immunodeficiencies, but it is a balance of probabilities as to the most likely cause. He is unlikely to have SCID (D) as this usually presents earlier in life and may have been fatal by 3 years of age if undiagnosed. Their mother is HIV negative which means vertical transmission of HIV is excluded and he is unlikely to have acquired HIV (E). He is lacking in other features which are suggestive of DiGeorge's syndrome (A) (cleft palate, midfacial hypoplasia, cardiac anomalies (including Tetralogy of Fallot), VSD) and hypocalcaemia. Complement deficiency (B) can present in a spectrum of phenotypic characteristics, but commonly in meningococcal infections. The fact that two brothers both have the propensity to infections should raise the suspicion of an X-linked condition (irrespective of the paternity of the brothers). The lack of B cells, and therefore immunoglobulins, predisposes to bacterial infection, particularly of the respiratory tract but also the CNS, making (C) the most likely.

Complement deficiency

10 B The complement pathway is important in detecting and eradicating these organisms early on and, without effective complement systems, overwhelming infection may develop. The complement cascade involves a series of proteins which can opsonize and create and insert a membrane attack complex into the organism, which aims to eradicate it. Deficiencies along the pathway have been noted: protein C3 resulting in recurrent pyogenic infection, protein C1, C2 and C4 associated with autoimmunity and proteins C5–9 with a risk of getting infections with *N. meningitidis* (B). Children with sickle cell disease (functional asplenia) or other children without a functioning spleen are at risk of infection with encapsulated organisms such as (A) or (C). Patients who are immunocompromised (secondary to HIV or immunosuppressive therapy, e.g. steroids or chemotherapy), are at risk of (D) or (E).

SECTION 16:
RESPIRATORY

QUESTIONS

1. Asthma

A 5-year-old boy was diagnosed with asthma aged 3 years. He presented to accident and emergency with shortness of breath, increased work of breathing and a 1-week history of coryzal illness and fever. On examination he is tachypnoeic 60/ min, tachycardia 160 bpm and has minimal air entry bilaterally. He has intercostal recession, tracheal tug and is too breathless to complete a sentence. Oxygen saturation is 90 per cent in air. What is the initial management of this boy?

    A. Immediate intubation and ventilation
    B. High flow oxygen through non-rebreather mask
    C. IV salbutamol and magnesium sulphate infusion
    D. Back to back salbutamol and Atrovent though oxygen driven nebuliser
    E. Trial of continuous positive airway pressure support

2. Chronic cough

A 3-year-old child presents to the GP with a chronic cough for the last month. He had previously been fit and well since he suffered a severe pertussis infection when he was 1 month of age. He has subsequently been fully immunized but was noted to be on the 0.4th centile for height. What is the most likely cause for his cough?

    A. Cystic fibrosis
    B. Recurrent pertussis infection
    C. Habit
    D. Asthma
    E. Bronchiectasis

3. Pneumonia

A 15-year-old boy attends his GP with a week of cough productive of yellow sputum, fever to 39°C and chest pain on the right side of the chest on coughing. There is no history of foreign travel or unwell contacts. On examination there is reduced air entry in the right lower zone with crepitations and bronchial breathing. You diagnose a right-sided chest infection. What is the most likely causative organism?

    A. *Staphylococcus aureus*
    B. *Mycobacterium tuberculosis*
    C. *Streptococcus pneumoniae*
    D. *Mycoplasma pneumoniae*
    E. *Chlamydophila pneumoniae (Chlamydia pneumoniae)*

4. Primary ciliary dyskinesia

A 4-year-old girl has recently moved to the area and is registering with you, her new GP. She has had a diagnosis of primary ciliary dyskinesia (PCD) made last week and the parents wish to know more about the complications. Which of the following is not a complication of PCD?

    A. Pancreatic insufficiency
    B. Infertility
    C. Sinusitis
    D. Bronchiectasis
    E. Dextrocardia

5. Breathing difficulties in a neonate

A 26 week, premature baby was born by emergency caesarean section due to maternal pre-eclampsia. He required ventilation until age 38 weeks corrected gestation and is still requiring oxygen to maintain his saturations. At 12 months of age he has poor vision and neurodevelopmental function, requires home oxygen and was admitted for a recent respiratory syncytial virus (RSV) bronchiolitis. What is the underlying diagnosis of his respiratory problems?

    A. Respiratory distress syndrome (hyaline membrane disease)
    B. Chronic lung disease (bronchopulmonary dysplasia)
    C. Cystic fibrosis
    D. Diaphragmatic hernia
    E. Pulmonary hypoplasia

6. Foreign body inhalation

John is a 2-year-old boy whose mother has been concerned about a cough for the last 2 weeks which started out of the blue. He has been previously fit and well with no respiratory or cardiac problems from birth. There is no family history of illness. He is thriving and eating as normal, but has a persistent cough, recently productive of yellow and slight blood stained sputum. You suspect that John may have a pneumonia and lung collapse secondary to an inhaled foreign body. Which is the most likely location of this boy's foreign body?

    A. Left lower lobe
    B. Right upper lobe
    C. Right middle lobe
    D. Left upper lobe
    E. Right lower lobe

7. Cystic fibrosis

A couple who are known to both be carriers of cystic fibrosis ask to see you. They had genetic counselling but declined antenatal diagnostic testing and their baby has now been born and is ready to be discharged home. The parents are now keen to get the baby tested so that if treatment is required it can be initiated early on. What initial test do you suggest for the baby?

- A. Newborn blood spot screening
- B. Chest x-ray
- C. Faecal elastase
- D. Genetic testing
- E. Sweat test

8. Bronchiolitis

A 5-week-old baby was admitted today to the children's ward with bronchiolitis. The nasopharyngeal aspirate identified respiratory syncitial virus. He was saturating to 96 per cent in air this morning and was feeding two-thirds of his usual amount of formula milk. You are asked to review him as his work of breathing is worsening now it is night time. He has nasal flaring, intercostal and subcostal recession, tachypnoea and crepitations and wheeze heard bilaterally. What do you expect his capillary blood gas to show?

- A. pH 7.16 PCO_2 kPa 3.1 PO_2 10.0 kPa   BE −8 HCO_3^- 18 mmol/L
- B. pH 7.38 PCO_2 kPa 5.5 PO_2 12.0 kPa   BE +1 HCO_3^- 25 mmol/L
- C. pH 7.20 PCO_2 kPa 8.2 PO_2 8.3 kPa   BE +2 HCO_3^- 26 mmol/L
- D. pH 7.40 PCO_2 kPa 1.2 PO_2 7.5 kPa   BE +5 HCO_3^- 28 mmol/L
- E. pH 7.47 PCO_2 kPa 6.3 PO_2 11.0 kPa   BE +10 HCO_3^- 35 mmol/L

9. Muscular dystrophy

Clara is a 14-year-old girl who was diagnosed with muscular dystrophy when she was younger. She now mobilizes in a wheelchair and other co-morbidities include a scoliosis and cardiomyopathy. She is being seen for her annual review in clinic. Which of these would best represent the respiratory complications of muscular dystrophy?

- A. Normal FVC, low FEV1/FVC ratio
- B. Flattened diaphragms on chest x-ray
- C. Morning dips in peak expiratory flow rate
- D. Extrathoracic obstruction on flow-volume loops
- E. Reduced FVC, normal FEV1/FVC ratio

10. Rib fractures

A 10-month-old baby boy is brought to accident and emergency with inconsolable crying. His mother says he is a miserable baby and even after feeding he does not settle. He has recently started to cruise around furniture, but is not yet walking. His crying has been worse today and both his parents had been awake all night due to his incessant crying. On examining the baby, you note that he is more upset when being handled and is a bit better when lying on his front. You do a chest x-ray which shows three posterior rib fractures; his mother states he fell down some steps yesterday. What is the likely diagnosis and appropriate management strategy?

A. Birth trauma; no intervention necessary as they will heal spontaneously

B. Accidental injury; ensure no pneumothorax present, reassure and discharge home

C. Accidental injury; ensure no pneumothorax present and admit for observation

D. Non-accidental injury (NAI); advise the parents you will refer to social services and discharge home

E. NAI; discuss with social services and paediatric consultant and admit the child to a place of safety

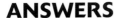

ANSWERS

Asthma

1 D Asthma management follows the British Thoracic Society guidelines which have a step-wise approach to the management of both chronic and acute asthma. According to his symptoms he has life-threatening asthma, but initial management still requires the use of back to back salbutamol nebulizers (D). He is hypoxic in room air, so giving oxygen driven nebulizers will be of benefit compared to inhalers or oxygen alone (B). If after three doses of salbutamol and one of Atrovent nebulizer he is not improving, he may require IV salbutamol or aminophylline and magnesium sulphate, but not first line (C). Although he does require high flow oxygen, this alone will not help the underlying problem. If he is not responding to intravenous therapy then intubation and ventilation will be required with intensive care support (A). Continuous positive airway pressure (E) is not used in the management of asthma, as it does not provide ventilatory support.

Chronic cough

2 E A severe respiratory infection in early childhood can present later in life with bronchiectasis (E) caused by dilatation and poor mucociliary clearance, predisposing to further infection. Any chronic illness may impact on the growth and development of a child. Other important causes of chronic cough include (D) asthma (though usually associated with nocturnal cough, atopy and eczema) and (A) cystic fibrosis (can present with respiratory and gastrointestinal involvement due to pancreatic insufficiency), and a thorough history is needed, but bronchiectasis (E) is still more likely given the history. Once the initial pertussis infection is treated it is unlikely that he will have further infections (B), and having been immunized this provides some protection, though immunity does wane with time and infected adults are likely the carriers of this disease. Coughs may become habitual (C) but his must be a diagnosis of exclusion.

Pneumonia

3 D The causative organisms of pneumonia can be categorized into typical (*Streptococcus pneumoniae, Staphylococcus aureus, Haemophilus influenzae, Moraxella catarrhalis*) or atypical (*Mycoplasma pneumoniae, Legionella* spp., *Chlamydia* spp.). *Streptococcus pneumoniae* (C) is the most common typical cause and would be more likely in under 4 year olds. *Mycoplasma pneumoniae* (B) is more common in older children presenting with pneumonia. The presentation of a lobar pneumonia and a short history is not consistent with tuberculosis (B) which may present with systemic features of weight loss, loss of appetite and a more indolent course. *Staphylococcus aureus* (A) and *Chlamydia pneumonia* (E) are possible but are less likely causes epidemiologically.

Primary ciliary dyskinesia

4 A   (A) Pancreatic secretions are not reliant on cilia for the expulsion of enzymes and pancreatic fluids. They travel along the pancreatic duct and are joined by biliary secretions in the ampulla of Vater. The respiratory tract (C) and (D) and reproductive organs (B) are both lined by cilia to ensure the movement of particles. Cilia are also necessary for the determination of the sites of the internal organs during development. These children can have dextrocardia alone or situs inversus (E).

Breathing difficulties in a neonate

5 B   Chronic lung disease is by definition an oxygen requirement at 36 weeks corrected gestation or at 28 days post-term (B). It occurs in premature babies as a consequence of barotraumas or volutrauma during the ventilation, surfactant deficiency and oxygen therapy, though the pathophysiology is complex. It can be minimized by using the lowest possible pressure and volume settings to optimize respiratory function in premature infants, but despite this there can be long-term consequences. These children are at risk of respiratory tract infections, particularly RSV for which the preventative paluvizumab monocloncal antibody can be given. (A) Respiratory distress syndrome is due to surfactant deficiency and may be present soon after birth; however, if the clinical manifestations persist, these children may also develop chronic lung disease. (C) Cystic fibrosis does not present in this way, and is more likely to cause meconium ileus or prolonged jaundice in the neonatal period. (D) Diaphragmatic hernia and renal abnormalities can both result in pulmonary hypoplasia (E) and then respiratory difficulties at birth.

Foreign body inhalation

6 C   The right middle lobe is the terminal one of the three branches of the right main bronchus (the other being the right upper lobe and right lower lobe). The right main bronchus is the widest, shortest and most vertical of the bronchi and hence the most likely for a foreign body descent (path of least resistance). The right middle lobe is the most direct anatomically likely location for the foreign body; therefore (A), (B), (D) and (E) are incorrect.

Cystic fibrosis

7 A   Newborn blood spot screening (NBSS) is a national screening programme to target early diagnostic testing for cystic fibrosis, hypothyroidism, phenylketonuria (and sickle cell disease and medium chain acyl dehydrogenase deficiency in some areas). The NBSS (A) is a blood spot sample and for cystic fibrosis tests for immune reactive trypsin; if positive, the sample will be sent for further genetic analysis to try to identify the gene mutation (D). The child will then require a sweat test, the gold standard test, to confirm the diagnosis (E). A chest x-ray in the newborn will not be useful (B). Faecal elastase (C) is useful to detect pancreatic insufficiency secondary to cystic fibrosis, but not all children will have pancreatic involvement so is not a diagnostic test.

Bronchiolitis

8 C He has increased work of breathing causing him to tire. He has an infective process in his lungs resulting in inflammation and an inability to oxygenate effectively. Therefore he will develop type 2 respiratory failure as seen in (C) with hypoxia and hypercapnia producing respiratory acidosis. The blood gas in (D) may represent his situation before he becomes exhausted, with hyperventilation resulting in low PCO_2 and hypoxia, but with metabolic compensation. (A) is a metabolic acidosis which may be secondary to sepsis. (B) is a normal blood gas. (E) is a metabolic alkalosis.

Muscular dystrophy

9 E Muscular dystrophy causes a restrictive pattern of respiratory disease (E). This may be due to weak intercostals and diaphragmatic muscles and scoliosis, resulting in a reduced capacity for lung and chest wall expansion. Spirometry can be used in a clinic setting to assess lung function. (A) is an obstructive pattern as may be seen with asthma, and morning dips (C) are characteristic of asthma. Flattening of the diaphragms is typical of hyperinflation and air trapping, for example bronchiolitis (B). There is no indication from the history of an extrathoracic obstruction (D), for example chest pain, cough, or lymphadenopathy.

Rib fractures

10 E Posterior rib fractures are highly suspicious of NAI, hence (B) and (C) are less likely to be correct. This child is 10 months old and the injuries he has sustained are not consistent with his development or proposed mechanism. The baby may be inconsolable, particularly after feeding, if he has symptoms of gastro-oesophageal reflux. It may be inferred that the parents in their fatigue and frustration may be responsible for the injuries. If you suspect NAI, then a detailed history and examination are needed, discussion with a senior paediatrician and social services to fully investigate the situation to safeguard the child (E) while (D) is not a safe protocol to follow. Birth should not result in rib fractures (A), though clavicular fractures can be seen after shoulder dystocia or forceps deliveries.

SECTION 17: CARDIOVASCULAR

QUESTIONS

1. Congenital heart disease (1)

What is the most common congenital heart defect?

- A. Coarctation of the aorta
- B. Ventricular septal defect (VSD)
- C. Atrial septal defect
- D. Patent ductus arteriosus
- E. Transposition of the great arteries

2. Congenital heart disease (2)

Which of the following is not a presenting symptom or sign associated with congenital heart disease?

- A. Respiratory distress with feeds
- B. Cyanosis
- C. Hepatosplenomegaly
- D. Vomiting with feeds
- E. Sweating with feeds

3. Innocent murmurs

Which of the following is not a feature of an innocent murmur?

- A. Systolic murmur
- B. Diastolic murmur
- C. Asymptomatic
- D. Heard only at the left sternal edge
- E. No heaves or thrills

4. Croup in child with murmur

You are asked to see a 2-year-old child with difficulty in breathing, a runny nose and a barking cough. His mother tells you he had a heart defect repaired as a baby and he still has a murmur. On examination he has noisy breathing with mild subcostal recession. He is apyrexial with a respiratory rate of 44 breaths per minute and heart rate of 152 beats per minute; capillary refill is 1–2 seconds. His throat is red and the tonsils are enlarged with no exudate. On his chest you see a midline sternotomy scar with a drain scar and a right thoracotomy scar. On auscultation the lung fields are clear, but he has an ejection systolic murmur in the left upper sternal edge which radiates to the back. He does not have a gallop rhythm. There are transmitted upper airway sounds only on the lung fields and the abdomen is soft with no organomegaly. What is the most appropriate management?

    A.   Admit for IV antibiotics
    B.   Give IV furosemide and admit
    C.   Admit for observation
    D.   Send home on oral antibiotics
    E.   Give oral dexamethasone and observe

5. Diagnosis of congenital heart disease

A 3-day-old baby is brought to accident and emergency with acute respiratory distress. She is tachypnoeic, tachycardic, cyanosed and her capillary refill is 5 seconds centrally. You note she has a flat nasal bridge, down sloping palpebral fissures and epicanthic folds. On auscultation there is a loud ejection systolic murmur at the left sternal edge. What is the most likely diagnosis?

    A.   Coartation of the aorta
    B.   VSD
    C.   Transposition of the great arteries
    D.   Tetralogy of Fallot
    E.   Patent ductus arteriosus

6. Duct-dependent congenital heart disease

You are doing a baby check on the post-natal ward on a baby who is 23 hours old. His mother tells you that he is not feeding well. On examination he is unsettled with a respiratory rate of 76 and a heart rate of 182. You think his hands and feet look blue and there is a soft systolic murmur heard at the left upper sternal border. You ask the midwives to check his saturations which are 85 per cent in air and start some oxygen. You explain to the mother that he needs to be managed on the neonatal unit. What is the next step in your management?

    A.   Stop the oxygen as this may drive the closure of the ductus arterioles
    B.   Give prostaglandin intravenously to open the duct while organizing an echocardiogram
    C.   Give antibiotics and prostaglandin intravenously while organizing an echocardiogram
    D.   Give indomethacin intravenously to open the duct while organizing an echocardiogram
    E.   Give indomethacin and antibiotics intravenously while organizing an echocardiogram

7. Rhythm disorders (1)

A 7 year old with a 3-day history of upper respiratory tract infection is brought to accident and emergency by his mother because he suddenly went pale and sweaty and seems to be working hard to breath. The triage nurse calls you to see him urgently because his heart rate is 200 beats per minute. You take him round to the resuscitation area, give him oxygen and connect him to the cardiac monitor. The electrocardiogram (ECG) shows a narrow complex tachycardia with a rate of 180 beats per minute. He remains alert, with a respiratory rate of 40. What is the most appropriate initial diagnosis?

    A.   Supraventricular tachycardia (SVT)
    B.   Wolff–Parkinson–White syndrome
    C.   Ventricular fibrillation
    D.   Atrial fibrillation
    E.   Ventricular tachycardia

8. Rhythm disorders (2)

What is the first step in management?

    A.   Non-synchronized shock
    B.   Adenosine
    C.   Adrenaline
    D.   Vagal manoeuvres
    E.   Synchronized shock

9. Prolonged fever with tachycardia

A 2-year-old child is referred to hospital by the GP after his third visit that week; he now has a rash and the GP is worried he has meningitis. He has had a fever for 5 days up to 39.5°C or above every day and is not eating or drinking well. On examination, he has a temperature of 38.5°C, heart rate of 150, respiratory rate of 30 and is miserable. He has a blanching macular rash on his torso, swollen hands and feet, red eyes, red cracked lips, large tonsils with no pus, and a left-sided 2 cm × 3 cm cervical lymph node which is mobile. There is no photophobia or neck stiffness. His chest is clear with normal heart sounds and his abdomen is soft with a palpable liver edge. You note his BCG scar is inflamed. What is the most likely diagnosis?

    A.   Viral tonsillitis
    B.   Bacterial tonsillitis
    C.   Meningitis
    D.   Hand, foot and mouth disease
    E.   Kawasaki's disease

10. Heart disease in a foreign national

A 14-year-old refugee from Afghanistan who has lived in the UK for 2 years comes to see you complaining of increasing fatigue and breathlessness on exertion. On examination she appears cyanosed and has bilateral basal fine crepitations and a soft pansystolic murmur with a displaced apex beat. She has never been in hospital and has no surgical scars. You urgently refer her for a cardiology review. What is the most likely diagnosis?

    A. Bacterial endocarditis
    B. Tetralogy of Fallot
    C. VSD producing a left-to-right shunt
    D. Eisenmenger's syndrome
    E. Ebstein's anomaly

11. Rheumatic fever

The major criteria for rheumatic fever include all of the following features except?

    A. A new murmur
    B. Swollen right knee for the past 8 days
    C. A geographic shaped rash with central pallor on the abdomen
    D. Involuntary movements of the arms
    E. Fever

12. Hypertension

A 5-year-old child was admitted overnight awaiting surgical repair of a broken right ankle and was noted to have a raised blood pressure consistently above 130/90 mmHg despite adequate analgesia. On examination he has a plaster on his right foot and appears comfortable at rest. On auscultation there is a soft systolic murmur heard at the right upper sternal edge. His femoral pulse is difficult to find, but present bilaterally. When felt with the radial pulse, the impulse in the femoral pulse occurs slightly later. His abdomen is soft and there are no bruits heard. The blood pressure done in the right arm is 136/92 mmHg but the left arm gives a reading of 124/80. What is the most likely diagnosis?

    A. Normal blood pressure in the left arm with a spurious result from the right
    B. Coarctation of the aorta
    C. Renal artery stenosis
    D. Phaeochromocytoma
    E. White coat hypertension

13. Signs of cardiovascular insufficiency/heart failure

Which of the following is not a feature of cardiac insufficiency?

    A. Scattered wheeze on auscultation of the chest
    B. Central cyanosis
    C. Sacral oedema
    D. Tachypnoea with the apex beat palpable in the 7th intercostal space just lateral to the mid-clavicular line
    E. Hepatomegaly

14. Down's syndrome

Forty per cent of children with trisomy 21 have congenital heart defects. Which of the following is not associated with Down's syndrome?

    A. Tetralogy of Fallot
    B. Atrioseptal defect (ASD)
    C. VSD
    D. Atrioventricular septal defect (AVSD)
    E. Transposition of the great arteries

15. Syncope

A 14-year-old girl was seen in accident and emergency following her third collapse this year and referred to cardiology for review of a low rumbling murmur heard at the left upper sternal edge. Her ECG in accident and emergency was normal. Her blood sugar was 5.3 mmol/L. Urea and electrolytes were normal. The most recent collapse occurred at school while waiting for exam results to be given out. Previously they occurred while watching a parade all afternoon standing in a crowded street, and at a party. On all three occasions she felt dizzy beforehand, was unconscious for less than 10 seconds and fully alert following the episode, but did feel nauseous. Her echocardiogram today is normal. What is the most likely diagnosis?

    A. Venous hum murmur and vasovagal syncope
    B. Innocent murmur and epilepsy
    C. Wolff–Parkinson–White syndrome
    D. Patent foramen ovale and sick sinus syndrome
    E. Neurocardiogenic syndrome

ANSWERS

Congenital heart disease (1)

1 B One-third of all congenital heart defects are VSDs (B). All others are much less common. The second most commonly seen is the patent ductus arteriosis (D) which makes up just over 10 per cent. Atrial septal defects (C), coarctation of the aorta (A) and transposition of the great arteries (E) each make up approximately 5 per cent.

Congenital heart disease (2)

2 D Congenital heart disease may be diagnosed antenatally on the anomaly ultrasound or at the baby check if a murmur is heard. However, if the signs are not present or seen at these time points, it is important to know the possible symptoms and signs that may evolve over the next few weeks or months that might be associated with congenital heart disease. Classically, children become breathless (A) and sweaty (E) with feeds. The effort of feeding burns calories and tires the child so that growth becomes restricted and the child may fail to thrive. Infants with heart failure may develop hepatomegaly and potentially splenomegaly, as a result of back-pressure secondary to right-sided heart failure (C). This sign is more helpful than looking for jugular venous distension in an infant, since the neck is short and the jugular veins are difficult to observe. Any cardiac defect with a right-to-left shunt may present with cyanosis (B). It would be unusual for congenital heart disease to be associated with vomiting (D) unless there were other illnesses such as gastro-oesophageal reflux or pyloric stenosis as well.

Innocent murmurs

3 B Characteristics of an innocent murmur include: a soft blowing systolic murmur (A), localized to the left sternal edge (D), with no radiation, and no diastolic component (B) or parasternal thrill (E) and normal heart sounds in an asymptomatic patient (C).

Croup in child with murmur

4 E This child has had corrective cardiac surgery and has a residual murmur of pulmonary stenosis. The most likely explanation for this acute presentation is croup, which should be treated with dexamethasone as for any other child. His breathing and observations should have improved before he goes home (E). This child does not have a fever and there is no pus on the tonsils to suggest a bacterial infection. Croup is largely due to viral upper respiratory infections, and dexamethasone should be all that is required. He does not need antibiotics ((A) and (D)). Admission for observation (C) would not be unreasonable as a tachycardic child should not be sent home without careful evaluation, but it is not the best answer because you should treat his respiratory distress due to the croup with dexamethasone (E) and admit if no improvement. He is not in heart failure (no gallop rhythm, no crackles in his lung fields, and no hepatomegaly) and he therefore does not need furosemide (B).

Diagnosis of congenital heart disease

5 D This is a presentation of a duct-dependent type of congenital heart defect. The ductus arteriosus is a short vessel connecting the pulmonary artery to the aortic arch. It allows most of the blood from the right ventricle to bypass the fetal lungs which are filled with fluid. Within hours or at the most a few days following birth, the duct closes to form the ligamentum arteriosum. However, any congenital heart defect that results in decreased blood flow from the heart to the lungs, or decreased oxygenated blood on reaching the systemic circulation, will depend on blood flowing through the ductus arteriosus to compensate for the abnormal anatomy. When the duct closes, that circulation stops and infants with Tetralogy of Fallot (D), pulmonary atresia, tricuspid atresia, transposition of the great arteries (C) and total anomalous pulmonary venous drainage will go blue. These duct-dependent lesions require urgent re-opening of the duct with prostaglandin. This situation is the opposite of a patent ductus arteriosus (E). The other information you are given describes dysmorphic features of Down's syndrome (trisomy 21). Down's syndrome is associated with atrioventricular septal defects, VSDs and Tetralogy of Fallot (D). Coarctation of the aorta (A) does not produce central cyanosis, although the left arm and lower limbs may have reduced blood pressure and saturations depending on the severity of the stenosis. VSDs (B) produce a left-to-right shunt (thus the infant is not cyanosed) unless they are left untreated, when Eisenmenger's syndrome develops, typically in the teenage years where pulmonary hypertension results in a right-to-left shunt and cyanosis. This process develops slowly and does not present in infancy.

Duct-dependent congenital heart disease

6 C The correct answer is to cover the baby for sepsis with antibiotics and to maintain the patency of the ductus arteriosus while organizing an echocardiogram to elucidate the underlying cardiac anatomy (C). A blue baby with a murmur should be treated as a duct-dependent anomaly until proven otherwise. A septic baby could be mottled and present with a flow murmur and until the echocardiogram has been performed it is difficult to rule out sepsis; thus not covering with antibiotics would be wrong (B). You should always administer oxygen to a cyanotic child (A) unless specifically told not to by the cardiology team, and in this situation there would be clear guidelines to maintain the saturations between an upper and lower limit, typically in the 80s. Indomethacin is wrong ((D) and (E)); this is used to close the duct in children who have a persistent ductus arteriosus resulting in significant respiratory distress or impaired systemic oxygen delivery.

Rhythm disorders (1)

7 A The ECG shows a narrow complex tachycardia with a rate of 180 beats per minute. At this rate it is hard to say if P waves are present or not; however this history of a child with an intercurrent illness suddenly becoming unwell with a tachycardia is suggestive of an SVT (A). SVTs may be triggered by Wolff–Parkinson–White syndrome (B), a re-entry tachycardia due to an accessory pathway between the atria and the ventricle. Once the rhythm has slowed down there will be a delta wave visible in all QRS complexes, which is a slanting upstroke of the R wave, and this is associated with a short PR interval. All that can be said of this child is that the QRS complexes are narrow and fast, suggesting a supraventricular origin. Ventricular fibrillation (C) would be characterized by a fast wide irregular complex on ECG, with no discernible P waves. Ventricular tachycardia (E) will be characterized by a regular wide complex tachycardia with no visible P waves. Atrial fibrillation (D) would have the classical saw toothed baseline of P waves with a slower rate of QRS complexes superimposed.

Rhythm disorders (2)

8 D The first step in management for a child who is still alert would be vagal manoeuvres (D) such as asking a child to blow a syringe like a balloon, unilateral carotid massage or putting the head in ice. Ideally, these should be carried out while the child is on recorded cardiac monitoring to assess the response. If these do not work, adenosine (B) would be the next step. Failing these actions, sedated synchronized cardioversion (E) is indicated while the patient remains alert. If a patient becomes cardiovascularly compromised, for example is losing consciousness, then the synchronized cardioversion should be carried out urgently without waiting for sedation. Adrenaline (C) would not be used unless the patient loses output. Non-synchronized cardioversion (A) is only indicated for ventricular fibrillation (VF) or ventricular tachycardia with no cardiac output; this is because in all other situations if the shock lands on the QRS complex it may cause VF.

Prolonged fever with tachycardia

9 E The most likely diagnosis is Kawasaki's disease (E) as he fulfils the diagnostic criteria (5 out of 6): 1) fever for more than 5 days, 2) bilateral non-purulent conjunctivitis, 3) rash, 4) oral changes such as dry, cracked, red lips, strawberry tongue, 5) erythema and oedema of the hands or feet and 6) cervical lymphadenopathy. Inflammation at the BCG scar is common but is not a diagnostic criterion. Kawasaki's disease is a vasculitis of unknown aetiology that typically affects young children and is complicated by coronary aneurysm formation. Treatment is with intravenous immunoglobulin and high dose aspirin. By 5 days the fever caused by a viral tonsillitis (A) should be settling, even though other symptoms such as cough may persist for some time. This child could have a bacterial tonsillitis (B) and covering with antibiotics would be prudent, but it would be unusual to have conjunctivitis and swollen hands and feet with bacterial tonsillitis. You might expect to see pus on the tonsils if it is due to a bacterial infection. Hand, foot and mouth disease (D) produces a mild coryzal illness, mouth ulcers and painful papules on the hands and feet in young children and is caused by a coxsackie virus infection. He has no signs of meningism – neck stiffness or photophobia and his rash is blanching – making meningitis (C) or meningococcal septicaemia less likely.

Heart disease in a foreign national

10 D This child grew up in an area without resources for congenital cardiac corrective surgery. She likely has a large VSD which has led to left ventricular hypertrophy and failure, to the extent that she now has pulmonary hypertension and a right-to-left shunt resulting in cyanosis, i.e. Eisenmenger's syndrome (D). There are no infective features to suggest bacterial endocarditis (A). Without surgical correction, a child with Tetralogy of Fallot (B) would not survive to their teens. Young children with a VSD have a left-to-right shunt (C) with blood flowing from the high pressure left ventricle to the right ventricle and this does not produce cyanosis. Ebstein's anomaly (E) is another congenital heart defect that would not survive without surgery and is a combination of an abnormal tricuspid valve, hypoplastic right ventricle and pulmonary stenosis.

Rheumatic fever

11 E Rheumatic fever is one of the post-infectious complications of group A streptococcal infection and classically occurs after an episode of tonsillitis. Diagnosis is made on the presence of two major, or one major with two minor, criteria, plus evidence of streptococcal infection such as a throat swab or positive antistreptolysin titre. Major criteria include: pancarditis such as endocarditis – murmur (A) or valvular dysfunction, myocarditits – heart failure, pericarditis – rub, effusion or tamponade; polyarthritis common in the knees (B), wrists, and ankles and may flit from joint to joint, lasting for more than 1 week in total (to distinguish this from reactive arthritis); Sydenham's chorea results in involuntary movements (D) starting 2–6 months after the infection; erythema marginatum (C) is an early feature which is a flat erythematous rash on the trunk or limbs that expands with a topographical map-like border and fades from the centre; subcutaneous nodules are painless pea sized nodules on the extensor surfaces. Minor criteria include fever (E); arthralgia; family or personal history of rheumatic fever; raised inflammatory markers; and ECG changes such as a prolonged PR interval.

Hypertension

12 B This child is hypertensive in both arms but there is a discrepancy between the right and left arm with a radio-femoral delay and a systolic murmur heard in the aortic area, supporting a diagnosis of coarctation of the aorta (B). This is likely to be a mild stenosis which is why it was not picked up earlier. The restricted blood flow to the abdomen and kidneys results in feedback loops producing hypertension to maintain perfusion. The blood pressure in the left arm is still high (A) but it is lower than the right arm because of the coarctation restricting blood flow to the left and lower body. There is no bruit heard on examining the abdomen and other findings point to coarctation, making renal artery stenosis (C) unlikely, but to rule it out an abdominal ultrasound with Doppler would be required. Phaeochromocytoma (D) is a rare cause of hypertension caused by an adrenal tumour producing catecholamines and imaging would be required to diagnose this; therefore it is extremely unlikely to be the correct answer. White coat hypertension (E) is raised blood pressure associated with anxiety, induced by the presence of medical professionals. There is an underlying reason found on examination for his hypertension; therefore (E) is not the correct answer.

Signs of cardiovascular insufficiency/heart failure

13 B All of these may be present in cardiovascular disease. However, while cyanosis (B) may either be due to lung pathology or a right-to-left cardiac shunt, it is not, in itself, a sign of heart failure. Both wheeze (A) or bi-basal crackles are features of heart failure due to pulmonary oedema. Dependent oedema (C) is a feature of heart failure and in an infant who mostly is lying down this will collect on the back as well as the feet. Tachypnoea and a displaced apex beat suggestive of left ventricular hypertrophy are suggestive of cardiac failure (D). Hepatomegaly (E) occurs in heart failure due to back pressure in the venous system resulting in congestion in the portal vein.

Down' syndrome

14 E Forty per cent of cardiac defects in children with Down's syndrome are AVSDs (D). Thirty per cent have a VSD (C), 10 per cent an ASD (B) and 6 per cent have Tetralogy of Fallot (A). While transposition of the great arteries (E) is often associated with ASDs or VSDs, it is not classically associated with trisomy 21 and is therefore the correct answer.

Syncope

15 A A low rumbling murmur heard above the nipple line with a normal echocardiogram is a venous hum and a normal finding in children. In light of all her cardiovascular investigations being normal, the most likely diagnosis is vasovagal syncope (A), associated with prolonged standing or anxiety. You have not been given an electroencephalography report and there is no suggestion that she was convulsing or post-ictal following her collapses, making epilepsy unlikely (B). Wolff–Parkinson–White (C) syndrome would have delta waves on the ECG, whereas her ECG is normal. A patent foramen ovale would be seen on echocardiogram and sick sinus syndrome would show bradycardia on the ECG (D). Neurocardiogenic syndrome (E) could be diagnosed on a tilt table test, which has not been mentioned, and would not typically have prodromal symptoms.

SECTION 18:
NEPHROLOGY

QUESTIONS

1. The febrile child

A 1-month-old baby attends accident and emergency with a 2-day history of fever to 38.8°C measured at the GP surgery. He has been vomiting, with no diarrhoea, rash, cough or coryza. A clean catch urine has leukocytes +++ and ketones, no nitrites, blood or protein. An urgent microscopy shows >200 cells/µL white cells. What is the most appropriate course of action?

    A. Discharge home with 3 days of trimethoprim
    B. Admit for a course of IV antibiotics to cover a urinary tract infection (UTI)
    C. Admit for a lumbar puncture, blood cultures and chest x-ray, IV antibiotics
    D. Organize an urgent DMSA scan
    E. Discharge home with reassurance and advice to return if fever persists

2. Generalized oedema

A 5-year-old boy presents to his GP with a 3-day history of puffy eyes. He has been unwell with a coryzal illness for the last week. His mother states he has had no new medications and no hayfever, allergies or asthma. On further examination he has generalized oedema and scrotal oedema. He is tachycardiac and has cool peripheries, no skin rashes or erythema. What is the most likely diagnosis?

    A. Periorbital cellulitis
    B. Allergic reaction
    C. Nephrotic syndrome
    D. Nephrotic syndrome with hypovolaemia
    E. C1 esterase deficiency

3. Blood pressure management

A 12-year-old girl presents to her GP with a UTI. She has no past medical history of note and is not taking any medication. On testing her routine observations, her blood pressure was 140/90 mmHg with a manual sphygmomanometer. You are concerned this may be high for her age. She has no headaches, visual disturbance, vomiting, chest pain, dyspnoea or neurological signs. What is your next course of action?

    A. Repeat the blood pressure on three different occasions
    B. Discuss the blood pressure reading with a paediatric nephrologist
    C. Commence sodium nitroprusside
    D. Repeat the blood pressure measurements with an automated machine
    E. Discharge home with reassurance

4. Haematuria

A 6-year-old girl presents to hospital with a large right-sided abdominal mass. It does not cross the midline. On further questioning she has had macroscopic haematuria and weight loss of 4 kg over the last 4 months. She has reduced appetite and lethargy. Her blood pressure is 125/73 mmHg, heart rate 120 bpm. Which of the following is not a complication of this malignancy?

    A.   Malnutrition
    B.   Hypertension
    C.   Renal impairment
    D.   Urinary catecholamines
    E.   Metastatic spread

5. Purpura

James is an 8-year-old boy who recently attended accident and emergency with a swollen left ankle. He had an x-ray and was discharged home and told there was no fracture. He has now developed a dark purple rash on his legs, which does not disappear with a glass pressed on. He was brought back to the department today vomiting, with abdominal pain. His observations and urine dipstick are all within normal limits. What is the most likely diagnosis?

    A.   Diabetic ketoacidosis
    B.   Viral gastroenteritis
    C.   Meningococcal sepsis
    D.   Idiopathic thrombocytopenic purpura
    E.   Henoch–Schönlein purpura

6. Post-infectious complications

A 7-year-old boy presented to accident and emergency with diarrhoea and vomiting for the past week. He had no history of foreign travel and but had been to a zoo recently on a school trip. He was discharged home, after providing a stool sample, with rehydration advice as he was less than 5 per cent dehydrated and tolerating oral fluids. The stool had grown 'Escherichia coli 0157' which was phoned from the microbiology laboratory to the on-call doctor 48 hours later. What is the most serious complication?

    A.   Acute kidney injury
    B.   Haemolytic uraemic syndrome
    C.   Severe hypernatraemic dehydration
    D.   Henoch–Schönlein purpura
    E.   Post-gastroenteritis syndrome

7. Renal impairment

A 5-year-old girl was brought to hospital at midnight by her mother with 5 per cent partial thickness burns to her chest and abdomen. Her mother states that she pulled on the kettle at 2 pm and the boiling water scalded her. On examination she is tachycardic, and drowsy with cool peripheries. Her initial blood tests: sodium 150 mmol/L, potassium 7.8 mmol/L, urea 10.2 mmol/L, creatinine 104 μmol/L, haemoglobin 14 g/dL. What is the most likely aetiological factor to account for these results?

    A. Post-renal cause of acute kidney injury
    B. Poisoning
    C. Renal cause of acute kidney injury
    D. Dehydration
    E. Pre-renal cause of acute kidney injury

8. Bladder outflow obstruction

A 10-day-old baby boy was brought to accident and emergency with a distended abdomen. On questioning, he was born at term with no antenatal concerns. Until 2 days ago he had been feeding well and not vomiting, he had been wetting nappies, but mother has not witnessed a good urinary stream. On examining the child, you find a mass, dull to percussion, arising out of the pelvis, and he has had no wet nappies for the last day. You suspect he may have posterior urethral valves. Which one test will help to diagnose this underlying condition?

    A. DMSA scan
    B. Renal biopsy
    C. Computed tomography (CT) abdomen
    D. Micturating cystourethrogram
    E. Renal ultrasound

9. Renal transplant

A 12-year-old boy who was born with multicystic dysplastic kidneys. He had a renal transplant when he was 7 years old due to chronic kidney disease stage V after having peritoneal dialysis for 1 year. Which of the following would you not expect him to be taking?

    A. Septrin
    B. Tacrolimus
    C. Diclofenac
    D. Growth hormone
    E. Erythropoietin

10. Polycystic kidney disease

An 11-year-old girl presents to the out of hours GP while on holiday in England with abdominal pain. She tells you she has polycystic kidney disease which was diagnosed early in life. She has bilateral palpable kidneys and hepatosplenomegaly, with visible distended veins on the abdomen and ascites. Abdominal ultrasound shows liver fibrosis. What is the inheritance of this condition?

    A.   Autosomal dominant

    B.   X-linked

    C.   Sporadic mutation

    D.   Autosomal recessive

    E.   Microdeletion

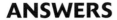

ANSWERS

The febrile child

1 C This child has a non-specific presentation. The differential diagnosis of vomiting in children is broad including infection, surgical, reflux and raised intracranial pressure. This child is febrile which increases the suspicion of infection; however, in children under 3 months a febrile presentation requires a thorough search for the cause. Therefore this child needs a septic screen which includes, blood culture, urine cultures, cerebrospinal fluid cultures, chest x-ray and C-reactive protein – (C) and not (E). Although the urine has leukocytes, these are not sensitive on their own or in infants. This child should not be discharged until a focus has been found for the infection (A). If the urine culture grows >105 colony-forming units per millilitre of a single organism, the diagnosis of a UTI can be made and then (B) would be correct. These children will require imaging of the renal tract with ultrasound, DMSA and micturating cystourethrogram depending on age (see NICE guidelines on UTI in children), though a DMSA scan is done at least 6 weeks after the infection (D) as it can be misleading in the acute situation of infection.

Generalized oedema

2 D Nephrotic syndrome (triad of proteinuria, hypoalbuminaemia and generalized oedema) presents with puffy eyes, which could also be a feature of any of the above diagnoses. However, the examination findings of generalized oedema make periorbital cellulitis (A) (in the absence of a fever) and allergic reaction (in the absence of skin rash, wheals, flares) (B) unlikely. The diagnosis of nephrotic syndrome (C) precipitated by an intercurrent infection in this case is correct, but with tachycardia and cool peripheries this suggests this child additionally has hypovolaemia, due to increased interstitial fluid collection due to reduced oncotic pressure (D). Rarely, C1 esterase deficiency (E) can present with generalized oedema following an intercurrent illness.

Blood pressure management

3 A Blood pressure measurements in children need the same considerations as for adult patients. There may be external factors influencing the reading such as pain, anxiety, incorrect cuff size and poor technique. Manual measurements are preferable to automated ones (D). The blood pressure should be repeated on at least three occasions (A) and if still high investigations and management should be initiated with guidance from paediatric nephrologists (B). Sodium nitroprusside (C) is the treatment of choice for malignant hypertension, which is not consistent with the history. Causes of hypertension in children include: essential hypertension, renal (renal artery stenosis, chronic kidney disease, Wilms' tumour), cardiac (coarctation of the aorta), endocrine (Cushing's syndrome, phaeochromocytoma, neuroblastoma) and metabolic (hyperaldosteronism, congenital adrenal hyperplasia). Therefore, simple discharge home is not acceptable without considered exploration (E).

Haematuria

4 D Wilms' tumour can result in hypertension (B) and renal impairment (C), dependent on the functioning of the contralateral kidney. General complications of malignant disease include metastases (E) and malnutrition (A) due to poor appetite, vomiting and increased metabolic demands. Sympathetic nervous system stimulation does not occur with Wilms' tumours but with neuroblastoma, an important differential diagnosis, due to catecholamine production from the tumour which originates from the adrenal medulla. Catecholamines can be detected in urine samples.

Purpura

5 E Henoch–Schönlein purpura (E) is a diagnosis based on a set of symptoms including arthralgia, rash (urticarial to purpuric), abdominal pain and renal involvement (hypertension, nephrotic syndrome). It is a common paediatric condition affecting 3–10 year olds and usually follows a viral illness. It is a vasculitis process which can cause severe gastrointestinal and renal complications but is usually benign and self-limiting. Any child with abdominal pain and vomiting should have their glucose checked as they may be presenting for the first time with diabetic ketoacidosis (A). Viral infections can precipitate a reactive arthritis, though this follows the primary infection (B). Meningococcal sepsis (C) is always a concern in children with a purpuric rash and this must be considered and excluded and, in this case, is less likely with the normal heart rate, blood pressure and respiratory rate (observations within normal limits). Idiopathic thrombocytopenic purpura (D) may present with the rash, but the other symptoms are unusual with this condition and the platelet count would be low, whereas in Henoch–Schönlein purpura the platelet count is normal.

Post-infectious complications

6 B Haemolytic uraemic syndrome (B) is a serious complication of particularly *E. coli* and *Shigella* gastroenteritis. It is caused by a verocytotoxin produced by these bacteria which initiates an inflammatory reaction in vascular endothelium and neutrophil activation. It is recognized by a triad of microangiopathic haemolytic anaemia, acute kidney injury and thrombocytopenia. The morbidity and mortality results from the renal impairment which may require dialysis or progression to chronic kidney disease (A). Children with severe gastroenteritis of any cause may suffer from dehydration and if water loss is greater than salt loss, this may cause hypernatraemia (C). Children may also suffer with food intolerances (i.e. lactose intolerance) after an episode of gastroenteritis due to damage to the mucosal enzyme activity (E). Henoch–Schönlein purpura often follows a viral infection and is characterized by arthralgia, purpuric rash on the extensor surfaces of the lower limbs, abdominal pain and renal involvement (D).

Renal impairment

7 E This girl has presented with a scald injury. The accident happened 10 hours before presentation which may arouse suspicion of non-accidental injury, but at present the more concerning feature is the acute kidney injury in a child with clinical shock. Burns damage the protective skin barrier, which allows excessive fluid and electrolyte loss. She may have been losing fluid through the damaged skin during the day, causing worsening dehydration (D); however she is now so fluid depleted that she has pre-renal acute kidney injury and hypovolaemia (E). This may subsequently result in acute tubular necrosis and thus a renal cause of acute kidney injury (C), but the primary cause is (E). The high sodium and haemoglobin would also support the diagnosis. Causes of post-renal acute kidney injury (A) are obstructive, such as ureteric stones, bladder outflow obstruction and neuropathic bladder. Poisoning (B) should be considered in children with drowsiness, especially in the context of non-accidental injury, and clues in the history such as access to illicit substances or medicines.

Bladder outflow obstruction

8 D This presentation of an enlarged, palpable bladder and anuria for 24 hours is suggestive of bladder outflow obstruction. This, in conjunction with a poor urinary stream, would make the diagnosis of posterior urethral valves likely. This is diagnosed using micturating cystourethrogram (D). DMSA (A) and renal biopsy (B) would provide information about the kidney. CT abdomen (C) would image the enlarged, fluid-filled bladder but possibly not the urethral valves. Renal ultrasound (E) will show the enlarged bladder and possibly show evidence of hydroureter and hydronephrosis with backflow from the bladder.

Renal transplant

9 C After renal transplantation there are many medications that are required. These children are susceptible to opportunistic infections and septrin (A) is used as prophylaxis to *Pneumocystis carinii* (*Pneumocystis jiroveci*), they are also particularly at risk of cytomegalovirus, varicella zoster virus and fungal infection. Immunosuppression is necessary to avoid rejection of the transplanted organ, including tacrolimus (B), ciclosporin and mycophenolate mofetil. Children with chronic renal disease may have impaired growth which can respond to growth hormone (D). They are often anaemic due to defective renal erythropoietin production and supplementation is beneficial (E). Diclofenac (C) should not be used in renal impairment as it and other non-steroidal anti-inflammatory drugs are nephrotoxic.

Polycystic kidney disease

10 D This girl has polycystic kidney disease, of which there are two types. The autosomal recessive type (D) presents in childhood with bilateral renal masses, respiratory distress due to pulmonary hypoplasia and congenital hepatic fibrosis with pulmonary hypertension. It is due to tubular dilatation of the distal collecting system. Renal function is impaired and progressively deteriorates, requiring renal replacement therapy (dialysis or transplant). The autosomal dominant (A) type may present in older children or adults. The cysts are grossly dilated nephrons which compress normal renal tissue. It affects renal, liver and cerebral vasculature.

SECTION 19: HAEMATOLOGY

QUESTIONS

1. Sickle cell disease

An 11-year-old girl was brought to accident and emergency in December with pain in her left leg. She is known to have sickle cell disease and her baseline haemoglobin is 7.0 g/dL. She has been admitted in the past with painful leg and chest crises. She has a cough and coryza. Today her blood results show: haemoglobin 6.8, white cell count (WCC) 12×10^9/L, platelets 209×10^9/L, C-reactive protein (CRP) 20 mg/L. What is not part of the appropriate initial management?

  A. IV fluids
  B. 15 L oxygen through a non-rebreather mask
  C. Exchange transfusion
  D. IV antibiotics
  E. Oramorph

2. Limping child

A 4-year-old boy is brought to accident and emergency with a limp for 1 day. He was unhappy to weight bear on his right leg. He had been with his grandparents all day and his mother brought him to hospital when she returned from work that evening. He was afebrile with a heart rate of 110 bpm but had had a cold last week. Mum reports no history of trauma. What is the most important diagnosis to exclude?

  A. Behavioural
  B. Acute leukaemia
  C. Reactive arthritis
  D. Soft tissue injury
  E. Septic arthritis

3. Idiopathic thrombocytopenic purpura

A 14-year-old girl was diagnosed with idiopathic thrombocytopenic purpura (ITP) last week after she attended the children's assessment unit with recurrent epistaxis. She had a platelet count of 16×10^9/L last week and now re-presents to accident and emergency with further episodes of epistaxis, haematemesis and petechiae. She had a heart rate of 110 bpm and her blood pressure is 100/70 mmHg. What is the next best management step?

  A. Give a platelet transfusion and red cell transfusion
  B. Arrange an urgent upper gastrointestinal endoscopy
  C. Give IV immunoglobulin and steriods
  D. Admit and monitor the haemodynamic status and administer a fluid bolus
  E. Discharge home with advice to return if the symptoms continue for
      more than 24 hours

4. Acute myeloid leukaemia (AML)

A 14-year-old girl went to her GP with a sore throat and cervical lymphadenopathy. She had a blood test done and you are called later that day with results. Haemoglobin 6.0 g/dL, WCC 230×10^9/L, neutrophils 0.9×10^9/L, platelets 77×10^9/L; blood film showed blasts and Auer rods. What is the most important management priority for this child in the first 24 hours from diagnosis?

    A. Overwhelming sepsis
    B. Febrile neutropenia
    C. Heart failure
    D. Uncontrollable bleeding
    E. Tumour lysis syndrome

5. Haemophilia

A 2-year-old boy is admitted to the paediatric ward with a swollen, painful left knee. He has been afebrile and has a history of minor trauma to his knee earlier today. His mother is a haemophilia carrier and his father is not affected. You are keen to rule out haemophilia in this child. Which two clotting factors should you test for?

    A. Factor VII and IX
    B. Factor VII and VIII
    C. Factor V and VI
    D. Factor VIII and IX
    E. Factor X and XI

6. Complications of childhood oncological disease

A 20-year-old man presents to the infectious diseases department with a large 7 cm × 8 cm swollen painful lump in the left anterior triangle of his neck. He has night sweats, 10 kg weight loss and a dry cough for the last month. He was treated with surgery and radiotherapy for a high grade astrocytoma when he was 8 years old. Which of the following is not a recognized complication of his childhood condition and its treatment?

    A. Finger clubbing
    B. Haematological malignancy
    C. Educational difficulties
    D. Short stature
    E. Infertility

7. Bleeding disorder

A 12-year-old girl has been seeing her GP for the last year with heavy periods and had suffered with bleeding gums when she was younger. She is otherwise well and lives with her adoptive parents who now have parental responsibility. Her coagulation tests reveal normal prothrombin time (PT) and activated partial thromboplastin time (APTT), low factor VIII, low von Willibrand factor (vWF), abnormal platelet aggregation and increased bleeding time. What is the likely inheritance of her condition?

    A.   Autosomal dominant
    B.   Autosomal recessive
    C.   X-linked
    D.   Robertsonian translocation
    E.   Sporadic mutation

8. Thrombocytopenia

A 4-year-old girl has just returned from holiday in France where she visited a petting farm. She has had diarrhoea for 2 days, and her mother noticed fresh red blood mixed with the stools. She has also been vomiting. On admission to hospital her blood tests showed: Hb 5 g/dL, WCC 15×10^9/L, platelets 55×10^9/L, urea 19 mmol/L, creatinine 110 μmol/L. Her stool culture is pending. What is the most likely diagnosis?

    A.   Platelet disorder
    B.   Inflammatory bowel disease (IBD)
    C.   Severe dehydration
    D.   Henoch–Schönlein purpura (HSP)
    E.   Haemolytic uraemic syndrome (HUS)

9. Anaemia

An 18-month-old boy presented to the GP with a history of eating soil. He had been in the garden this afternoon as his mother put the washing out. She found him eating the soil and took him straight inside. On examination, he is well and alert but has pale conjunctivae. He is not tachycardic or tachypnoeic. His diet consists of predominantly of breast milk. What is the most likely result of his haemoglobin and haematinics?

    A.   Hb 10 g/dL, MCV 80 fl, ferritin normal, iron normal, vitamin B12 and folate normal
    B.   Hb 6.5 g/dL, MCV 100 fl, ferritin normal, iron normal, vitamin B12 and folate low
    C.   Hb 5.5 g/dL, MCV 55 fl, ferritin low, iron low, vitamin B12 and folate normal
    D.   Hb 7 g/dL, MCV 70 fl, ferritin normal, iron normal, vitamin B12 and folate normal
    E.   Hb 6.8 g/dL, MCV 65 fl, ferritin normal, iron low, vitamin B12 and folate normal

10. Haemolytic anaemia

A 9-month-old boy presented to his GP with lethargy and a prominent forehead. He is pale on examination and has yellow sclerae. He is the first child of his non-consanguineous parents. His haemoglobin is 6.5g/dL, WCC 5.0×10^9/L, platelets 300×10^9/L. His blood film shows evidence of haemolysis, no spherocytes, no sickle cells and a good reticulocyte count. Direct antiglobulin test (DAT) is negative. What is the most likely diagnosis?

    A.   Beta thalassaemia
    B.   Sickle cell disease
    C.   ABO incompatibility
    D.   Hereditary spherocytosis
    E.   G6PD deficiency

ANSWERS

Sickle cell disease

1 C   (C) is correct. This child has a painful crisis caused by vaso-occlusion of small blood vessels supplying the bones in her leg. This leads to pain, which can require analgesia with morphine (Oramorph or patient controlled pumps). Painful crises may be triggered by cold weather, infection, hypoxia or dehydration. Therefore, the initial management of painful crises includes rectifying these triggers with analgesia (E) (opiates may be required), rewarming, antibiotics (D), oxygen (B) and IV fluids (A). If there is a marked drop in haemoglobin, top up transfusion may be required. Exchange transfusion is indicated for sickle chest crisis, stroke and priapism.

Limping child

2 B   Acute leukaemia (B) can present with a limp due to bone pain secondary to dissemination of the disease. It is important to do a full blood count (FBC) and blood film on these patients to look for pancytopenia and the presence of blast cells. The other diagnoses are also of importance to investigate for, but may be more or less likely depending on the history. There is no reported history of trauma so (D) is unlikely, but note that he has been with a different carer throughout the day than the one presenting with him now. He may need a plain x-ray of the hip and femur to exclude traumatic injury. The presence of a fever with limp or restricted movement of a joint must raise suspicion of septic arthritis (E), which in the hip is a medical emergency due to potential interruption of blood flow with increasing pressure in the joint. Reactive arthritis (C) can present after a viral illness and may show evidence of inflammation (raised WCC and CRP) but not to the extent as with septic arthritis.

Idiopathic thrombocytopenic purpura

3 D   This girl has ITP, characterized by low platelets and mucosal bleeding. It usually occurs a few weeks after a viral illness. It is caused by immune-mediated destruction of circulating platelets within the reticuloendothelial system. It typically occurs in children between 2 and 10 years of age. The management depends on the severity of the presenting symptoms. The course of the illness is self-limiting, and if there is no continued bleeding, they may be monitored as an outpatient. However, this girl has continued episodes of bleeding and is tachycardic and hypotensive. She cannot be discharged (E) as she is medically unstable and needs close monitoring and a fluid bolus (D). Platelet transfusion (A) is not usually required as these platelets will be destroyed too, but in life-threatening bleeding with low platelets they may be required. An urgent endoscopy (B) would help to identify a gastric or oesophageal lesion, but given the previous history and low platelets this is not required and may cause harm if it were to cause further bleeding. IV immunoglobulins and steroids (C) can be used for children with continued bleeding, to try to reduce the underlying immune destruction, but a bone marrow aspirate should be carried out prior to commencing steroids to exclude malignancy.

Acute myeloid leukaemia (AML)

4 E She has a diagnosis of AML, as suggested by Auer rods on blood film. There is a very high WCC, predominantly due to blast cells in the bone marrow. This results in a reduction in the other cell line production producing a pancytopenia. Although anaemia can result in heart failure (C), low platelets can result in bleeding (D) and low neutrophils can result in increased susceptibility to infection (B) and overwhelming sepsis (A). The most important initial management step is to prevent tumour lysis syndrome. As the treatment for AML begins, a large number of cells break down which can cause complications such as hyperkalaemia, hyperphosphataemia, gout, fluid overload or dehydration, raised urea and creatinine, known as tumour lysis syndrome (E). Prophylactic hyperhydration, allopurinol or rasburicase and monitoring of electrolytes is required from the time of diagnosis.

Haemophilia

5 D Haemophilia A and B are X-linked inherited conditions. Haemophilia A is due to a deficiency in clotting factor VIII. Haemophilia B is due to a deficiency in clotting factor IX. There is a spectrum in severity of the disease based on the extent of the deficiency and proportion of functional factor:

Mild 10–50 per cent, moderate 2–10 per cent, severe <2 per cent

Haemophilia can be treated with replacement of factors VIII or IX for haemophilia A and B, respectively. Desmopressin can be useful to stimulate production of clotting factors. Consideration of the clotting function is needed during times of elective and emergency surgery. Physiotherapy is important to minimize the complication of arthritis in the affected joint.

Complications of childhood oncological disease

6 A Children with malignancies may present later in life with problems including secondary malignancy due to high levels of radiation during radiotherapy, commonly leukaemias and lymphomas (B). Educational difficulties (C) may be multifactorial in aetiology, with long periods missed from school due to ill health or poor ability to concentrate, seeing or hearing depending on the extent of the malignancy. Radiotherapy can affect the spine and growth hormone, both of which can contribute to growth problems (D). Irradiation and chemotherapy can also render gonadal tissue dysfunctional (E). Egg harvesting for females and sperm storage for males should be considered prior to therapy. Clubbing (A) is not a recognized complication of radiotherapy or chemotherapy. The causes of clubbing include cystic fibrosis, bronchiectasis, cyanotic congenital heart disease, inflammatory bowel disease and liver cirrhosis.

Bleeding disorder

7 A This girl has von Willebrand's disease (vWD) and presents with a picture of mucosal bleeding which can be associated with platelet disorders (of actual number or function). This would suggest the mild phenotype of vWD, type 1 with partial deficiency of vWF. There are three types as follows:

- Type 1 – partial deficiency of vWF
- Type 2 – defective vWF
- Type 3 – complete deficiency of vWF

vWD type 1 and 2 are autosomal dominant (A) (type 3 is autosomal recessive) and a family history may be useful in the history. Haemophilia A and B are X-linked disorders (C). Platelet disorders are often secondary to other causes (consumption, destruction, defective production in bone marrow) but aplastic anaemias such as Fanconi's anaemia are inherited in an autosomal recessive (B) manner. Robertsonian translocations (D) (fusion of two acrocentric chromosomes near the centromere with resultant loss of the short arms) can result in Down's syndrome or recurrent pregnancy loss. Sporadic mutations (E) are not known to be associated with the development of vWD.

Thrombocytopenia

8 E HUS (E) is a microangiopathic haemolytic anaemia consisting of acute kidney injury, haemolytic anaemia and thrombocytopenia. It occurs secondary to *Escherichia coli* or *Shigella* gastroenteritis due to an endotoxin initiating an inflammatory response. Treatment is largely supportive fluid management but may require renal replacement therapy. Renal impairment may resolve but a few can develop chronic kidney disease. IBD (B) is unlikely in this age group but can present with bloody diarrhoea, anaemia, abdominal pain and weight loss. Severe dehydration (C) may result in a pre-renal cause of acute kidney injury leading to raised urea and creatinine (though the urea may be disproportionately high). However, this would not explain the abnormalities of the full blood count. Platelet disorders (A) can lead to mucosal bleeding including haematemesis, haematuria, per rectum (PR) or per vaginam bleeding, and epistaxis. However, it does not explain the renal impairment. HSP (D) is a syndrome consisting of purpuric rash, arthralgia, abdominal pain and renal involvement. It may present with PR bleeding and diarrhoea due to gut vasculitis and renal failure, but there is no evidence of rash or joint involvement.

Anaemia

9 C   This child is exhibiting pica, a phenomenon of eating substances that are not food, secondary to severe iron deficiency anaemia consistent with microcytic anaemia with low iron stores (ferritin) as well as low circulating iron (C). The most likely cause is due to prolonged breastfeeding and delayed weaning. Children have sufficient iron stores for 4 months after birth. After this time they require supplementation which usually comes from the introduction of pureed and solid foods. Delay in weaning can lead to iron deficiency anaemia, hypocalcaemia and poor weight gain. (A) shows a normal study, with no evidence of anaemia and normal haematinics. (B) shows a macrocytic anaemia with vitamin B12 and folate deficiency (megaloblastic anaemia). (D) shows a microcytic anaemia with normal iron, suggesting another cause such as thalassaemia or sideroblastic anaemia. (E) is a macrocytic anaemia with normal vitamin B12 and folate, suggesting another cause such as hypothyroidism, liver disease, myeloproliferative disorders.

Haemolytic anaemia

10 A   Beta thalassaemia (A) is a haemolytic anaemia of autosomal recessive inheritance. Thalassaemia presents with anaemia after 6 months of age, when HbA is starting to be produced. Thalassaemia is present in Mediterranean and Asian populations and is due to a defect in the production of haemoglobin beta chains or alpha chains (beta and alpha thalassaemia, respectively). Patients can be homozygous (disease) or heterozygous (carriers). They present with anaemia and jaundice and may show evidence of extramedullary haemopoeisis (frontal bossing and maxillary overgrowth). Bloods tests will show a normocytic anaemia with hyperbilirubinaemia. A reticulocyte response would be expected with normal bone marrow function. Other non-immune haemolytic anaemias include other haemoglobinopathies such as sickle cell disease (B) (HbSS on Hb electrophoresis and sickle cells on blood film), red cell membrane defects (spherocytosis (D) and elliptocytosis seen on blood film) and red cell enzyme defects (G6PD deficiency (E) and pyruvate kinase deficiency, enzyme testing required for diagnosis), which usually present with acute crises which can be haemolytic, aplastic or with chronic anaemia and jaundice, splenomegaly due to increased red cell destruction. Immune-mediated haemolytic anaemias include ABO (C) or rhesus incompatibility. Carefully examine the mother's blood group (more likely if she is O and the child is A or B, and rhesus negative) and the DAT which may be positive.

SECTION 20:
SKIN DISORDERS

QUESTIONS

1. Eccyhmosis

A 3-year-old is brought into accident and emergency on a Monday morning because she has developed several bruises on her buttocks, left leg and right arm. She is seen with her nanny who reports finding the bruises when she was getting her dressed this morning. Recently the girl has not been herself. She has had several colds over the past 2 months and has been more lethargic lately. The nanny is worried she is losing weight. On examination she appears withdrawn, pale and has a bruise on the left buttock which is 5 cm × 8 cm. She has three other bruises on her left leg and right arm which are of varying colours. She also has some fine petechiae on her neck and cheeks. She has a runny nose and a cough but the chest is clear. What is the most likely diagnosis?

    A.   Non-accidental injury
    B.   Leukaemia
    C.   Idiopathic thombocytopenia
    D.   Henoch–Schönlein purpura
    E.   Accidental injury

2. Newborn rash (1)

On the day 1 baby check a mother is very concerned about a rash on her baby's face. Over the right eye, forehead and temple there is a pink-red, flat area of erythema. He is opening the eye, and his eye movements seem intact. The child's observations and rest of the examination are normal. What should you tell the mother?

    A.   This is a strawberry naevus and it may get bigger before it goes away by about 5 years of age
    B.   This is a port wine stain and the baby needs an MRI scan to check for intracranial involvement
    C.   This is a capillary haemangioma (stork mark) and is normal; it will fade over the first year or so of life
    D.   This is orbital cellulitis and he needs intravenous antibiotics
    E.   This is erythema toxicum which is a normal baby rash and will go away within the first few weeks

3. Eczema

A mother brings her 6-month-old, formula-fed baby to see the GP complaining that the olive oil she is using is not helping his persistent cradle cap and worsening rash on his face and arms. On examination he has extensive cradle cap and eczematous changes on his cheeks, neck, chest and arms. The neck skin creases are red and oozing with yellow crusts. He is miserable and feels warm to touch. What is the most appropriate management?

A. Advise using emollients and a soap substitute

B. Start emollients with a topical antibiotic

C. Refer to hospital for intravenous antibiotics

D. Recommend a trial of switching to soya based formula as he may be cow's milk protein allergic

E. Start topical steroids on the inflamed areas, and intensive emollient treatment

4. Petechiae (1)

A 4-year-old is brought into accident and emergency by very anxious parents. She has had a bad cough which makes her vomit and a fever for 2 days. She has now developed a rash on her face which does not pass the 'glass test', in that the spots are still visible when a glass is pressed against the skin. On examination she is alert and comfortable at rest, with fine petechiae on her cheeks and neck which are non-blanching. She has red, enlarged tonsils without pus and the chest is clear. What is the most likely cause of her rash?

A. Meningococcal sepsis

B. Idiopathic thrombocytopenia

C. Henoch–Schönlein purpura

D. Non-accidental injury

E. Capillary rupture secondary to raised pressure in the superior vena cava distribution

5. Petechiae (2)

A 2 year old was seen in accident and emergency by the senior house officer with a short history of fever, malaise and now vomiting. She had a blanching rash on her arms and abdomen. She looked unwell but had no clear focus for her fever. She was tachypnoeic but her chest was clear. A urine sample was requested which showed a trace of leukocytes and two plus of ketones. Forty-five minutes later the paediatric registrar came to review the child who appears lethargic with a capillary refill centrally of 6 seconds and the rash on her abdomen is now non-blanching. What is the most likely diagnosis?

A. Urinary tract infection (UTI)

B. Idiopathic thrombocytopenia

C. Meningococcal sepsis

D. Human herpes virus 6 infection

E. Diabetic ketoacidosis

6. Burns

A 2 year old is brought in by ambulance after pulling a pot of boiling water off the stove down on top of himself. He has significant burns to the whole of his face, torso and right arm. Estimate the percentage body surface area affected.

A. 20 per cent
B. 30 per cent
C. 40 per cent
D. 50 per cent
E. 60 per cent

7. Erythema nodosum

Which of the following is not a cause of erythema nodosum?

A. Oral contraception
B. Tuberculosis infection
C. Hepatitis B infection
D. Streptococcal infection
E. Sarcoidosis

8. Papules

A 3 year old is brought to see the GP with multiple pearly raised papules with central umbilications. They have been there for more than a month on his torso and upper legs. His mother is worried he has warts. What is the most likely diagnosis?

A. Molluscum contagiosum
B. Congenital warts
C. Scabies
D. Melanocytic naevi
E. Guttate psoriasis

9. Newborn rash (2)

On a newborn baby check of an Asian, 36-hour-old baby you note a large bruise coloured area on the buttocks and lower back which seems non-tender. The mother does not know how it got there. He is handling well and the rest of the baby check is unremarkable. What is the most likely explanation?

A. Non-accidental injury
B. Mongolian blue spot
C. Neonatal sepsis with disseminated intravascular coagulation
D. Idiopathic thrombocytopenic purpura
E. von Willebrand's disease

10. Newborn rash (3)

A 5-day-old baby is brought to see the GP because she has had a rash for the past 3 days which started on her chest, is spreading to her face and getting worse. On examination she handles well and is alert. There is an erythematous rash on her face, torso and right arm with little pustules. What is the most likely diagnosis?

A. Infected eczema
B. Neonatal sepsis
C. Neonatal acne
D. Molluscum contagiosum
E. Erythema toxicum

ANSWERS

Eccyhmosis

1 B This child is presenting with bruising on the buttocks and limbs as well as petechiae which raise alarm bells that the child may have low platelets. The two options on the list with low platelets are idiopathic thrombocytopenia (ITP) (C) or leukaemia (B). This child has a background of being unwell with a suggestion of weight loss which points to leukaemia as the most likely diagnosis (B). Henoch Schönlein purpura (D) does not produce low platelets but could produce the bruising on the buttocks: this would normally be associated with joint and abdominal pains as well as haematuria. It is a small vessel vasculitis which typically occurs 1–2 weeks after a throat infection. ITP (C) also is often triggered after a viral infection and it would be unusual for the child to be unwell at presentation with the bruises. If the full blood count comes back normal that would raise concerns of non-accidental injury (A). The petechiae in the head and neck could be produced by strangulation and the bruises of multiple ages as well as sited on the buttocks is unusual for an accidental injury (E); combined with a withdrawn child this should raise the suspicion of non-accidental injury (A). As you have not been given the full blood count results and the child is unwell with weight loss and recurrent illnesses, the single best answer is leukaemia (B).

Newborn rash (1)

2 B This is likely to be a port wine stain or naevus flammeus (B) which is a capillary vascular malformation in the dermis, present from birth and will persist for life. When present in the trigeminal distribution, a small proportion of children will have underlying brain involvement (Sturge–Weber syndrome) and should have an MRI brain to look for this as the child will be at risk of seizures and developmental problems. A strawberry naevus (A) or cavernous haemangioma is not usually present at birth and typically appears in the first month. Strawberry naevi will grow larger before shrinking and disappearing, typically before the age of 5 years. They may compress neighbouring structures as they grow and sometimes ulcerate with troublesome bleeding. They are not flat. A capillary haemangioma or 'stork bite' (C) is a pink macule found on the eyelids, central forehead or nape of the neck which is due to distension of the dermal capillaries; they mostly fade over the first year. Those on the neck may persist but will be covered by hair. They are not found on the lateral face; therefore this is not the right answer. The child is well, with normal observations, making cellulitis (D) very unlikely. In addition you have been given no information on whether the lesion feels warm, which you would expect in infection. Erythema toxicum (E) is a common innocent rash of the newborn which has an erythematous base with small pustules. It comes and goes all over the body for the first few weeks of life.

Eczema

3 C This child has infected eczema, characterized by red inflamed skin with yellow crusts which suggests a staphylococcal infection (but eczema herpeticum also needs to ruled out). He is systemically unwell, with misery and most probably a fever. He therefore needs intravenous antibiotics and must be referred to hospital (C). If he was not unwell, starting emollients with oral antibiotics would be appropriate, but topical antibiotics are to be avoided since they may rapidly select for resistant organisms and they may themselves be sensitizing (B). This child's eczema is severe and exploring other contributory factors such as cow's milk protein sensitivity is part of good management, but a trial of soya based formula without any clear history or investigations is inappropriate (D). He should be started on emollients and soap substitute (A) but this is not the best answer as he needs systemic antibiotics as well. Steroids (E) should not be started until the infection has been treated but he will require steroid creams to help treat his eczema once the infection has resolved.

Petechiae (1)

4 E This child's parents have done 'the glass test' by pressing a tumbler against the skin, to check if the rash is blanching or not. They are very anxious because they have been taught that a positive glass tests means meningitis, usually caused by meningococcal sepsis (A). However, she is well in herself making this less likely. It would be sensible to admit her for observation even if antibiotics are not started. She has petechiae in the superior vena caval distribution (E) which often occur in situations of raised pressure such as coughing or vomiting but can also be seen in shaken babies or strangulation injuries. In young children coughing bouts often trigger vomiting, but vomiting is a warning sign of meningitis, so she should be monitored. ITP (B) is often triggered about 1 week after a throat infection and it would be unusual for the child to still be unwell and only have petechiae on the face. A strangulation injury by an angry caregiver could produce this pattern of injury; however her coughing and vomiting give a plausible explanation of the lesion, making non-accidental injury (D) unlikely. Henoch–Schönlein purpura (C) is a vasculitis of the capillaries and typically causes a macular papular purpuric rash over the buttocks and extensor surfaces of the limbs, so the distribution of the rash in this case is wrong.

Petechiae (2)

5 C This child is rapidly becoming unwell with impending shock (capillary refill 6 seconds). The expanding rash quickly becomes non-blanching and suggests that she has disseminated intravascular coagulation, often seen with meningococcal sepsis (C). Idiopathic thrombocytopenia (B) is usually seen in well children following a recent upper respiratory tract infection. While the urine dipstick has a trace of leukocytes, this is most likely non-specific due to her being so unwell and in the absence of nitrites is not strongly suggestive of a UTI (A). Human herpes virus 6 infection is a very common cause of fever and rash in this age group, not infrequently associated with febrile convulsions, but it does not cause shock and the rash would remain blanching (D). Tachypnoea without chest signs is an indicator of acidosis but the urine dipstick did not have any glucose in it, so this presentation is not due to diabetic ketoacidosis (E).

Burns

6 C In children, the head represents a larger proportion of the body and the Lund–Browder chart is used to assess the burn percentage. The whole head would account for 18 per cent. This child has burned the anterior head = 9 per cent, the anterior torso = 18 per cent and the whole right arm = 9 per cent, which is not quite 40 per cent (C). In an adult, the whole head represents only 9 per cent of the body and therefore this same burn would be closer to 30 per cent (B). Just the torso would be about 20 per cent (A). Burns of 50 (D) or 60 per cent (E) are extremely extensive.

Erythema nodosum

7 C The oral contraceptive pill (A), tuberculosis (B), streptococcal infections (D) and sarcoidosis (E) are all known causes of erythema nodosum, which produces tender red nodules on the shins. Hepatitis B (C) does not cause erythema nodosum. It may produce non-specific rashes and jaundice.

Papules

8 A This child has a common condition of molluscum contagiosum (A) caused by a pox virus. They are usually self-limiting and will self-resolve within a year. Occasionally one may become superinfected with bacteria and require antibiotics. Particularly stubborn cases may be treated with cryotherapy to hasten resolution. 'Congenital warts' (B) is a term that usually refers to genital or anal warts, and the distribution and description of the lesions in this child are not consistent with this diagnosis. There is some controversy regarding the maximum incubation period for genital warts that are acquired from contact with maternal genital warts during delivery. These may take over a year or two to evolve and when they appear, child sexual abuse may erroneously be suspected. Scabies (C) cause itchy rashes due to the burrows of the mite in the skin, usually on the hands, axillae or groin and often involving the web spaces between the fingers. A melanocytic naevus (D) would be a hyperpigmented papule which would not usually have a central punctum. Guttate psoriasis (E) often follows an upper respiratory tract infection and produces raindrop-like scaly pink patches on the torso and arms.

Newborn rash (2)

9 B This is a Mongolian blue spot (B) and is more commonly found in darker skinned races. Mongolian blue spots are classically found on the buttocks and lower back and fade as the child grows up. It is not bothering the baby so it is unlikely to be an injury (A). The child is well on examination which makes sepsis with disseminated intravascular coagulation highly unlikely (C). Idiopathic thrombocytopenic purpura (D) is not seen in newborns as it requires a preceding infection to trigger the immune response, and maternal antibodies are protecting the baby. However, maternal autoantibodies against platelets could produce thrombocytopenia and purpura but this is not an answer choice. Von Willebrand's disease (E) is a clotting defect controlling the binding of platelets to damaged endothelium and typically presents with mucosal bleeding or menorrhagia.

Newborn rash (3)

10 E This is a typical presentation of erythema toxicum (E), a common innocent rash of the newborn which has an erythematous base with small pustules. It comes and goes all over the body for the first few weeks of life. The baby is well so an infection ((A) or (B)) is unlikely. Neonatal acne (C) is typically confined to the face and peaks at about 2 months. Molluscum contagiosum (D) does not have erythema or pustules, it produces pearly growths with a central punctum.

SECTION 21: ENDOCRINOLOGY

QUESTIONS

1. Type 1 diabetes

A 10-year-old girl was diagnosed with diabetes 1 year ago. She has been compliant with her insulin regimen and her HBA_{1c} is 6 per cent. She is attending her annual diabetic review and has been asking about why she has diabetes. What is the aetiology of type 1 diabetes?

    A. Inflammation of the pancreas causing exocrine and endocrine dysfunction
    B. Impaired glucose tolerance
    C. Secretory dysfunction of the pancreatic duct
    D. Autoimmune destruction of pancreatic islet cells
    E. Peripheral insulin resistance

2. Abdominal pain and vomiting

A 2-year-old girl was brought by her mother to accident and emergency after 4 days of vomiting and abdominal pain. She had brought her in 2 days ago after developing a cold and was discharged home and diagnosed with a 'tummy bug'. On examination, she was drowsy, had dry mucous membranes, deep heavy breathing, cool peripheries and tachycardia. Her mother reports a 1-month history of weight loss, excessive drinking and passing large volumes of urine prior to this episode. Her urine dipstick has ketones and glucose. Her blood gas shows the following: pH 7.10, PCO_2 kPa 2.1, PO_2 kPa 10.0, BE−12, HCO_3^- mmol/L 18. What is the most likely diagnosis?

    A. Severe dehydration secondary to gastroenteritis
    B. Sepsis secondary to gastroenteritis
    C. Diabetic ketoacidosis (DKA)
    D. Chronic kidney disease
    E. Hyperosmolar hyperglycaemic non-ketotic state

3. Prolonged jaundice

A 3-week-old baby is brought to the 'prolonged jaundice clinic'. His mother reports he has poor feeding, is not gaining weight appropriately and is more sleepy compared to her previous child. He opens his bowel once a day and is being mix breast and bottle fed. He is floppy, jaundiced, has a large, protruding tongue and a hoarse cry. He had a newborn blood spot screening test done at birth which was normal and he has no dysmorphic features. What is the most likely diagnosis of this child?

    A. Beckwith–Wiedemann syndrome
    B. Congenital hypothyroidism
    C. Down's syndrome
    D. Normal baby
    E. Prader–Willi syndrome

4. Hyperthyroidism

A 10-year-old girl with Graves' disease attends her GP with worsening of her symptoms. She was well controlled on carbimazole and has had relatively few symptoms for the past 6 months. She now has sweats, weight loss, diarrhoea and tremors which are affecting her school performance. What is the next management step?

    A. Review in 3 months
    B. Radioisotope therapy
    C. Stop carbimazole and start propranolol
    D. Optimize carbimazole dose and add propanolol
    E. Referral for thyroidectomy

5. Corticosteroid side effects

A 4-year-old boy was diagnosed with nephrotic syndrome 6 months ago and has required a long course of oral corticosteroids to maintain remission of the condition. He has developed truncal obesity and you are concerned he may be developing Cushing's syndrome. Which of the following is not a complication of Cushing's syndrome?

    A. Osteoporosis
    B. Short stature
    C. Gastric irritation
    D. Hypertension
    E. Hypoglycaemia

6. Short stature

A 13-year-old girl has presented to her GP with her mother with concerns that she is the shortest in her class at school. She has always been 'on the small side' according to her mother, despite eating well. When you examine her you find she is hypertensive but has no cardiac murmur. Respiratory and abdominal systems are normal. She has no signs of pubertal development and you notice she has widely spaced nipples and a low hair line. You are considering the diagnosis of Turner's syndrome. What is the most appropriate diagnostic investigation?

A.   Mid-parental height
B.   Echocardiogram
C.   Four limb blood pressures
D.   Karyotype
E.   Fluorescence *in situ* hybridization (FISH)

7. Tall stature

You are asked to examine a tall 15-year-old boy. His height is above the 98th centile for his age and he has other concerns about the development of breast tissue. He was told this was normal as he develops through puberty but his father states he has no facial or underarm hair. Jake allows a brief examination of his genitalia and you note he has a small penis and testicular volume. He has no arachnodactyly or visual problems. What is the most likely diagnosis?

A.   Delayed onset of puberty
B.   Klinefelter's syndrome
C.   Precocious puberty
D.   Marfan's syndrome
E.   Normal variation

8. Delayed puberty

A 16-year-old boy attends your GP clinic for the first time with his father. He has recently moved to the area. His father is concerned that he is shorter than his peers at school and he frequently complains about being bullied. On further questioning there is no evidence of chronic illness or familial illness and he eats a balanced diet. His weight is on the 25th centile and his height is on the 10th centile. On examination he has no evidence of facial, axillary or pubic hair, his testes are both descended and are <4 mL volume. What is the most likely cause of his delayed puberty?

A.   Anorexia nervosa
B.   Hypothalamo-pituitary dysfunction
C.   Kallmann' syndrome
D.   Cryptorchidism
E.   Constitutional delay

9. Precocious puberty

A 6-year-old girl has presented to her GP with a rapid increase in growth. Her mother is also concerned that she seems to have developed pubic and axillary hair and breast development prior to this but thought it would go away. She has no history of trauma and has reported problems with her vision. Her levels of gonadotrophin-releasing hormone (GnRH), follicle-stimulating hormone (FSH), luteinizing hormone (LH) and oestrogen are high. You are concerned that she may have a pituitary tumour. What is the likely visual field defect?

    A.   Monocular blindness
    B.   Central scotoma
    C.   Homonymous hemianopia
    D.   Bitemporal hemianopia
    E.   Myopia

10. Chronic steroid use

A 9-year-old girl presents to accident and emergency with fever, vomiting and dysuria. She is wearing a steroid bracelet and has a steroid card stating she is on daily prednisolone for severe asthma and eczema and is therefore at risk of adrenal suppression. She is tachycardic at 140 bpm and you are concerned that her blood pressure is low. Her capillary glucose is 3.0 mmol/L. What is the single most important investigation?

    A.   Cortisol
    B.   Full blood count
    C.   Renal function tests
    D.   Urine culture
    E.   Blood culture

ANSWERS

Type 1 diabetes

1 D Type 1 diabetes is due to autoimmune destruction of the B cells of the islets of Langerhans in the pancreas. This leads to absolute insulin deficiency and a state of catabolism, particularly lipids, in the absence of insulin. These children are dependent on exogenous insulin for life. Type 2 diabetes is due to reduced production of insulin but also peripheral resistance in tissues (E). Diabetes may be acquired with other conditions such as chronic pancreatitis (A), corticosteroid use (B) or cystic fibrosis (C).

Abdominal pain and vomiting

2 C This girl has the classical history of developing polyuria and polydipsia with weight loss, now with a viral illness precipitating DKA (C). Abdominal pain and vomiting are common in DKA and the disease process is triggered by insulin deficiency leading to lipolysis and ketone production. This results in the acidosis along with glycosuria osmotically increasing water losses in urine and leads to dehydration, worsening the acidosis. She will likely have high blood sugar which should also be measured in the laboratory as the bedside tests are inaccurate at very high levels. Gastroenteritis ((A) and (B)) can cause both profound dehydration and sepsis (with bacteraemia or viraemia), with ketonuria but there should not be glycosuria. Children with polyuria should have renal function checked (D), but in this setting with acute illness and ketonuria and glycosuria suggestive of DKA, diabetes is a better explanation of polyuria. Hyperosmolar hyperglycaemic non-ketotic state (E) occurs as a complication of type 2 diabetes, which is rare in childhood and does not present with ketonuria, though the incidence is increasing with childhood obesity.

Prolonged jaundice

3 B This child has many features of hypothyroidism (B). Children with prolonged jaundice should have their thyroid function tested. The newborn blood spot tests for high thyroid-stimulating hormone (TSH) levels in response to low thyroxine, which should detect most congenital hypothyroidism. Rarely, in children with panhypopituitarism, there is low TSH and therefore low thyroxine. Babies with Down's syndrome (C) can also have hypotonia (floppiness), poor feeding and weight gain, macroglossia and hypothyroidism but with typical facial features which are not present here. Other conditions causing macroglossia include Beckwith–Wiedemann syndrome (A) (other features would include: fetal macrosomia, hypoglycaemia secondary to hyperinsulinaemia, hemihypertrophy, abnormal ear development). Other conditions causing hypotonia and poor feeding include Prader–Willi syndrome (obesity and learning difficulties in later life) (E). This is not a normal baby (D) as jaundice beyond 2 weeks is pathological.

Hyperthyroidism

4 D   Hyperthyroidism is due to raised thyroxine which may be due to high pituitary stimulation (high TSH) or endogenous thyroid production (low TSH). The symptoms are multisystemic and include tachycardia, heat intolerance, diarrhoea, weight loss, amenorrhoea, tremor and psychosis. Carbimazole acts to suppress thyroxine production and therefore reduce symptoms. This girl has got worsening symptoms and therefore the first course of action would be to optimize the dose of carbimazole to reduce the production of thyroxine, and then add propranolol which can be given for symptomatic relief, especially for tremors (D). Propranolol is not a replacement for carbimazole as it does not directly affect thyroxine production (C). Radioisotope treatment (B) and surgery (E) would be considered as further management strategies. (A) is not correct as she is symptomatic and therefore requires treatment to become clinically euthyroid.

Corticosteroid side effects

5 E   Oral corticosteroids are required for many inflammatory or autoimmune conditions to suppress the immune response and provide symptomatic relief for patients. We can minimize the effects of steroids by ensuring we give the minimum required dosage, alternate day prescribing and weaning at the end of the treatment course. Steroids have many side effects including: hypertension (D), glucose intolerance and tendency to hyperglycaemia, not hypoglycaemia (E), weight gain causing truncal obesity and a subscapular fat pad, short stature (B), osteoporosis (A), cataracts, gastric irritation (C), striae, thinning of skin and increased bruising, proximal myopathy, increased susceptibility to infection and adrenal suppression. The truncal obesity and thin myopathic limbs is characteristic of patients on long-term steroid therapy.

Short stature

6 D   Turner's syndrome results from the genotype 45X0. Therefore a karyotype would be diagnostic (D). FISH (E) is used to diagnose conditions caused by microdeletions in conditions such as DiGeorge' syndrome, cri du chat syndrome and Williams' syndrome. The four limb blood pressure (C) and an echocardiogram (B) may be useful in coarctation of the aorta and aortic stenosis which can occur as part of Turner's syndrome but are not important in the diagnosis itself. Mid-parental height (A) is important to note in children who are short, as one of the differentials to consider is familial short stature. It is calculated by the sum of the parents' height in centimetres, divided by 2, then +7 cm for a boy or –7 cm for a girl.

Tall stature

7 B Both Klinefelter's and Marfan's syndromes (D) can result in tall stature (though associated features with Marfan's syndrome include high arched palate, myopia, lens dislocation, arachnodactly, arm span > height, hypermobility, aortic arch abnormalities, mitral valve prolapse, chest wall deformity). Precocious puberty (C) leads to tall stature initially but ultimate height is often shorter than peers as the growth spurt occurs earlier. He also has signs of delayed puberty with small testicular volume (<4 mL) and no adrenarche. Delayed puberty (A) (in boys no pubertal development by the age of 15 years) alone would usually be associated with short rather than tall stature. The tall stature, hypogonadism and delayed puberty with gynaecomastia is suggestive of Klinefelter's syndrome (B) and a karyotype should be done, showing 47XXY. This is not a normal variation (E) as failure to develop signs of puberty by the age of 15 years in boys requires investigation.

Delayed puberty

8 E The most common cause of delayed puberty is constitutional delay (E), although this is a diagnosis of exclusion. Delayed puberty is more common in boys. He does not have cryptorchidism (undescended testes) (D) on examination. Although there is a history of bullying which may in turn lead to psychological problems including anorexia nervosa (A) (rare in boys, but should be considered), his weight centile is greater than his height, making this unlikely though a body mass index should be calculated too (weight/height squared). Kallmann's syndrome (C) is characterized by low luteinizing hormone-releasing hormone and anosmia, which is not mentioned but this disease is rare (1 in 10000–86000). It is important to exclude hypothalamo-pituitary dysfunction (B) by measuring GnRH, LH and FSH but it is not the most likely cause.

Precocious puberty

9 D This girl has features consistent with precocious puberty, which is the onset of puberty at <8 years in girls and <9 years in boys. The causes may be central or gonadal. Central causes will have raised GnRH, FSH and LH levels which stimulate the gonads to produce oestrogen or testosterone. Gonadal causes have low GnRH, FSH and LH due to negative feedback from excessive endogenous production of oestrogen or testosterone. Central causes may include a pituitary tumour which can lead to excessive production of the pituitary hormones (FSH, LH, melanocyte-stimulating hormone, adrenocorticotrophic hormone, prolactin, growth hormone, oxytocin, antidiuretic hormone). The pituitary is in close proximity to the optic chiasm, where the optic tracts decussate from the nasal visual fields. As the chiasm is compressed by the tumour, these tracts are affected leading to a bitemporal hemianopia (D). The other visual disturbances would not be directly related to a pituitary tumour. Monocular blindness (A) may be due to unilateral disease in front of the optic nerve or involving the optic nerve itself, e.g. cataracts, vitreous haemorrhage, retinoblastoma. Central scotoma (B) can result from multiple sclerosis or optic nerve gliomas. Homonymous hemianopia is due to lesions of the optic radiation posterior to the lateral geniculate body, such as stroke or cerebral palsy. Myopia (E) or short-sightedness is common and may be related to syndromes such as Marfan's syndrome.

Chronic steroid use

10 C This girl is having an Addisonian crisis. She has been on long-term corticosteroids and is therefore at high risk of having developed adrenal suppression. She has subsequently developed a urinary tract infection and the physiological response would be to increase endogenous steroid production. However, with her hypothalamic-pituitary-adrenal axis down-regulated due to her exogenous steroid use, this is not possible. She therefore is steroid depleted. She has hypotension, hypoglycaemia and is likely to develop hyperkalaemia and hyponatraemia. Cortisol (A) is likely to be low, but this will not change your management of her condition. Full blood count (B), urine culture (D) and blood culture (E) may help to elucidate the cause of the deterioration and treat it, but will not provide information about the Addisonian crisis. Renal function (C) is important to identify hyponatraemia and hyperkalaemia which may require treatment. Hydrocortisone and IV dextrose would be the initial treatment of choice, with antibiotics.

SECTION 22:
BONE AND
RHEUMATOLOGY

QUESTIONS

1. Immobile child (1)

A 3 year old is brought to accident and emergency by his parents because he has not been walking for the past day and refuses to stand. He is normally fit and healthy but he did have antibiotics for tonsillitis 2 weeks ago. They do not think he has had any injuries but he attends daycare and something could have happened there. He is up to date with his immunizations and his parents have no concerns with his development. On examination he looks well, is apyrexial, with a heart rate of 120 and respiratory rate of 26 with no bruising. His knees are normal on examination and the hips have a full range of movement except he cries on external rotation of the right hip. There are no deformities seen on x-ray of the hips and knees. After some paracetamol he manages to stand and take a few antalgic steps with encouragement, limping on the right leg. What is the most likely diagnosis?

    A.   Reactive arthritis
    B.   Non-accidental injury
    C.   Growing pains
    D.   Osteomyelitis
    E.   Septic arthritis

2. Joint pains

A 6-year-old girl is taken to see her GP because she is complaining of knee and elbow pains frequently. Her mother thinks it is worst after her ballet classes and when she gets home from school. She denies stiffness or pain in the mornings. Her mother has been administrating paracetamol several times a week and is worried that this is too much to be giving a child. On examination, the child looks well and has full range of movement of her joints with evidence of hyperextension. There are no swollen joints or effusions present and she is non-tender on examination. What is the most likely diagnosis?

    A.   Repetitive strain injury
    B.   Marfan's syndrome
    C.   Hypermobile joints
    D.   Osteoarthritis
    E.   Juvenile idiopathic arthritis (JIA)

3. Slipped femoral epiphysis

A 14-year-old slightly overweight boy is brought into accident and emergency from a football match where he slipped and fell but was unable to get back up due to pain in his right leg, which is now looking shortened and externally rotated. X-rays show the right femur to be disconnected from the femoral head almost completely at the level of the epiphysis. What is the most appropriate management?

A. Analgesia, nil by mouth until emergency internal fixation can be performed
B. Antibiotics and nil by mouth while waiting for an open reduction operation
C. Analgesia and bed rest with traction until healed
D. Analgesia and a hip spica cast
E. Reassure and mobilize with physiotherapy as tolerated

4. Greenstick fracture

What is a greenstick fracture?

A. The classic pattern of vertebral column fractures associated with abuse by being hit with a cane or 'green stick'
B. A fracture of the distal radius and ulna with dorsal displacement associated with a fall on the outstretched hand
C. A fracture of the distal radius and ulna with ventral displacement
D. A fracture of the long bones in young children where only one cortex is broken and the other is buckled
E. A fracture of the long bones in young children where the cortex is buckled on one side of the bone with no cortex separation on the opposite side

5. Recurrent fractures

A 2-year-old boy is brought to accident and emergency for the sixth time and is found to have a right-sided non-displaced transverse fracture of his tibia. His parents state that he was running in the living room and tripped landing on a toy truck. He has broken his other leg twice, several fingers and his right arm previously. He appears healthy, is well dressed and his growth is normal. His mother is very upset, she is 5 months pregnant with their second child and her anomaly scan yesterday suggested the baby has a broken leg. What is the most likely explanation for these fractures?

A. Osteogenesis imperfecta
B. Domestic violence and child abuse
C. Osteopetrosis
D. Achondroplasia
E. Clumsy child

6. Non-accidental injury

A 2-month-old baby is brought in by the babysitter because he has been crying since she arrived to look after him and his right leg looks swollen. He is the only child living in the household. She does not think he is moving it and is worried it is injured. On examination he is miserable, his heart rate is 160, respiratory rate of 56, and capillary refill is less than 2 seconds. He has a swollen right thigh. He cries more when that leg is examined. You note a yellow bruise on his left thigh and two purple bruises on either arm. X-rays show a fracture of the right femur but the arms appear intact. A chest x-ray shows three healing posterior rib fractures. You are highly suspicious of non-accidental injury. What is the most appropriate management?

- A. Give analgesia and plaster the leg fracture. Ask the babysitter to bring him back with the parents because he needs to be admitted
- B. Give analgesia. Call the duty social worker on-call to get permission to discharge him once his leg has been plastered
- C. Give analgesia and plaster the leg fracture. Contact the parents and inform them that he needs to be admitted. Ask them to come to the hospital and inform social services once they have arrived and been updated
- D. Give analgesia and plaster the leg fracture. Call the police to bring the parents to hospital
- E. Give analgesia and plaster the leg fracture. Call the police to arrest the babysitter for child abuse

7. Congenital hip dysplasia

On a newborn baby screening examination, you see a baby girl born by elective caesarean section for breech presentation. This is her mother's first child. The examination is normal except for a clunk felt on Barlow's test and a relocation click on Ortolani's manoeuvre on the right side. What is the next step in management?

- A. Refer to orthopaedics
- B. Arrange an ultrasound for 6 weeks of age
- C. Refer to physiotherapy
- D. Ask a midwife to put on a plaster hip spica
- E. Explain to the parents a watch and wait management is most appropriate as most self-resolve

8. Juvenile idiopathic arthritis

Which of the following is not a correct match?

- A. Systemic JIA – acute illness with daily fevers, malaise, failure to thrive, rash, muscle and joint aches for greater than 6 weeks associated with raised inflammatory markers

B. Extended oligoarthritis – an arthritis originally affecting one or two joints for the first 6 weeks and over time has spread to multiple joints

C. Psoriatic arthritis – presents with interphalangeal joint swelling, scaly skin rash, nail pitting and dactylitis

D. Polyarticular arthritis – more common in boys, affecting multiple small joints for more than 6 weeks

E. Enthesitis-related arthritis – associated with HLA-B27 tissue type, and presents in older boys with large joint arthritis, swollen tender tendons, sacro-iliitis and bamboo spine on x-ray. It is associated with anterior uveitis which if left untreated may cause blindness

9. Immobile child (2)

A 4 year old is brought to accident and emergency acutely unwell and refusing to walk for the past 2 days. Her parents are not aware of any recent injuries. On examination, she is pyrexial (T = 39.2°C), capillary refill 3 seconds centrally, heart rate 150 beats per minute, respiratory rate 40 breaths per minute. Her right thigh is swollen and slightly erythematous but too tender to examine fully. An x-ray of the hip and femur shows soft tissue swelling surrounding the proximal femur but the bones look normal. An urgent MRI shows a periosteal reaction in the proximal femur with extensive inflammation in the surrounding soft tissues. What is the most likely diagnosis?

A. Osteomyelitis
B. Non-accidental injury
C. Cellulitis
D. Reactive arthritis
E. Juvenile idiopathic arthritis

10. Weakness

A 5-year-old is referred to paediatrics due to concerns initially raised by his school teacher that he is weak and clumsy. On examination he has wasting of his quadriceps and walks in a waddling gait. His blood creatine kinase is 1600 mmol/L (normal is 24–190). What is the most likely diagnosis?

A. Muscular dystrophy
B. Neglect with failure to thrive
C. Malnutrition with failure to thrive
D. Acute myositis
E. Spinal muscular atrophy

ANSWERS

Immobile child (1)

1 A   The most likely answer is reactive arthritis (A) which typically follows an upper respiratory tract infection 1–2 weeks later, usually affecting the large weight bearing joints. This is unlikely to be osteomyelitis (D) or septic arthritis (E) because he is well and apyrexial. Having said this, a full blood count and differential and acute phase markers should be checked before concluding this is reactive arthritis. Growing pains (C) are usually more troublesome at night and do not stop children from weight bearing. Non-accidental injury (B) should always be kept in mind; however, he has no physical evidence of injury and the x-ray shows no fractures, making this less likely.

Joint pains

2 C   Her joint pain does not stop her from activities and she has normal joint assessment except for hyperextension of the joints, making the most likely cause of her joint pain being simply hypermobile joints (C). Sometimes physiotherapy may be helpful to strengthen the muscles supporting joints. While Marfan's syndrome (B) may feature hypermobile joints, it is not the most prominent feature and tall stature, high arched palate and long limbs should be present to suggest this as a possible diagnosis. There is no history to support repetitive strain injury (A) and a child's ballet class should not cause this. There are no swollen joints on examination to support a diagnosis of osteoarthritis (D) or JIA (E).

Slipped femoral epiphysis

3 A   This child has presented with a slipped upper femoral epiphysis, which is more common in teenage boys who are obese and often occurs with a minor injury. The management requires internal fixation (A) typically with a pin. It is rare for open reduction (B) to be used as this approach is associated with an increased incidence of avascular necrosis of the femoral head. Bed rest and traction (C) are not the best option as the risk of avascular necrosis is too high. The femur needs to be urgently pinned to the femoral head and therefore mobilization (E) is wrong. A hip spica cast (D) is used for developmental hip dysplasia.

Greenstick fracture

4 D   In young children the bones are soft and flexible so a forceful impact may bend the bone rather than break it. This results in a buckle in the cortex. In a torus fracture (E) only buckling of the cortex is seen just on one side of the long bone whereas in a greenstick fracture (D) a buckle is seen on one side with the opposite cortex interrupted. The greenstick fracture takes longer to heal than the torus fracture. A Colles fracture (B) results in the distal end of the ulna and radius sliding backwards and shortening; it is unusual in children and would more commonly occur through the growth plate, known as a Salter–Harris fracture. The reverse of a Colles fracture occurs in a Smith's fracture (C) with ventral displacement of the radial fragment. There is no classic fracture pattern of the spine associated with child abuse (A).

Recurrent fractures

5 A   Osteogenesis imperfecta (A), also known as brittle bone disease, is a collagen metabolism disorder which is typically autosomal dominantly inherited and has variable penetration where the most severe forms may develop fractures *in utero*. While risks for child abuse (B) should always be explored in any injury and repeated injuries are a worrying sign, this does not explain the fetus with a broken bone. Osteopetrosis (C) is an autosomal recessive disorder of dense brittle bones associated with frequent fractures, failure to thrive, recurrent infections, hypocalcaemia and thrombocytopenia. This is not the correct answer, as his growth is normal. Achondroplasia (D) results in short stature due to marked shortening of the limbs but is not associated with fractures. Stating that a child is clumsy (E) is not an adequate diagnosis to explain repeated injuries; either there is an underlying diagnosis as to why the child is so unsteady and injuring themselves repeatedly, or there is a bone abnormality or there is child abuse, all of which need to be investigated.

Non-accidental injury

6 C   The most appropriate action is to bring the parents to the hospital to take a full history (C). The child's safety is paramount and he should not be discharged until a full safety assessment is made and all of his injuries have been assessed and treated. Once the parents are there and have been updated it is then important to inform them of the social services referral, but they cannot refuse it. The child must be kept in a place of safety so discharge is not an option (A). The parents should be informed prior to social services referral (B) unless there are other children in the community that may also need protection, in which case, social services need to be informed and will liaise with the police to bring those children in to a place of safety. It would be inflammatory and counter-productive to bring the parents into hospital by police, although the police will be involved as part of child-safeguarding enquiries (D). There are injuries of several different ages on this child, different colour bruises and healing rib fractures making it unlikely that the babysitter is at fault (E), although it is important to keep an open mind regarding potential perpetrators. An accurate, well-documented history from each person who has cared for the child is crucial.

Congenital hip dysplasia

7 B   This child has several risk factors for developmental hip dysplasia: female, first child, breech presentation. Other risk factors include clubbed foot, family history of hip dysplasia, oligohydramnios and macrosomia. Barlow's examination of the hips involves pushing the flexed hip backwards testing for dislocation while the Ortolani test starts with the hips flexed and abducted: the examiner's fingers lift the greater trochanters forward in an attempt to relocate a dislocated hip; if a click is felt, the test is positive. The most appropriate management is to request an ultrasound as an outpatient follow-up at 6 weeks of age (B). This is a sensitive test, and waiting until 6 weeks improves the specificity as many unstable hips self-resolve. If the ultrasound is positive then a referral to orthopaedics (A) would be appropriate at that time. First line therapy would be a Pavlik harness which is put on by specially trained physiotherapists (C) and worn for 6 weeks. Midwives are not trained in administering plasters and a hip spica would be put on post-surgery when first line therapy has failed. Many services would ultrasound all babies with breech presentation even without clinical findings to support hip dysplasia. Left untreated this child may walk with a limp, never walk or develop avascular necrosis of the femoral head and therefore should be actively managed. A watch and wait management plan (E) is therefore inappropriate.

Juvenile idiopathic arthritis

8 D   All of the above definitions are true except for polyarticular arthritis (D) which is more common in girls and presents with symmetrical arthritis of the wrists, hands, ankles and knees. Occasionally the spine and jaw may be affected as well. By definition, polyarticular arthritis affects more than four joints at presentation for more than 6 weeks. Oligoarthritis (B) presents with less than five affected joints in the first 6 weeks and even if other joints become involved later it is still referred to as oligoarthritis but becomes extended. If the oligoarthritis persists beyond 6 months without extension to five or more joints it is called persistent. Option (A) is a classic description of systemic juvenile idiopathic arthritis, which should be considered in the differential diagnosis of prolonged fever in children, even when minimal or no joint symptoms or signs are evident. Option (C) is a classic description of the findings in psoriatic arthritis. Enthesitis-related arthritis (E) is also called juvenile spondylitis, and refers to inflammation of the entheses, which are the areas where tendon and other connecting tissues join to bone.

Immobile child (2)

9 A   This child's presentation is worrying for osteomyelitis (A) or septic arthritis, in view of the high fever, tachycardia, tachypnoea and a swollen painful leg. This is why the MRI was arranged so quickly. X-rays do not show osteomyelitis changes until about 2–3 weeks later, but the soft tissue swelling may be noticed. An MRI is required to see the inflammatory bone changes early on, which include periosteal reactions. If her x-ray showed a fracture with no known history of trauma, that would raise concerns of non-accidental injury (B), which would need to be explored further. This is not just cellulitis (C) as there is extensive involvement of the soft tissues and bone on the MRI. A reactive arthritis (D) would not present with a high fever and a systemically unwell child. If the hip were involved this would be a septic arthritis. The history is too short for juvenile idiopathic arthritis (E), which requires a 6-week history with no infection identified, and no MRI periosteal reactions supporting osteomyelitis.

Weakness

10 A   This child presents with a waddling gait and wasting of proximal muscles which points to a muscular dystrophy (A), which is strongly supported by the raised creatine kinase. You would expect a positive Gower's sign, in which the child is unable to get up from the floor without walking his hands up his legs for support. Spinal muscular atrophy (E) would present in infancy with decreased tone and the child would never be able to walk. There is no information in the question stem about the child's growth, and unless you are given serial weights and centiles it is impossible to say there is failure to thrive ((B) and (C)). There is no mention of pain, which makes acute myositis (D) an unlikely diagnosis.

SECTION 23:
NEUROLOGY

QUESTIONS

1. Febrile convulsion

A 3 year old is brought into accident and emergency by ambulance following a generalized tonic clonic seizure that lasted 2 minutes. She did not require any treatment to stop the seizure but on arrival the ambulance crew measured her temperature as 39.2°C and gave paracetamol. She is now apyrexial with a heart rate of 140, respiratory rate of 30 and capillary refill less than 2 seconds. On examination she has red enlarged tonsils with no pus, no neck stiffness or rash. What is the most appropriate management?

    A. Oral penicillin
    B. Lumbar puncture and IV ceftriaxone
    C. Explain that this was a febrile convulsion and discharge home
    D. Start phenytoin
    E. Discharge home with rescue buccal midazolam for future seizures

2. Altered consciousness

A 7 year old is referred to neurology due to frequent episodes of day-dreaming at school where she is unresponsive. She is falling behind in her work because of this. An electroencephalograph (EEG) shows three spike waves per second activity in all leads. What is the most likely diagnosis?

    A. Temporal lobe epilepsy
    B. Absence epilepsy
    C. Day-dreaming
    D. Benign Rolandic epilepsy
    E. Narcolepsy

3. Fainting

A mother brings her 2-year-old daughter to the GP on a Monday morning. Over the weekend she became very upset on being told 'no'. She was screaming and then held her breath, went blue and fainted. She woke up quickly and seemed okay afterwards. However, it has just happened again this morning when she found some scissors and her mother took them away. On this occasion she had a brief generalized convulsion lasting about 10 seconds. What is the most likely explanation?

    A. Breath holding attacks
    B. Reflex anoxic seizures
    C. Absence epilepsy
    D. Wolff–Parkinson–White syndrome
    E. Vasovagal syncope

4. Complications of emergency delivery

A mother with known placenta praevia with heavy vaginal bleeding was rushed into the labour ward and delivered by emergency caesarean section at 35 weeks' gestation. Pre-delivery the fetus was bradycardic and after birth APGARs were three at 1 minute, five at 5 minutes and nine at 10 minutes. Thirty-six hours later on the special care baby unit the baby is irritable and requiring nasogastric tube feeds as he is not sucking well. The tone in his upper limbs is reduced and an EEG showed seizure activity which has been controlled by intravenous phenobarbitone. His cranial ultrasound is normal. His blood sugar monitoring is between 3.5 and 5 mmol/L, C-reactive protein (CRP) was less than 5 mg/L and is 7 mg/L today. He is apyrexial. What is the most likely diagnosis?

    A.   Intraventricular haemorrhage
    B.   Group B streptococcal meningitis
    C.   Hypoglycaemia
    D.   Mild hypoxic ischaemic encephalopathy (HIE)
    E.   Moderate HIE

5. White matter lesions

A 15-year-old girl comes to accident and emergency complaining of sudden right arm weakness and double vision. Last week she was incontinent of urine twice. She is normally fit and well. On examination she has a left-sided 6th nerve palsy and four out of five power in her right arm. The examination is otherwise unremarkable. An MRI head shows multiple hyperintense, inflammatory, white matter lesions. What is the most likely diagnosis?

    A.   Brain metastasis
    B.   Multiple sclerosis
    C.   Tuberous sclerosis
    D.   Tuberculous meningitis
    E.   Neurofibromatosis

6. Depression/self-harm

A 15-year-old girl is brought into accident and emergency from school having disclosed to a friend that she took 10 paracetamol tablets last night. Her blood level of paracetamol is below the treatment line, her liver function tests and clotting are normal. Her father died of a brain tumour 3 years ago and her mother is being treated for reactive depression. The girl tells you that she has been feeling low lately, particularly because she does not think she will do well in her up-coming exams. She regrets taking the tablets and does not think she will do it again. What is the most appropriate management?

A. Admit for monitoring of liver function and Child and Adolescent Mental Health Services (CAMHS) assessment
B. Refer to CAMHS as an outpatient and discharge as not currently suicidal
C. Refer to Social Services
D. Start antidepressant – fluoxetine
E. Start IV Parvolex

7. Upper motor neuron (UMN) lesion

Which of the following is not a feature of a UMN lesion?

A. Slow-relaxing Achilles tendon reflex
B. Brisk reflexes
C. Increased tone
D. Decreased power
E. Up-going plantar reflex

8. Raised intracranial pressure (ICP)

Which for the following is not a feature of raised ICP?

A. Headache
B. Morning vomiting
C. Sun setting eyes
D. Bulging anterior fontanelle
E. Papilloedema

9. Sickle cell disease

A 10-year-old girl with sickle cell disease presents to her GP on Monday morning complaining of weakness in her right leg. She says she collapsed on Saturday afternoon and has not felt right since. What is the most likely diagnosis?

A. Sickle cell painful crisis
B. Parvovirus B19 infection
C. Aplastic crisis
D. Cerebral infarction
E. Osteomyelitis of the right femur

10. Cerebral palsy

A 6-year-old boy is registering with a new GP, having just moved to the area. He is in a wheelchair but is able to mobilize with a fast scissoring gait over short distances. He has increased tone in his legs and has scars from previous tendon release surgeries. His upper limbs are normal. His mother says that his school performance is good and he is writing well. She thinks he was going to have a Statement of Special Educational Needs assessment before they moved. As the GP, what is the most appropriate next step in management?

A. Reassure his mother that as he is doing well at school he does not need a statement
B. Refer to a community paediatrician
C. Refer to the physiotherapists and occupational therapists
D. Liaise with his new school teacher to make sure the school is able to support his physical needs
E. Refer to an educational psychologist

11. Headaches (1)

A 6-year-old boy is taken to see the GP by his mother because he has been getting severe abdominal pains, sometimes with vomiting and yesterday with a headache as well. He has no diarrhoea or constipation. His growth and examination are normal. He has no significant past medical history. In his family history, his maternal grandfather recently died of gastric cancer and mum's migraines have been worse since his death. She is worried her son is getting gastric cancer too. What is the most likely diagnosis?

A. Crohn's disease
B. Brain tumour
C. Somatization disorder
D. Gastric cancer
E. Coeliac disease

12. Anti-epileptic medication

Which of the following is not the correct side effect of anti-epileptic medicine?

A. Sodium valproate – aplastic anaemia
B. Carbamazepine – visual disturbance
C. Lamotrigine – rash
D. Vigabatrin – behavioural disturbance
E. Levetiracetam – anorexia

13. Headaches (2)

A 13-year-old Somali girl presents to accident and emergency with a 1-month history of headaches, weight loss and night sweats. Her father is concerned that she seems confused and is more unwell with her headache despite paracetamol. She was born in the UK and has had all her immunizations. She travelled to Somalia 6 months ago. The rest of the family is well although dad has a cough. On examination she is thin and looks unwell but is neurologically intact with no abnormal findings on clinical examination. Which diagnosis needs to be ruled out first?

A. Brain tumour
B. Tuberculous meningitis
C. Pulmonary tuberculosis

D. Migraines
E. HIV infection

14. Infantile spasms

A 4-month-old baby being investigated for infantile spasms is noted to have an ash leaf macule on his back under Wood's light. His EEG shows hypsarrythmia. The report of his MRI brain states there are subependymal nodules. What is the diagnosis?

A. Neurofibromatosis type I
B. Neurofibromatosis type II
C. West's syndrome
D. Tuberous sclerosis
E. Tay–Sachs disease

15. Neurocutaneous syndromes

A 3 month old is brought into accident and emergency with a generalized tonic clonic seizure. She is apyrexial and the seizure stopped after 15 minutes with rectal diazepam given by the ambulance crew. Her heart rate is 130, respiratory rate of 36 and capillary refill is less than 2 seconds. On examination she is drowsy, has a port wine stain on her forehead but is otherwise normal on examination. What is the most likely cause of her seizure?

A. Sturge–Weber syndrome
B. Tuberous sclerosis
C. Neurofibromatosis type I
D. Meningitis
E. Neurofibromatosis type II

ANSWERS

Febrile convulsion

1 C This is a typical febrile convulsion which are associated with rapid rises in temperature. The child is now stable and likely has a viral tonsillitis as the focus of infection. Parents need reassurance and explanation that febrile convulsions are not usually associated with later epilepsy but may recur in future febrile illnesses. Typically, children do not continue to have febrile convulsions beyond the age of 5 years. Management should be regular anti-pyretics and dress the child lightly during febrile illnesses. Oral penicillin (A) should be prescribed for bacterial tonsillitis, either with pus or if the child is unwell clinically. IV ceftriaxone and lumbar puncture (B) would be for suspected meningitis but this 3-year-old child has a clear focus for the fever, no neck stiffness or rash making this unlikely. In children having their first febrile convulsion under the age of 12 months, it is mandatory to rule out meningitis. Phenytoin (D) would be used for status epilepticus (seizure lasting longer than 30 minutes). Buccal midazolam (E) is used in the community for children who have seizures lasting longer than 5 minutes; febrile convulsions are usually short and unless a child has had a prolonged seizure they would not be sent home with rescue medication.

Altered consciousness

2 B This is a typical presentation of absence epilepsy (B). This form of epilepsy often does not affect school performance, but frequent seizures interrupt the directions or information she receives at school and may contribute to her falling behind in her work. The EEG shows three spike waves per second in all leads, which is diagnostic for absence seizures. Temporal lobe epilepsy (A) would show an EEG with seizure activity in the temporal lobes and classically presents with a warning aura or sensation, impaired consciousness or unresponsiveness, and a focal seizure which may spread to become a generalized tonic clonic seizure. In day-dreaming (C), the person is responsive if called. Benign Rolandic epilepsy (D) causes partial seizures which usually occur in the early morning and affect young children, typically resolving in the teens. Narcolepsy (E) is a sleep disorder where affected persons spontaneously fall asleep at inappropriate times.

Fainting

3 A Breath holding attacks (A) are not uncommon in toddlers at times of temper tantrums. They grow out of them and no treatment is required. Parents need to be reassured that the brief seizure is not harmful. A reflex anoxic seizure (B) typically occurs when a child is frightened or hurt, such as a bump to the head. The child goes pale and faints, hypoxia may cause a short seizure, but the child quickly recovers. Absence epilepsy (C) presents with short vacant periods where the child is unresponsive, followed sometimes by a brief period of confusion when they are aware they have missed something. Wolff–Parkinson–White syndrome is associated with a spontaneous onset re-entry tachycardia or supraventricular tachycardia which may lead to dizziness, shortness of breath and sometimes fainting. An ECG would show a delta wave. Vasovagal syncope, or a simple faint, is associated with standing for long periods of time in warm environments.

Complications of emergency delivery

4 E   This child has experienced an hypoxic insult perinatally during his mother's haemorrhage and is now showing signs of HIE: poor feeding, altered tone and seizure activity on EEG. Mild HIE (D) presents with irritability, startle responses, poor feeding and hyperventilation. Moderate HIE (E) also has altered tone or reduced movement and seizure activity. While ischaemic changes early on may be difficult to see on cranial ultrasound, intraventricular haemorrhage (A) is easily seen and is associated with both hypoxic insults and a cause of seizures in the neonate. This child's cranial ultrasound was normal. Group B streptococcal meningitis (B) is a serious and life-threatening illness for the neonate and may cause seizures. It is therefore routine practice to treat unwell neonates with antibiotics, but the exposure for this infant is reduced as the delivery was a caesarean section and the CRP has been normal twice, making this an unlikely explanation for this illness. Hypoglycaemia (C) is also a cause of seizures in neonates but the definition is lower in this age group (below 2.5 mmol/L) so this child is not hypoglycaemic.

White matter lesions

5 B   She has presented with neurology consistent with multiple lesions. All of the options may cause more than one lesion in the brain but multiple sclerosis (MS) (B) classically affects the white matter with demyelinating lesions which are inflamed, as seen in this case. Brain metastasis (A) and tuberculosis (D) would typically cause space occupying lesions with surrounding oedema. In tuberous sclerosis (C), the MRI typically shows subependymal calcifications and hypointense white matter lesions or tubers. Neurofibromatosis (E) may cause gliomas or acoustic neuromas which would be seen as a space occupying lesion. The MRI taken together with a history of intermittent and sudden changes in neurological function, especially vision and urinary incontinence, point towards the diagnosis of MS.

Depression/self-harm

6 A   She should be admitted for observation until CAMHS have assessed her (A) and created a follow-up plan. As she presented after the window of intervention for her overdose, her liver function should be monitored.

While she denies feeling suicidal now, it is important that she be risk-assessed by mental health services and be discharged with a safety net that she can access if her feelings are driving her to repeat self-harm activities. She should therefore not be discharged (B). Social Services (C) may be required if it is felt that the mother's depression is leading to issues of neglect, and sometimes Social Services and CAMHS will see patients together but this is more common with illicit drug or alcohol misuse. An antidepressant would not be the first line treatment for adolescent depression and she should first be assessed by CAMHS. Parvolex (E) is used to treat and reverse the toxicity of paracetamol; however it is ineffective beyond 15 hours post-overdose.

Upper motor neuron (UMN) lesion

7 A   Slow-relaxing reflexes may be a sign of a systemic illness such as hypothyroidism or lower motor neuron diseases such as Guillain–Barré syndrome. Increased reflexes (B) and tone (C), decreased power (D) and up-going plantar responses (E) are all features of UMN lesions.

Raised intracranial pressure (ICP)

8 D   All of these options are associated with intracranial pathology but a bulging anterior fontanelle occurs when there is increased fluid in the brain in a young child before the fontanelle closes; thus there will be no raised ICP as the open fontanelle provides a space for the extra fluid. In an older child with the same underlying pathology and a closed fontanelle, the result is raised ICP. Symptoms and signs may include: headache (A), morning vomiting (B), sun setting eyes (C) (a late sign of raised ICP caused by pressure on cranial nerves III, IV and VI) and papilloedema (again a late sign of raised ICP).

Sickle cell disease

9 D   Here the worrying and important diagnosis to rule out is a stroke (D). Sickle cell patients are at risk of stroke, especially if their sickle cell percentage is above 30 per cent of the total red blood cell population. She is not complaining of pain in her leg, just weakness; therefore this is not a painful crisis (A) or osteomyelitis (E). Sickle cell patients with parvovirus B19 infection (B) are at risk of an aplastic crisis (C) with associated secondary infections, bleeding and severe anaemia, but these would not explain her symptoms.

Cerebral palsy

10 B   This child has diplegic cerebral palsy and needs multidisciplinary support to manage his care. He should have a formal statement to create a plan of what physical support he will need for school, so (A) is wrong. The community paediatrician (B) is best placed to coordinate this process, although assessments by physiotherapists and occupational therapists (C), liaison with the school (D), and educational psychology (E) reports will be needed. In addition he will need to be referred to orthopaedic specialists and possibly Social Services to assess eligibility for grants to adapt the home.

Headaches (1)

11 C This child presents with abdominal pain, sometimes with vomiting or associated headache, with a family history of migraine and distinct psychological triggers, making the most likely diagnosis a somatization disorder (C). This term encompasses various different descriptive terms such as abdominal migraine, recurrent abdominal pain, non-organic pain, functional pain and irritable bowel syndrome. Children may experience migraines as abdominal pain and as they get older they develop more classical migraine headaches. Crohn's disease (A) would usually present in an older child (but can occur in this age group) with changes in bowel habit and failure to thrive. There is often a family history, which is not present in this case. A brain tumour (B) would be more likely to present with headaches rather than abdominal pain as well as having neurological signs and symptoms. Gastric cancer (D) is very rare in children but would have features of poor appetite and weight loss as well. Coeliac disease (E) usually presents with abdominal distension, diarrhoea and failure to thrive.

Anti-epileptic medication

12 A Sodium valproate (A) side effects include increased appetite, weight gain, hair loss and liver failure, but not aplastic anaemia. Carbamazepine (B) is associated with lupus erythematosus syndrome, dizziness and visual disturbances. Lamotrigine (C) is associated with rash, behavioural changes and irritability. Vigabatrin (D) side effects include behavioural changes, retinopathy, sleep disturbance and weight gain. Levetiracetam (Keppra) is associated with anorexia, abdominal pain, vomiting, diarrhoea, behavioural changes and thrombocytopenia.

Headaches (2)

13 B A brain tumour (A) is unlikely with a normal neurological examination. She has weight loss and night sweats which should raise a suspicion of tuberculosis (TB), which is particularly common in the Somali community. There is no specific history of cough and more concerning is her headache and confusion, making the most likely diagnosis tuberculous meningitis (B). She should have a lumbar puncture, provided there are no signs of raised ICP. A chest x-ray would be performed routinely in this case to look for pulmonary TB (C). While migraines (D) may be very troublesome and frequent, they do not cause weight loss and night sweats and investigations for lymphoma or tuberculosis should always be carried out when these symptoms are present. Patients diagnosed with TB should be screened for HIV (E) co-infection, but this does not need to be done immediately as it will not change the initial management.

Infantile spasms

14 D Ash leaf macules are a skin manifestation of tuberous sclerosis (D) and the typical MRI findings of this are subependymal nodules. Tuberous sclerosis is a cause of infantile spasms, associated with hypsarrythmia on EEG, which are treated with vigabatrin. Seizures do occur in neurofibromatosis ((A) and (B)) but are much less common and not usually associated with any imaging changes. West's syndrome (C) is a syndrome of infantile spasms and developmental regression, one cause of which is tuberous sclerosis. As you are given no information on this child's development, West's syndrome is not the best answer when there is clear evidence to support the cause as tuberous sclerosis. Tay–Sachs disease (E) is an autosomal recessive deficiency of hexosaminidase A and presents with seizures, developmental regression, deafness, progressive loss of motor function and increased tone, which is most common in Ashkenazi Jewish populations.

Neurocutaneous syndromes

15 A A port wine stain is a flat purple haemangioma which is present from birth. Any baby born with a port wine stain in the trigeminal region or in the hair should have an MRI brain to look for intracranial haemangiomas as they are at risk of epilepsy. This is called Sturge–Weber syndrome (A). Tuberous sclerosis (B) causes infantile spasms which are brief tonic movements sometimes called 'salaam attacks' as a description of the movement and often mistaken for infant colic. Neurofibromatosis ((C) and (E)) rarely causes seizures so this would not be the most likely cause. A child with meningitis (D) which has caused a seizure would be unwell with fever and possibly evidence of shock, whereas this child has a normal capillary refill, a normal heart rate and is apyrexial.

PART III
PSYCHIATRY

SECTION 24: PSYCHOPATHOLOGY AND CLASSIFICATION IN PSYCHIATRY

QUESTIONS

1. Disturbances of memory (1)

A 79-year-old woman with a diagnosis of Alzheimer's disease is causing concern as she is constantly getting lost on the way back from the local shop to her home, which is only a short walk and one that she has done nearly every day for 20 years. What sort of memory disturbance does this represent?

    A.   Autobiographical memory
    B.   Episodic memory
    C.   Procedural memory
    D.   Semantic memory
    E.   Topographical memory

2. Disturbances of memory (2)

A 72-year-old woman who suffers from Alzheimer's disease is asked who the Prime Minister was during the Second World War, to which she replies 'Winston Churchill'. She is then asked where she lived during the war, to which she answers 'Winston Churchill'. What phenomenon is being described here?

    A.   Confabulation
    B.   Déjà vu
    C.   Ganser's syndrome
    D.   Jamais vu
    E.   Perseveration

3. Disturbances of perception (1)

A young woman wakes from a nightmare and sees her dressing gown hanging from the door, which she mistakes as an assailant. What is being described here?

    A.   Affect illusion
    B.   Completion illusion
    C.   Pareidolic illusion
    D.   Tactile hallucination
    E.   Visual hallucination

4. Disturbances of perception (2)

A young man with schizophrenia describes how he can hear the secret service in their base in Finland discussing their plans to assassinate him. What is this phenomenon known as?

A. Extracampine hallucination
B. Functional hallucination
C. Hypnagogic hallucination
D. Hypnopompic hallucination
E. Reflex hallucination

5. Disorders of thinking (1)

A 28-year-old man is diagnosed with schizophrenia, with the belief that he has
been targeted for extermination by a religious cult who have implanted tiny
electrical 'ants' into his fingernails. When asked when he knew this, he said he had
seen a magazine story 3 months ago on 'retiring to the country' and immediately
felt this was a covert message from the cult that he should be 'retired'. There was
no evidence of delusions prior to this. What is being described here?

A. Autochthonous (primary) delusion
B. Autoscopy
C. Delusional atmosphere
D. Delusional memory
E. Delusional perception

6. Disorders of thinking (2)

A 48-year-old man with poorly controlled schizophrenia is admitted to the ward.
He appears confused and he is difficult to interview. On asking him why he is in
hospital, he replies, 'Jealousy, the Collaborative, collaborate and dissipate. What's
in my fridge? It isn't my time'. How would you describe this type of thinking?

A. Circumstantial
B. Derailment
C. Flight of ideas
D. Pressure of speech
E. Thought blocking

7. First-rank symptoms of schizophrenia

Which of the following is not a first-rank symptom of schizophrenia as described
by Schneider?

A. Delusional perception
B. Persecutory delusions
C. Running commentary — 3rd order   hallucination
D. Somatic passivity
E. Thought alienation

8. Disorders of speech

A 72-year-old man with Parkinson's dementia is seen in clinic. He is asked how he is feeling, to which he replies, 'I feel fantastic...tic...tic...tic...tic...'. What is the name for this type of speech abnormality?

    A.   Alogia
    B.   Dysarthria
    C.   Echolalia
    D.   Logoclonia
    E.   Neologism

9. Disorders of body image

A 26-year-old man is seen by his GP. For the last few months, he has become increasingly concerned about a mole on his cheek, which he feels has got bigger and people are noticing it more. Over the last week he has become convinced that people are laughing at it when he passes them. He has a thought in his head of 'you're so ugly, look at the size of that mole'. The patient does not feel he knows where the thought comes from, but it does not seem to be his. He wonders if someone has planted the thought there. The GP does not feel the mole is in any way abnormally sized or has other unusual features. What is the most likely aetiology of these symptoms?

    A.   Compulsion
    B.   Delusion
    C.   Hallucination
    D.   Rumination
    E.   Somatization

10. Symptoms of depression

Which of the following is not a core symptom of depression as defined by ICD-10?

    A.   Anergia
    B.   Anhedonia
    C.   Anorexia
    D.   Hyperphagia
    E.   Insomnia

11. Classification of stress disorders (1)

A 42-year-old man sees his GP after witnessing a horrific motorway pile-up. For the last 6 weeks he has been experiencing recurrent and intrusive images of the event where he relives what happened, both at night and during the day. At night he is also having vivid nightmares about the crash which is now stopping him from going to sleep. He has not driven his car since, although he himself was not involved in the crash. Every time a car starts he jumps and becomes extremely upset. His mood is low and he feels disconnected from his wife and children and he has been thinking about killing himself. What symptom is not being described here?

A. Avoidance
B. Detachment
C. Insomnia
D. Increased arousal
E. Night terrors

12. Classification of stress disorders (2)

What is the most likely diagnosis in the case described in the previous question?

A. Acute stress reaction
B. Adjustment disorder
C. Depressive episode
D. Dissociative fugue
E. Post-traumatic stress disorder (PTSD)

13. Psychopathology of catatonia

A 49-year-old woman with schizophrenia is admitted to the psychiatric unit in a mute state. She is staring blankly ahead and not responding to any commands. She is not eating or drinking and looks dehydrated. Which of the following is the least likely to be observed in catatonia?

A. Catalepsy
B. Clanging
C. Echolalia
D. Negativism
E. Stupor

14. Classification systems in psychiatry

Which of the following statements regarding the two classification systems in psychiatry (ICD-10 and DSM-IV) is false? Note this refers specifically to the section in ICD-10 related to psychiatry and mental health.

A. Dementia cannot be classified in either of the two systems
B. DSM-IV uses a multiaxial system
C. Homosexuality is no longer a diagnostic category in the two systems
D. ICD-10 was developed by the World Health Organization (WHO)
E. The first categories in ICD-10 are those related to organic disorders

15. Psychopathology of thought and speech

Which of the following would be the best definition of the term 'loosening of associations'?

A. A decrease in the amount of words produced by a patient
B. An incompleteness of the development of ideas or thoughts, leading to a lack of logical relationship between them

C. Difficulty in verbalizing names of objects, despite being able to describe their function
D. Talking in a roundabout manner before finally answering a question
E. The creation of a new word with particular meaning to the patient

ANSWERS

Disturbances of memory (1)

1 E As the name suggests, the inability to orientate oneself represents a failure of topographical memory (E) which is fairly common in dementia. Autobiographical memory (A) refers to specific events and issues related to oneself such as one's 60th birthday or the birth of one's grandchild. Episodic memory (B) is essentially analagous to autobiographical memory. Procedural memory (C) is also known as 'implicit memory' (whereas autobiographical would be 'explicit') and refers to the memory or knowledge of 'how to do things'. These are accessed unconsciously – motor skills (such as driving) would fall into this category for example. Semantic memory (D) refers to our 'knowledge base' and is unrelated to specific experiences or events – for example, knowing your nine times table or what the capital of Australia is.

Disturbances of memory (2)

2 E Perseveration (E) is seen almost exclusively in organic brain disease, for example dementia. It involves giving an appropriate response to a stimulus the first time but then giving the same response (incorrectly) to a different second stimulus. Note, it is not limited to verbal statements, but may also occur with, for example, motor activity. Confabulation (A) is the phenomenon whereby false memories occur and results in incorrect answers being given. It is a complex concept, may result from the sufferer trying to 'cover up' not knowing the real answer and may be confused with deliberate attempts to deceive, or as is often seen in organic brain disease, the sufferer inventing 'fantastical' answers, which may be difficult to separate from delusions. Déjà vu (B) refers to the phenomenon whereby the person feels the sense of familiarity of having encountered an event before, even though it is a new experience for them. It may be a feature of temporal lobe epilepsy but is seen in non-pathological states and does not always indicate organic disease. Ganser's syndrome (C) is an unusual phenomenon whereby people give 'approximate' answers, among other symptoms, such as, 'How many legs does a cow have?' 'Five'. It has caused considerable debate as to whether it represents an organic psychotic disorder or a dissociative disorder. Jamais vu (D) refers to the sensation that a familiar event or place has never been encountered before.

Disturbances of perception (1)

3 A An illusion is a misinterpretation of a perception, as opposed to a hallucination, in which a new perception is experienced in the absence of a stimulus. Illusions are not usually pathological. An affect illusion (A) is one in which a perception is altered depending on the mood state; in this case a frightened woman wakes suddenly and misinterprets a hanging piece of clothing for an attacker. A completion illusion (B) occurs when there is a lack of attention, and a perception is 'incorrectly' interpreted, for example skipping over a misprint in a book because we are tired. Pareidolic illusions (C) consist of shapes being seen in other objects – the classic example being seeing images such as animals in cloud formations. In contrast to other illusions, pareidolic illusions become more vivid with concentration. A tactile hallucination (D) refers to a tactile ('touch') sensation in the absence of a stimulus. This scenario does not represent a visual hallucination (E) as the stimulus is real (the dressing gown), but it has been misinterpreted. Had there been no dressing gown and the woman had still seen an assailant, this may then have represented a visual hallucination.

Disturbances of perception (2)

4 A   An extracampine hallucination (A) is one which occurs beyond the usual range of sensation, in this case, beyond the limits of audibility – there is no possibility that the patient would be able to hear anyone speaking from Finland. These are definite hallucinations as the patient is hearing them, rather than them constituting delusional beliefs. A functional hallucination (B) occurs when a hallucination is experienced only when an external stimulus is present in the same modality. An example may be a patient hearing voices only when he hears classical music. Note that although the stimulus and the hallucination are in the same modality, they do not have to take the same form, e.g. in the example just given the stimulus is music, while the hallucination is voices. Hypnagogic (C) and hypnopompic (D) hallucinations refer to those that occur on falling asleep and waking respectively, and may occur in non-pathological states. An example would be the feeling of falling off a cliff when falling asleep. Reflex hallucinations (E) are similar to functional hallucinations but the stimulus is in a different modality to the hallucination, for example, a woman with schizophrenia hearing voices every time her child looks at her.

Disorders of thinking (1)

5 E   A delusional perception (E) occurs when a normal perception (e.g. seeing a magazine cover) is invested with a delusional meaning (a cult is trying to kill me). The perception is given a whole new false, and usually bizarre, meaning that is specific to the patient and nearly always of monumentous importance. An autochthonous delusion (A) is one that arises out of the blue (and unlike delusional perception is not attached to a real stimulus). It should be distinguished from secondary delusions in which the beliefs are understandable in the context of the sufferer's mood or history (e.g. a mood-congruent depressive delusion). A primary delusion is by definition un-understandable in any context. Autoscopy (B) refers to the sensation of seeing oneself, although its aetiology and precise psychopathology is controversial. Delusional atmosphere (C), also known as delusional mood, refers to the state of perplexity or bewilderment in which sufferers feel that something is 'going on' but without being able to state exactly what. It often occurs prior to a delusion forming and the sufferer will often describe feeling odd and that everything around them has new 'meanings' and significance to them in particular. Delusional memory (D) is when a patient recalls an event from the past and interprets it with a delusional meaning. Although this may seem similar to the answer 'E', the difference is that the event at the time will not have been invested with a delusional interpretation; it is only afterwards that this occurs.

Disorders of thinking (2)

6 B Derailment (B) is a type of formal thought disorder in which there are disjointed thoughts with no meaningful connections. It is commonly seen in schizophrenia, but also presents sometimes in other disorders. Circumstantial thinking (A) is somewhat difficult to describe but occurs when the person talks around a subject exhaustively with only loosely relevant associations. They will usually return to the point but only after many detours of almost irrelevant (or certainly over-inclusive) information. Flight of ideas (C) occurs when thinking is accelerated – associations between ideas are logical to an extent, but the 'goal' of thinking changes rapidly, usually because of poor attention as a result of a manic state. Pressure of speech (D) is the 'verbal' description of this acceleration (whereas flight of ideas refers to the speed of thoughts as opposed to speech). Thought blocking (E) occurs most commonly in schizophrenia and manifests as the patient suddenly stopping in mid-sentence without them being able to explain why. It is not the same as thought withdrawal, in which the patient believes an external agency is removing thoughts from their head.

First-rank symptoms of schizophrenia

7 B Persecutory delusions (B) are certainly seen in schizophrenia but they do not form part of the core of 'first-rank' symptoms that Schneider described as core to the diagnosis. It should be noted that these symptoms are not pathognomonic of schizophrenia as they have also been observed in other disorders (e.g. 20 per cent of those with biploar disorder). Not everyone with schizophrenia has 'first-rank' symptoms. Delusional perception (A) has been described above and is a first-rank symptom. Running commentary (C) refers to third-person auditory hallucinations in which one or more voices discuss in great detail what the person is doing as they do it. Other types of auditory hallucination designated as first-rank include audible thoughts, in which the patient's thoughts are 'spoken out loud', and voices heard arguing with each other. Somatic passivity (D) is the symptom whereby patients feel that their body is being controlled by an external source. While it may be present along with somatic or tactile hallucinations, in itself it is a delusional belief, not a hallucination. Other first-rank passivity phenomena include passivity of emotions or impulses. Thought alienation (E) is similar to the above but involves the patient's thoughts rather than impulses or feelings. People may feel that their thoughts are being planted (thought insertion), taken away (thought withdrawal) or played out loud (thought broadcasting).

Disorders of speech

8 D   Logoclonia (D) describes the symptom of repeating the last syllable of a word repeatedly and is often seen in Parkinson's disease. It has a different aetiology to stammering or the tics seen in Tourette's syndrome. Alogia (A) is the phenomenon of 'not having any words' and refers to extreme poverty of speech. It is commonly seen in severe negative schizophrenia or dementia. Dysarthria (B) refers to a difficulty in the manufacture of speech, and is usually caused by structural lesions either in the vocal cords or the brainstem. Echolalia (C) is the phenomenon whereby words or sentences that the patient hears are repeated back, sometimes continuously and incessantly. It often has an organic cause such as dementia or brain injury but may also be seen in functional disorders such as schizophrenia. Neologisms (E) are new words created by the patient that have a specific meaning for them, usually involved with their delusional beliefs. It is not the same as using a known word in a different way (known as metonymy). For example, when describing the machine used to trace his whereabouts, a man with schizophrenia referred to it as a 'Labulizer'.

Disorders of body image

9 B   This is a difficult question, but actually one that is seen with some regularity by GPs and psychiatrists. The key features here that make this most likely to be a delusion (B) is the thought that people are looking at him excessively, coupled with the intrusive thought that is not his own. In a rumination (D), the patient would recognize the thought as being their own. It is not a hallucination (C) because the thought is not spoken out loud. A compulsion (A) represents a repetitive act, driven by obsessive anxiety. Somatization (E) refers to physical symptoms that manifest as the result of intrapsychic anxiety with no adequate physical explanation. Usually these patients end up having exhaustive negative medical investigations and refuse to accept that there is nothing physical to be found. The important point of this question is that it would be easy to mistake this for obsessive–compulsive disorder or dysmorphophobia. Always assess for more 'sinister' symptoms such as psychosis as they can sometimes be hidden beneath more obvious diagnoses.

Symptoms of depression

10 D Hyperphagia (D), or increased consumption of food, is not a core symptom of depression according to ICD-10, although it certainly can be seen in depressive disorders, and forms part of the criteria for atypical depression. Anergia (A), or lack of energy, is a core symptom of depression, although obviously is non-specific. Anhedonia (B), or lack of enjoyment or inability to experience pleasure, is perhaps even more common than anergia. Anorexia (C) as a symptom means lack of appetite and most certainly does occur in depression – this should not be confused with anorexia nervosa which is a specific condition. Insomnia (E), particularly in the form of early morning wakening, is a common and extremely distressing symptom of depression. Do not underestimate how disabling lack of sleep can be for depression sufferers.

Classification of stress disorders (1)

11 E Night terrors (E) are not the same as nightmares, and they do not occur in rapid eye movement sleep – the sufferer (who is usually a child) does not tend to remember any bad dreams, but will awake from sleep in a state of abject terror and confusion, often shouting and sometimes lashing out. Hypnopompic hallucinations are common on waking, particularly seeing insects. Avoidance symptoms (A) are evident here in the form of the patient not wanting to drive his car. Detachment (B) is also present in feeling disconnected from his wife and children. A feeling of derealization or depersonalization may also occur, in which the sufferer feels in some way removed from the world around him or even from his own body. Insomnia is present (C) as the patient is purposefully not sleeping from fear of the nightmares. Note insomnia may be 'induced' by the patient in this way, it does not necessarily mean the person is trying to sleep. There is evidence of increased arousal (D) in terms of jumping at the sound of car engines.

Classification of stress disorders (2)

12 E Note that the symptoms have been present for more than 1 month which is required for a diagnosis of PTSD (E). The criteria for diagnosis include exposure to a potentially life-threatening event, re-experiencing of the event in various ways such as nightmares or flashbacks, avoidance of stimuli that recall the event (e.g. driving) and increased arousal such as hypervigilance, increased startle reaction, insomnia and sometimes irritability and anger. Depressive symptoms (C) are also extremely common, but the diagnosis here is clearly one with a stressful precipitant. An acute stress (A) reaction must subside within hours or days of a stressful event and results in disorientation and confusion in response to the stressor. Panic and other symptoms of anxiety commonly occur. Adjustment disorders (B) occur in response to a significant and stressful change in life circumstances or events, such as bereavement or emigration. The main symptoms are those of depression or anxiety along with an inability to cope with daily tasks. A dissociative fugue (D) is one of the dissociative or conversion disorders, in which either the body or mind in some way lose their normal integration. They usually resolve after weeks or months and are manifestations of intrapsychic stress. They were originally known as 'hysterical' disorders but the term is no longer used because of its sexist overtones. In a dissociative fugue, the sufferer will have a period of amnesia during which he or she will travel, often for long distances, and certainly beyond their usual range of travel. Despite this they often appear normal to passers-by.

Psychopathology of catatonia

13 B Clanging (B) is a form of thought disorder whereby words are used based on their similar sounds or rhyming and the meaning becomes unimportant. For example, 'A cat pat on my hat sack, ate the bait and skated'. It is seen in schizophrenia but would not be a typical feature of catatonia. Catatonia is a state of either stupor in which a patient is entirely unresponsive (E) or excited. It is associated with various conditions, not just schizophrenia, and its exact cause is not known. It appears to be less common than 50 years ago, but the reason for this is not clear. Catatonia can be associated with various symptoms, including catalepsy (A), in which the limbs become rigid. Sometimes patients' limbs can be moved into unusual positions and will remain in place even if extremely uncomfortable. This is known as waxy flexibility. Catalepsy should not be confused with cataplexy, in which there is sudden and transient loss of muscle tone resulting in collapse. Echolalia (C) is the phenomenon whereby sufferers repeat the words of those speaking to them. Remember that not all catatonic patients are mute, and echolalia is often found in these patients. Negativism (D) is the symptom whereby catatonic patients will appear to automatically do the opposite of what they are asked to do. This is not just resisting instructions or movement but actually attempting to perform the opposite instruction or movement.

Classification systems in psychiatry

14 A Dementia (A) can certainly be classified in both ICD-10 and DSM-IV, although the various subtypes of dementia are not necessarily accurately definable. For instance, Lewy body dementia is not represented in ICD (or at least not in the section related to psychiatric disorders, it is mentioned in the neurological disease section, but this is not usually used in mental health settings). DSM-IV is a multiaxial system (B), in other words a diagnosis will be made up of several different axes. These are: Axis 1 – clinical disorders, Axis 2 – personality disorders and learning disability, Axis 3 – acute medical conditions and physical disorders, Axis 4 – psychosocial and environmental factors contributing to the disorder, and Axis 5 – global assessment of functioning. In this way it differs from ICD-10 which uses only a single category per diagnosis. Homosexuality was, to many people's surprise, still included in the ICD (European) system until 1990 and the DSM (American) system until 1986. It can still be found vestigially as a category relating to 'ego-dystonic sexual orientation' in ICD-10. ICD-10 (D) is a WHO system of coding diseases, symptoms, social circumstances and injuries. The first categories in ICD-10 (E) are related to organic disorders (F00–F09). There has been some attempt by ICD-10 to classify disorders 'hierachically', with organic disorders needing to be excluded first and therefore placed first. This, however, is just one of the many various controversies surrounding the classification systems used currently in psychiatry, the scope of which is well beyond this book.

Psychopathology of thought and speech

15 B Loosening of associations (B) is seen in schizophrenia. It has various definitions but fundamentally describes a form of thought disorder in which links between ideas become illogical. (A) describes alogia and is seen in chronic schizophrenia among other disorders. (C) is a definition of nominal dysphasia, seen in dementia, stroke and other organic disorders. (D) refers to circumstantiality, often seen in hypomanic states. (E) is the definition for a neologism, which is most usually seen in schizophrenia.

SECTION 25:
ORGANIC PSYCHIATRY

Questions

QUESTIONS

1. Causes of delirium

A man is admitted to accident and emergency after being found semi-conscious in the street. He is unkempt and does not have any information on his person; he appears to be street homeless. In accident and emergency he has a tonic clonic seizure which is self-limiting after 3 minutes. The man is post-ictal for a short time but soon becomes restless, tremulous and sweaty. His speech is rambling, and he complains about the bed sheets being filthy and 'filled with mites'. He is tachycardic with a blood pressure of 186/114 mmHg. What is the most likely diagnosis?

    A.   Alcoholic hallucinosis
    B.   Delirium tremens
    C.   Cocaine withdrawal
    D.   Diabetic ketoacidosis
    E.   Opiate overdose

2. Investigation of delirium

You order a full set of bloods on this man. Which of the following results would be most indicative of the underlying cause of his delirium?

    A.   Elevated serum glucose
    B.   Elevated serum potassium
    C.   Low mean corpuscular volume (MCV)
    D.   Low serum vitamin B12
    E.   Raised platelets

3. Management of delirium

A 73-year-old woman is admitted to hospital with an infective exacerbation of chronic obstructive pulmonary disease (COPD). Apart from COPD and hypertension she has no other medical problems. On the third day of her admission, she becomes acutely confused. During the night she is awake, shouting constantly for her husband, claiming that the nurses are prison guards and that they are keeping her against her will. She is slightly calmer the day after. You are the FY1 on call and are asked to come and see her over the weekend as the nurses are worried it will happen again at night. What should your initial management be?

    A.   Prescribe clozapine 25 mg bd regularly
    B.   Prescribe haloperidol 2 mg intravenously immediately
    C.   Prescribe lorazepam 0.5 mg orally just before bedtime

    D.   Prescribe lorazepam 0.5 mg orally twice daily regularly

    E.   Prescribe nothing at this stage

4. Pharmacological causes of organic depression

Which of the following medications is most likely to be associated with an organic depressive disorder?

    A.   Prednisolone

    B.   Sertraline

    C.   Thyroxine

    D.   Tramadol

    E.   Tryptophan

5. Focal cerebral disorders

A 27-year-old man is involved in a road traffic accident. During rehabilitation his family have become very upset as they feel he has 'changed'. They report that his concentration is poor and at times he is saying very hurtful things to his wife, which they say is extremely out of character. He has also begun eating large quantities of junk food, whereas before he was extremely fit and careful with his diet. Which part of the brain is most likely to have suffered an injury?

    A.   Basal ganglia

    B.   Frontal lobe

    C.   Limbic structures

    D.   Parietal lobe

    E.   Occipital lobe

6. Neurological signs and psychiatric symptoms

A 28-year-old woman is admitted to hospital systemically very unwell, with a reduced level of consciousness, headache, fever, nausea and vomiting and dysphasia. This is followed by several seizures. Initial cerebrospinal fluid (CSF) analysis shows the CSF is clear, with raised protein, raised mononuclear cell count, no polymorphs and normal glucose. Her partner says that for the preceding few days she had been acting strangely, seeing things that were not there, accusing him of leaving the gas on and getting very agitated. She then became drowsy and he called the ambulance. Your initial management should be based on which being the most likely diagnosis?

    A.   Bacterial meningitis

    B.   Herpes simplex encephalitis

    C.   Neuropsyphilis

    D.   Sporadic Creutzfeld–Jakob disease (CJD)

    E.   Temporal lobe epilepsy

7. Metabolic causes of psychiatric symptoms

A 76-year-old man with squamous cell lung carcinoma attends accident and emergency with his wife who is his full-time carer. She has become concerned as he has become extremely depressed over the last couple of weeks, along with being extremely thirsty and having little energy. Up until then he was coping very well with his diagnosis. What is the most likely cause of these symptoms?

A. Hypercalcaemia
B. Hypocalcaemia
C. Hyperkalaemia
D. Hypokalaemia
E. Hypophosphataemia

8. Movement disorders and psychiatric symptoms

A 14-year-old boy, with no prior psychiatric or medical history, is noted to be seriously slipping in his A-level course work, after previously being a 'Grade A' student. He has also started behaving recklessly, going out late whereas previously he had been shy with few friends. He is getting into frequent fights at school. Other changes include the onset of tremor and strange writhing movements in his arms. His mother has also noticed that his skin appears to have taken on a yellow tinge. What is the most likely diagnosis?

A. Huntington's disease
B. Multiple sclerosis
C. Multiple system atrophy
D. Wilson's disease
E. Young-onset Parkinson's disease

9. Stroke and psychiatric symptoms

Which of the following is the most common psychiatric manifestation following stroke?

A. Anxiety symptoms
B. Delusions
C. Depressive symptoms
D. Hallucinations
E. Obsessive–compulsive (OCD) symptoms

10. Cerebral tumours and psychiatry

A 38-year-old man is admitted with a several week history of rapidly deteriorating memory, which he covered to some extent with extensive confabulation. He was also found to be sleeping, drinking and eating excessively. On examination he was pyrexial. His blood work showed a markedly raised serum osmolality. An MRI shows an intracranial mass. Where is the most likely anatomical location for this lesion?

A. Around the third ventricle
B. Cerebellum
C. Corpus callosum
D. Frontal lobe
E. Pons

11. Autoimmune disorders and psychiatry

A 34-year-old woman presents to accident and emergency claiming that the devil has returned to earth and is hunting her through her neighbours, who are recording her every movement. The psychiatric assessment shows florid delusions and auditory hallucinations. She has no past psychiatric history. Her husband tells you that she was fine up until 2 weeks ago. Her hands have also been shaking and she has complained that the devil has been torturing her muscles. She has widespread lymphadenopathy and an enlarged spleen. An unusual rash is present across her cheeks and nose, which she says is the brand of the devil. What is the most likely diagnosis?

A. Behçet's disease
B. CREST syndrome
C. Graves' disease
D. Systemic lupus erythematosus (SLE)
E. Wegener's granulomatosis

12. Dietary deficiencies and psychiatric symptoms

Which of the following vitamin deficiencies is most likely to lead to a triad of gastrointestinal disturbance, dermatological symptoms and a heterogeneous constellation of psychiatric symptoms?

A. Niacin
B. Vitamin A
C. Vitamin B1
D. Vitamin C
E. Vitamin D

13. Epilepsy and psychiatric symptoms

Which of the following statements regarding neuropsychiatric manifestations of epilepsy is correct?

A. Automatisms in epilepsy are usually pre-ictal
B. Epilepsy is usually associated with enduring personality difficulties
C. Psychosis is negatively correlated with epilepsy
D. Rates of suicide are higher in people with epilepsy than people not suffering with epilepsy
E. Temporal lobe epilepsy is usually associated with tonic clonic seizures

14. Early-onset dementia

Which of the following regarding early-onset dementia (or young-onset dementia (YOD)) is correct?

    A.   Alzheimer's disease in younger patients is not associated with a family history

    B.   Alzheimer's disease is an uncommon cause of YOD

    C.   Dementia is under-represented in Down's syndrome

    D.   Pick's disease is classically associated with personality changes

    E.   YOD is usually caused by prion diseases

15. Unusual causes of psychiatric symptoms

A 19-year-old white woman presents to accident and emergency with abdominal pain, arm weakness and diminished reflexes. She is also extremely agitated and is responding to auditory hallucinations. You are unable to get a history from her, and you call her GP – there is little of note in her history, although she has only been in the practice for a few months as she is a first year student. The only recent entry is a new prescription for the oral contraceptive pill (OCP). What is the most likely diagnosis?

    A.   Acromegaly

    B.   Acute intermittent porphyria

    C.   Diabetic ketoacidosis

    D.   Heroin intoxication

    E.   Sickle cell anaemia

ANSWERS

Causes of delirium

1 B   Delirium tremens (B) is a syndrome caused by alcohol withdrawal in patients with a long history of alcohol consumption, or more likely alcohol dependence. It is a medical emergency and is characterized by autonomic instability, nausea and vomiting, altered mental state ('delirium'), tremor ('tremens'), and sometimes seizures. The first symptoms usually appear within 6–12 hours of the last drink and peak at around 24–48 hours. Patients may also complain of hallucinations, usually visual, which take the form of seeing small insects. Note, this is not the same as formication, which technically is the physical sensation of feeling insects crawling over one's skin. This is commonly seen in cocaine intoxication, but rarely can also be seen in cocaine withdrawal (C). However, cocaine withdrawal is not usually associated with autonomic instability or fitting. Alcoholic hallucinosis (A) is a syndrome also caused by withdrawal from alcohol in those dependent on it. Hallucinosis can also occur in those that continue to drink, although this is rarer. Alcoholic hallucinosis is sometimes taken to mean a relatively rare condition where verbal auditory hallucinations occur alone and in clear consciousness, and is often mistaken for schizophrenia. Whichever definition is taken, the presence of autonomic instability and fits would rule out alcoholic hallucinosis. Diabetic ketoacidosis (D) may present with confusion, although sweating would be uncommon. Patients may complain of severe thirst, and possibly chest or abdominal pain. On examination, patients will appear dehydrated and may have a distinctive smell of ketones on the breath. Fits would be relatively uncommon compared to a decreased level of consciousness. Opiate overdose (E) would not present in this way – patients would exhibit respiratory and central nervous system depression.

Investigation of delirium

2 D   This question relates to the likely blood results in chronic alcohol misuse. Chronic alcohol dependence is associated with vitamin B12 deficiency (D), both as a result of poor nutritional intake and a direct toxic effect of alcohol on bone marrow. B12 is involved in DNA synthesis and this leads to an impairment in erythrocyte metabolism, resulting in larger cell volumes before they divide. This will be evident on a full blood count with a raised, not lowered, MCV (C). Other effects of alcohol on blood and blood chemistry include a decrease in platelet count, known as thrombocytopenia, as opposed to thrombocytosis (raised platelet count) (E). This results from both vitamin deficiency (B12/folate) and again a direct toxic effect of alcohol. The low platelet count is not usually symptomatic. Alcohol is also generally associated with hypoglycaemia as opposed to hyperglycaemia (A), although the latter can also occur. Therefore, serum glucose would be less helpful in diagnosing chronic alcohol abuse. Alcohol also causes hypokalaemia as opposed to hyperkalaemia (B). There may be numerous causes for this, such as decreased intake through poor nutrition or vomiting, but it is also thought to occur through decreased tubular reabsorption of potassium secondary to a low magnesium level.

Management of delirium

3 E   This is a clear case of delirium, or acute confusional state characterized by a recognized causative factor (infection), older age and fluctuating confusion. Acute confusional states are extremely common in medical inpatients (perhaps in the region of 30 per cent of those over 65 in hospital). It is extremely important that it is managed well – while it has traditionally been considered a transient syndrome with no sequelae, there is growing evidence that delirium leads to increased psychiatric and physical morbidity. When managing delirium, the first steps should be conservative (E) unless the patient is putting themselves or others at significant risk of harm. While this scenario is distressing (at least for the nursing staff), there is no evidence that this is the case. Therefore, initially patients should be treated with intensive nursing interventions. These may include nursing the patient in a side room, keeping lighting appropriate to the time of day, repeated reassurance, the use of prominently visible clocks to orient the patient. Only if the patient continues to become very distressed should medication be considered. The best treatment for delirium is contentious, but guidelines currently suggest that low-dose antipsychotics such as haloperidol (B) are the most appropriate. Haloperidol is a 'typical' antipsychotic with relatively few anticholinergic effects. This is thought to be useful as the cholinergic system has been implicated in the pathogenesis of delirium and anticholinergic drugs are a common cause of acute confusional states in older age. Newer, or 'atypical' antipsychotics may also be useful but have been studied far less than haloperidol. However, you would not use haloperidol intravenously unless patients were refusing medication via the oral route. Benzodiazepines ((C) and (D)) are second line agents, although they are probably the agents used most commonly in medical inpatient settings for treating delirium. They are prone to causing respiratory depression, and can cause a syndrome of 'paradoxical excitation' whereby the delirium appears to worsen with their use. If the delirium is caused by alcohol or benzodiazepine withdrawal, then they may be the most appropriate medication. The principles of using medication in delirium are to use the lowest dose possible, review regularly and remember to discontinue them after the delirium has resolved. The inconsistent use of medication as required, particularly benzodiazepines, may lead to falls – it is far better to use small doses regularly and review their effects. Clozapine (A) is a potent antipsychotic reserved for the management of treatment-resistant schizophrenia and therefore not an appropriate drug choice here.

Pharmacological causes of organic depression

4 A   Prednisolone (A) is a corticosteroid with numerous uses, including autoimmune and inflammatory disorders. It has long been observed that corticosteroids can cause psychiatric side effects. While this is most commonly thought of as mania ('steroid psychosis'), they also may cause depressive disorders. Mania is probably more common than depression, but the two may coexist. Depression may result from the acute use, chronic use or discontinuation of corticosteroids. This is thought to be mediated by the hypothalamo-pituitary adrenal axis, which has a complex but undoubted role in the regulation of mood – depression is commonly seen in Cushing's disease, probably as a direct result of a state of chronic hypercortisolism. Sertraline (B) is a selective serotonin reuptake inhibitor (SSRI), the most commonly prescribed class of antidepressants. There has been widespread debate about whether SSRIs cause an increase in suicidal thoughts. The NICE guidelines on depression indicate that there may be a small increase in suicidality in the very early stages of antidepressant use. However, it is important to note the following:

- There appears to be no higher risk with SSRIs compared to other antidepressants. The risk of clinically important suicidal behaviour is highest in the month before starting antidepressants and declines thereafter.
- There is no temporal association between antidepressant use and completed suicide. It has been observed that in the initial stages of antidepressant treatment, motivation and energy usually improve prior to improvements in low mood, which may in some part be attributable to the increase in suicidal thoughts.
- The increase in suicidal thoughts may in part be the result of those patients in whom side effects are troublesome, such as akathisia (restlessness), which is itself an independent predictor of suicidal behaviour.
- The risk appears to be slightly higher in adolescents and young adults.

Overall, it is recommended that those at potentially higher risk (younger, experiencing side effects, suicidal thoughts prior to starting medication) should be monitored with increased frequency. A medication with a low toxicity (e.g. SSRI) should be used to avoid the increased risk of death in overdose. Thyroxine (C) is not associated with depressive reactions. In fact, thyroxine is the first line treatment for hypothyroidism, which itself may be associated with depression. Tramadol (D) is an opioid analgesic. Opiates are not associated with depressive reactions, and as they cause central release of serotonin, they may in fact have antidepressant properties. There have been case reports of successful augmentation of usual antidepressant treatment with opioids in treatment-resistant depression. Trytophan (E) is an essential amino acid and a precursor of serotonin. It is therefore occasionally used as an augmentation strategy in treatment-resistant depression, although the evidence for its use is unclear.

Focal cerebral disorders

5 B   This man is exhibiting signs consistent with a frontal lobe (B) injury, and more specifically an orbitofrontal insult. The frontal lobe is extremely vulnerable in traumatic brain injury. Frontal lobe syndromes can take many forms, but often involve changes in personality including:

- Inappropriate or 'fatuous' affect
- Lability and irritability of mood
- Hypersexuality
- Hyperphagia, or overeating
- 'Childishness' or prankish joking (known as 'Witzelsucht')

There is usually no insight into this change in behaviour. Other changes include poor concentration and 'forced utilization' – a strange phenomenon when patients will use objects they see in front of them irrespective of whether they need to use them or not, e.g. patients may get undressed and go to bed on entering a bedroom in the middle of the day despite not being tired. There may also be the emergence of primitive reflexes, such as the grasp reflex. The basal ganglia (A) are deep grey matter (subcortical) structures with strong connections to the cortex and thalamus. They have complex roles in motor behaviour, but because of their strong connections to the frontal cortex there may also be neuropsychiatric symptoms in basal ganglia disorders. However, these are usually associated with 'negative' symptoms such as slowing of movement and lack of spontaneity. There may also be an increase in obsessional symptoms, and the basal ganglia are thought to be heavily involved in the pathogenesis of OCD. Given their anatomical location, contusions to the basal ganglia are uncommon, but they are very susceptible to cerebral hypoxia. The limbic system (C) involves deep structures such as the hippocampus, parahippocampal gyrus, the amygdala, the fornix, cingulate gyrus and the thalamus. They have varied functions, but are principally involved in pleasure responses and memory. Injury to the limbic system would almost certainly result in some sort of amnesic syndrome, which is not the case in this question. Lesions of the parietal lobe (D) are associated with visuo-spatial deficits – either 'agnosia' (inability to recognize objects) or 'dyspraxia' (inability to coordinate motor activities). There may also be dysphasias, either motor or sensory depending on the site of the injury. Gerstmann's syndrome is a particular syndrome of parietal lobe injury consisting of four components, namely:

1. 'Left-right' disorientation
2. Dyscalculia (inability to perform arithmetical tasks)
3. Finger agnosia (inability to distinguish the fingers on the hand)
4. Agraphia (inability to write).

Non-dominant parietal lobe injuries may lead to body image disturbances, such as anosognosia (inability to recognize injury to a particular limb) or 'hemisomatognosia' (the feeling that one side of the body is missing). Occipital lobe (E) injury tends to result in complex visual disturbances that are often baffling. There may be vivid visual hallucinations. A very odd situation, known as Anton's syndrome, can occur in bilateral occipital lobe injury, in which the patient is cortically blind but has no insight into this and continues to affirm adamantly that they can see.

Neurological signs and psychiatric symptoms

6 B While there are no pathognomonic features of herpes simplex virus (HSV) encephalitis (B), the clinical history is strongly suggestive of an encephalitic picture. It is important to have an extremely low threshold for treating presumed HSV encephalitis, in part because if left untreated there is an extremely high (approximately 70 per cent) mortality rate, and the treatment (intravenous aciclovir) is relatively non-toxic. HSV encephalitis nearly always targets the temporal lobes and orbitofrontal structures. This is the most likely explanation for the preponderance of unusual behaviour or psychotic symptoms in the early stages of the illness, as can be seen here. The woman accusing her partner of leaving the gas on is most likely an olfactory hallucination, which are common in temporal lobe disorders. The rapidly advancing neurological signs indicate a generalizing cerebral infection. The CSF analysis is also typical of viral encephalitis (or meningitis) – showing markedly raised protein, normal or slightly low glucose, a clear appearance and a preponderance of mononuclear cells. This is opposed to bacterial meningitis (A) in which the CSF is more likely to be turbid or purulent, with a preponderance of polymorphonuclear cells, raised protein, and very low CSF glucose. There are also no other signs consistent with bacterial meningitis in this case, such as the typical meningococcal rash, or other signs of meningism (neck stiffness, photophobia). While there is nausea and vomiting, this is non-specific and is often present in encephalitis as there will be some concomitant irritation of the meninges. Neurosyphilis (C) would be uncommon in a woman of this age, although certainly not impossible.

It is possible to have an early (usually within 2 years of the primary infection) acute syphilitic meningitis, but this would not fit with the history (as per bacterial meningitis above). The history is too quick to fit with subacute and chronic neuropsyphilis. Late neurosyphilis (tabes dorsalis and 'general paralysis of the insane') are extremely rare these days, but they must be borne in mind as causes of unusual pain symptoms in the former and atypical dementia in the latter. Sporadic CJD (D) would present with a rapid onset (over weeks or months) of dementia associated with mood symptoms, spasticity and blindness. There are certain features here that would be consistent with temporal lobe epilepsy (E). However, temporal lobe seizures are usually gradual in onset and are often characterized by a motionless stare and automatisms (unusual and unconscious motor behaviours such as chewing or hand-rubbing, but may be more complex such as actually cooking or driving). Auras (unusual sensations immediately preceding a seizure) are common and may mimic typical psychotic hallucinations. They may occur in any modality. The extreme deterioration following a few days' history of strange behaviour would therefore not fit with typical seizure activity.

Metabolic causes of psychiatric symptoms

7 A   Hypercalcaemia (A) is a common complication of squamous cell carcinoma. The likely cause of this is due to the tumour releasing large amounts of parathyroid-related peptide leading to increased bone turnover. There may also be direct bone destruction from tumour invasion. Hypercalcaemia typically results in the classic syndrome of 'stones' (kidney stones), 'bones' (bone pain), 'groans' (constipation), 'psychic moans' (depression, aesthenia, confusion). Thirst is also a common symptom exacerbated by osmotic diuresis, as are nausea, vomiting and anorexia. If depression is the main presenting feature, it is extremely important to rule out metabolic disturbances in patients with cancer. Do not assume that the depression is a psychological reaction to the diagnosis of cancer (although of course this is also extremely possible) – hypercalcaemia is very correctable and symptoms will reduce quickly as the calcium level drops. Hypocalcaemia (B) will more likely present with peripheral neurological signs, such as hyperactive deep tendon reflexes, tetany (such as main d'accoucher or Trousseaus's sign – carpal spasm occurring in the presence of a blood pressure cuff inflated above systolic pressure, and Chvostek's sign – facial tetany induced by tapping the ipsilateral angle of the jaw). Paraesthesia and bruising of the skin may also occur. There may be psychiatric symptoms associated with hypocalcaemia, but they do not appear to follow a particular pattern. Hyperkalaemia (C) does not tend to present with psychiatric symptoms, but will commonly result in diffuse muscle weakness and fatigue. Hypokalaemia (D) may also present with these symptoms, but there may also be depression and sometimes anxiety. Hypophosphataemia (E) usually results in a delirium-like picture along with a wide range of motor problems.

Movement disorders and psychiatric symptoms

8 D   Wilson's disease (D), also known as hepatolenticular degeneration, is a rare autosomal recessive disorder of copper metabolism. The mutation (of which there are over 200 described) occurs in a gene on chromosome 13q (designated *ATP7B*), which encodes for a protein that is responsible for transporting copper for excretion in bile. Dysfunction of this protein therefore leads to copper accumulation in numerous tissues in the body, particularly the liver (causing jaundice) and the nervous system. Another extremely suggestive feature is the presence of Kayser–Fleischer rings, which are greenish-gold or brownish rings in the cornea resulting from copper deposition. Note that Kayser–Fleischer rings are now no longer thought of as purely pathognomonic of Wilson's disease as they may occur in other disorders such as primary biliary cirrhosis. Neuropsychiatric consequences of Wilson's disease include aggression, reckless behaviour, disinhibition and sometimes self-harming behaviours. There are also prominent neurological symptoms, including the ones detailed above. Huntington's disease (HD) (A) is an autosomal dominant inherited movement disorder. The genetic defect in HD is an expansion of a CAG triplet repeat at the 5′ end of a gene on chromosome 4p. The protein product of this gene is known as huntingtin. Its physiological function is unknown, but the triplet repeat codes for a polyglutamine tract at the N-terminus of the intracellular protein. This causes the accumulation of inclusion bodies within the cell which lead to cell death. Neuropathologically, there is cell loss in the basal ganglia, substantia nigra and cerebellum. The clinical symptoms are choreoid and athetoid movements, dementia and personality changes. The disease usually has an onset in the 4th–5th decades, but the disorder does show the unusual phenomenon of anticipation, when the age of onset decreases with subsequent members of the pedigree affected. This is due to expansion of the CAG repeat. Multiple sclerosis (B) is an inflammatory disease of the central nervous system, characterized by demyelination. Its aetiology is unknown. It is either episodic or progressive, but is almost invariably fatal. It is characterized by a wide range of neurological, psychiatric and cognitive symptoms. Other organs are not involved. It usually begins somewhere in the 3rd–6th decades. The psychiatric symptoms may also take on diffuse forms, but often patients have been described as presenting with euphoric symptoms. Cognitive symptoms, including frank dementia, are very common and more stable than the psychiatric presentations. Multiple system atrophy (C) is a rare disease of unknown cause. It shows clinical similarities to Parkinson's disease (PD), but pathologically there is more involvement of the putamen and caudate nuclei. There are also no Lewy bodies present in the substantia nigra, unlike PD. Also unlike PD, patients do not tend to develop dementia. Sleep disorders and depression are common however. Juvenile or young-onset Parkinson's disease (E) is extremely rare (only approximately five per 100 000 under 40). Patients show similar symptoms to 'classic' PD but tend to have more dystonic symptoms. Depression may occur, but dementia, which is common in classic PD, would be almost unheard of in young patients.

Stroke and psychiatric symptoms

9 C   Depression (C) is extremely common in stroke, with estimates in the literature of a prevalence of either early or late depression at 1/3. This is higher than would be expected as a result of chronic disease alone and suggests some causative mechanism of the disease process itself. Of course, many of the symptoms of stroke may make the diagnosis more difficult (e.g. apathy, emotional lability, poor concentration). Equally, depression may easily be missed in aphasic patients, who will be particularly at risk because of the added isolation of being unable to communicate. There is of course now growing evidence about the phenomenon of 'vascular depression', in which depressive disorders are thought to be directly related to accumulative cerebrovascular disease rather than clinically significant or recognized episodes of stroke. Psychotic disorders, including the experience of delusions (B) or hallucinations (D), have been less studied than depression in stroke patients. However, they are thought to occur in approximately 1–2 per cent of stroke sufferers. In patients with co-morbid dementia, care must be taken when deciding on management of psychosis in stroke given the association of antipsychotics with increased risk of death in these patients. Anxiety symptoms (A) are common, and a generalized anxiety disorder may be seen in up to one-quarter of patients. Obsessive–compulsive symptoms (E) in stroke have not been particularly well studied, in part because anecdotally they are rare.

Cerebral tumours and psychiatry

10 A   The symptoms of amnesia and confabulation are very typical of tumours involving the wall or floor of the third ventricle (A). Structures around this region include the thalamus and hypothalamus, which would also explain the other symptoms of hypersomnia, hyperphagia, pyrexia and polydipsia. The raised serum osmolality points to cranial diabetes insipidus secondary to tumour effects on the hypothalamus. Tumours of the cerebellum (B) would present with fewer psychiatric symptoms, although given its location in the posterior fossa, raised intracranial pressure would be common, which may present with dementia-like symptoms, and therefore the memory problems and confabulation may fit – the other symptoms, however, point to the involvement of diencephalic structures. There may be involvement of brainstem structures, with vomiting and headache. Typical cerebellar signs obviously may also occur such as ataxia and nystagmus. Corpus callosum tumours (C) produce profound psychiatric problems and a rapid deterioration of higher functions. This may present as severe memory problems and an almost catatonic state. Frontal lobe tumours (D) would tend to cause changes in personality but often can be mistaken for dementia. Almost any psychiatric symptoms can occur, but neurological symptoms tend to be relatively scarce. Tumours of the pons (E) tend to be aggressive gliomas. They tend to present as in (B) with brainstem signs such as headache, nausea and vomiting, diplopia, drowsiness and dysarthria. There may also be hydrocephalus with the resultant deterioration in intellectual function.

Autoimmune disorders and psychiatry

11 D SLE (D) is an autoimmune connective tissue disorder that may affect any organ in the body. It commonly presents in women (9:1 female to male ratio), usually in the third or fourth decades. Neuropsychiatric symptoms may occur at the beginning of the natural course of the disorder, without any seeming involvement of other organ systems. Unexplained psychotic symptoms, which may closely resemble schizophrenia, may occur, as may a dementia-like illness or affective disorders. This woman is also displaying neurological signs, making a diagnosis of a functional psychiatric disorder unlikely. The presence of Parkinsonism, widespread muscle pain, lymphadenopathy and splenomegaly are all consistent with the diagnosis. The 'malar rash', which is highly indicative of SLE, is present in this woman but its absence does not negate the diagnosis. Behçet's disease (A) is an autoimmune disorder characterized by recurrent mouth ulcers, genital ulcers and uveitis. Neurological or psychiatric symptoms are uncommon and usually a late presentation. It also tends to present in the third or fourth decades, but tends to be more common in men. The CREST syndrome (B) is a form of systemic scleroderma characterized by the following five cardinal features from which the acronym is derived: calcinosis, in which there is calcium deposits in the soft tissue, usually under the skin; Raynaud's phenomenon, in which there is bilateral cyanosis of the hands in response to cold or stress; oesophageal atresia, which presents with symptoms of gastro-oesophageal reflux; sclerodactyly, in which there is thickening of the skin of the hands and feet, taking on a 'shiny' appearance; finally, telangiectasia, which are lesions caused by dilated blood vessels and usually present on the face or hands. Psychiatric complications have been little studied in this disorder, although depression certainly does occur. Graves' disease (C) is an autoimmune thyroiditis, which incidentally may occur co-morbidly with SLE, although the greatest association is with rheumatoid arthritis. The characteristic symptoms include those of hyperthyroidism, which in psychiatric terms may resemble an anxiety disorder, with tachycardia and palpitations. There may be unexplained weight loss. Systemic symptoms, such as malaise, are also common, as is exophthalmos and pretibial myxoedema ('orange peel' skin on the shin). The psychiatric symptoms tend to either resemble an anxiety disorder, or other affective symptoms. Like SLE, women are more commonly affected, and usually in their 20s or 30s. Wegener's granulomatosis (E) is an autoimmune vasculitis that typically affects the lungs, kidneys and nervous system. It affects males slightly more often with a slightly later peak of incidence (fourth and fifth decades). The typical presentations are with dyspnoea, cough, haemoptysis, nasal ulceration, sinusitis, systemic symptoms, haematuria, and neurological symptoms – typically peripheral neuropathy but sometimes strokes and seizures. Psychiatric complications have not typically been described except in case reports.

Dietary deficiencies and psychiatric symptoms

12 A Nicotinic acid, or niacin, deficiency (A) is also known as pellagra. It classically manifests with gastrointestinal symptoms, such as diarrhoea, anorexia and gastritis. The dermatological manifestations include symmetrical, bilateral bullous lesions in sun-exposed areas. The psychiatric symptoms initially manifest as apathy, depression, or irritability. However, in later stages there are more florid symptoms resembling delirium, psychosis or a Korsakoff-like presentation. If identified, treatment with nicotinic acid usually leads to prompt and dramatic improvements in mental state. Vitamin A deficiency (B) is associated with night-blindness, dry skin and hair and anaemia. Thiamine, or vitamin B1 deficiency (C) is known as beriberi. The classical symptoms of this disorder are neuropathy and heart failure. Acute depletion of thiamine, as seen in alcohol dependence, leads to Wernicke's encephalopathy. Vitamin C deficiency (D) leads to scurvy, characterized by anorexia, diarrhoea, irritability, anaemia, gingival haemorrhage, poor wound healing, leg pain and swelling over the long bones. Vitamin D deficiency (E) leads to rickets in children and osteomalacia in adults. There is now growing evidence of some link with vitamin D to cognitive functioning. There are speculations about its role in seasonal affective disorder whereby patients have normal mental function during the year but during a particular season, e.g. winter, will display a mood disorder such as depression year after year during that season.

Epilepsy and psychiatric symptoms

13 D Epilepsy has numerous and complex neuropsychiatric and psychological interactions. It is undoubted that rates of suicide are higher in people with epilepsy (D) than the general population. However, the degree of the association is not clear. Similar risk factors appear to exist for suicide in people with epilepsy than in the general population, such as co-morbid psychiatric illness (which is also over-represented in people with epilepsy). Epilepsy is not usually associated with enduring personality difficulties (B). Automatisms (A) are unusual and sometimes complex repetitive motor activities observed in nearly all forms of epilepsy, but commonly associated with complex partial seizures (such as temporal lobe epilepsy). They are nearly always observed during a seizure (ictal) or in the post-seizure delirium (post-ictal). Psychotic symptoms are positively correlated with epilepsy (C). This is particularly true of temporal lobe epilepsy, but probably is also over-represented in other types of epilepsy. Temporal lobe epilepsy (E) is associated with psychological and psychiatric symptoms such as aura, sensory disturbances and depersonalization or derealization. Unusual symptoms such as déjà vu or jamais vu may also occur.

Early-onset dementia

14 D   Pick's disease (D) is a relatively uncommon dementia, classified as one of the frontotemporal dementias. It commonly presents in the sixth decade of life, e.g. earlier than the typical onset of other neurodegenerative disorders such as Alzheimer's disease. Because of its predilection for frontal and anterior temporal parts of the brain, it tends to present with changes in behaviour and personality before amnesic symptoms are obvious. This can lead to devastating consequences for those affected and their families. Alzheimer's disease in younger people ((A) and (B)) is often associated with specific familial inherited genetic mutations. There are numerous mutations, affecting the *APP* gene on chromosome 21 and the presenelin 1 and 2 genes on chromosomes 14 and 1, respectively. Alzheimer's disease is still the major cause of YOD. Down's syndrome (C) confers a much greater risk of dementia, with a prevalence estimated at around 50 per cent of those with Down's syndrome in those aged 60 or above. Prion diseases (E) are certainly a cause of YOD, usually with a rapid clinical course. However, they are still rare, probably accounting for only about 1.5 per cent of the total of cases of YOD.

Unusual causes of psychiatric symptoms

15 B   The features described are typical of acute intermittent porphyria (B), a relatively rare autosomal dominant inherited disorder, typically presenting in the second to fourth decades. It is a disorder of haem metabolism resulting in a build up of porphyrins and their precursors. Attacks are usually precipitated by one of a number of factors, including menstruation, alcohol, poor nutrition and certain drugs, such as the OCP. Porphyria can often be mistakenly diagnosed as a primary psychiatric disorder. Abdominal pain in any patient with psychiatric symptoms should always prompt further investigation. Acromegaly (A) is a disorder caused by increased growth hormone secretion, usually by a growth hormone-secreting tumour of the pituitary. It would usually present slightly later than adolescence/early adulthood. There are no psychiatric disorders commonly associated with this condition. Diabetic ketoacidosis (C) could present with abdominal pain but peripheral neuropathy would be unusual in a person of this age. Psychosis itself would also be uncommon, although of course confusion and clouding of consciousness are very highly associated with ketoacidosis. Heroin intoxication (D) would not present in this way. Opiate withdrawal may present with abdominal cramps and muscle aches, but frank weakness and changes in reflexes would be uncommon. Sickle cell anaemia (E) often does present with abdominal crises. However, it would be very rare in a white individual and would normally have presented long before the age of 19. Vaso-occlusion causes widespread and numerous symptoms, including stroke, but the picture here does not fit that of sickle cell disease.

SECTION 26: SCHIZOPHRENIA AND PSYCHOSIS

QUESTIONS

1. Subtypes of schizophrenia

A 24-year-old student presents with a 3-month history of social withdrawal and low mood. She is difficult to interview because she talks about random themes and has difficulty answering questions. She has vague paranoid ideation. She is childish and pulls faces at you during the interview. The most likely diagnosis is:

A. Hebephrenic schizophrenia — *thynt tallable disorder*
B. Catatonic schizophrenia
C. Paranoid schizophrenia
D. Residual schizophrenia
E. Simple schizophrenia

2. Epidemiology of schizophrenia

What is the lifetime prevalence of schizophrenia in the UK?

A. 0.01 per cent
B. 0.1 per cent
C. 0.4 per cent
D. 4 per cent
E. 10 per cent

3. Genetics of schizophrenia

A 19-year-old identical twin is diagnosed with schizophrenia. His mother makes an appointment to see you at the GP practice and asks what the likelihood is of his twin developing schizophrenia. What should you tell her?

A. It is inevitable that schizophrenia will develop in the brother
B. There is no increased risk of developing schizophrenia
C. The risk is about one in 100
D. The risk is about one in 10
E. The risk is about one in two

4. Antipsychotics (1)

A 19-year-old man with schizophrenia is brought to accident and emergency by his sister as he has become unwell over the last few days. He has recently been started on risperidone. He is confused, sweaty and tremulous. On examination the signs include tachycardia, low blood pressure, pyrexia and lead-pipe rigidity. His Glasgow Coma Scale score is decreased at 12/15. What is the most likely diagnosis?

A. Acute dystonia
B. Malignant hyperthermia
C. Neuroleptic malignant syndrome
D. Serotonin syndrome
E. Tyramine reaction

5. Antipsychotics (2)

A 23-year-old man is diagnosed with schizophrenia. He has had florid persecutory beliefs and auditory hallucinations for the past 3 months. In terms of medical history he has poorly controlled insulin-dependent diabetes and is obese. On admission to hospital he was so distressed he required intramuscular rapid tranquilization. On administration of 5 mg of haloperidol, he developed an acute dystonia in his neck muscles which was excruciatingly painful. What would be the most appropriate drug to commence to control his schizophrenia?

A. Aripiprazole
B. Clozapine
C. Olanzapine
D. Oral haloperidol
E. Sertraline

6. Schizophrenia and the Mental Health Act

A 24-year-old man with a diagnosis of schizophrenia, last admitted 6 months ago under Section, is brought in by police to the Mental Health Unit under Section 136. He has been harassing his ex-girlfriend with constant threatening phone calls and turning up at her house. He says he believes she is twisting his bones at night, preventing him sleeping and causing him massive pain, through witchcraft. He states that he is going to kill her if it goes on one more night and has purchased a special knife from a 'witchcraft' shop on the internet. He is experiencing auditory hallucinations directing him in the best way to use the knife against her. Against the advice of his consultant he has recently stopped his medication, which usually keeps him well. His symptoms typically follow these themes of violence and the supernatural when unwell. He claims that being in hospital will just allow her to target him more easily and will not stay voluntarily. What Section of the Mental Health Act (MHA) is most likely to be appropriate in this case?

A. Section 135
B. Section 2
C. Section 3
D. Section 4
E. Section 5(2)

7. Emergency management of acutely psychotic patients

The man described above is admitted under Section 3 of the Mental Health Act. On admission to the ward, he is acutely disturbed and becomes violent towards others and himself. He has slapped a member of staff. Staff try to calm him down but it is felt that the risks are escalating. He was prescribed 2 mg lorazepam orally which he has spat into the nurse's face. He has no prior recorded adverse drug reactions. What is the most appropriate pharmacological management of the patient?

- A. Haloperidol decanoate (depot) 50 mg intramuscular
- B. Haloperidol 10 mg orally
- C. Lorazepam 2 mg intramuscular
- D. Lorazepam 2 mg slow intravenous injection
- E. Propofol 120 mg intravenous injection

8. Management of treatment-resistant schizophrenia

A 22-year-old man with paranoid schizophrenia has been treated with three different antipsychotics and remains unwell. His team decide to prescribe clozapine which he has now been on for 3 weeks. He comes in for his regular blood test and the nurse in the clozapine clinic asks the junior doctor to see him as he appears unwell. On examination, he is sweaty and tachycardic with a temperature of 38.5°C. He has no chest pain but is coughing purulent sputum. What would the most likely isolated abnormality be on blood testing?

- A. High eosinophil count
- B. High platelet count
- C. Low haemoglobin
- D. Low lymphocyte count
- E. Low neutrophil count

9. Chronic schizophrenia

A 54-year-old man with schizophrenia has been on depot antipsychotics for the last 27 years as he hates taking tablets and has stopped them in the past. He has not been unwell in terms of his schizophrenia for the last decade. His community psychiatric nurse notices that he has developed odd movements around his mouth over the last few months, where he purses and smacks his lips. It is causing him difficulty speaking and it is distressing for him and his family. Which is the most appropriate course of action for managing this symptom?

- A. Gradual decrease in depot medication
- B. Offer emotional support
- C. Start anticholinergic such as procyclidine
- D. Start 'second-generation' antipsychotic such as olanzapine
- E. Stop depot immediately to prevent further deterioration

10. Prognosis in schizophrenia

A 22-year-old single man is diagnosed with schizophrenia. This is followed by a very rapid psychotic breakdown characterized by well-defined persecutory delusions. There is no mood component to his symptoms. He has shown a poor response to treatment. Which of the following indicates a positive prognostic feature of this man's illness?

    A.   Absence of mood symptoms
    B.   Being male
    C.   Being young
    D.   Poor initial response to treatment
    E.   Rapid onset of symptoms

11. Other psychotic disorders

A 38-year-old single woman is arrested outside the house of a celebrity TV chef after shouting outside all night. On interview she claims that the man has declared his love for her several times but is being prevented from seeing her by his wife who is keeping him handcuffed inside. She states it is he that has made several advances to her by sending her special messages when he is cooking on television. What syndrome or symptom is being described here?

    A.   Capgras syndrome
    B.   de Clérambault's syndrome
    C.   Folie à deux
    D.   Othello syndrome
    E.   Querulant delusions

12. Side effects of antipsychotics

A 27-year-old man has been started on haloperidol, a 'first-generation' antipsychotic, for control of his symptoms of schizophrenia. A few weeks later he comes to his GP in a highly embarrassed state, claiming that the CIA are experimenting on him, turning him into a woman. When the GP asks how he knows this, the man states that he has noticed his chest growing into 'breasts' and he can no longer get an erection with his girlfriend. What is the most likely cause of these symptoms?

    A.   Alpha-blockade
    B.   Drug-induced hepatitis
    C.   Hyperprolactinaemia
    D.   New-onset diabetes
    E.   Prostatic hypertrophy

13. Diagnosis of schizophrenia

Which of the following is not recognized as a diagnostic feature of schizophrenia according to ICD-10?

A. Formal thought disorder
B. Grandiose delusions
C. Running commentary
D. Symptoms lasting at least 1 month
E. Thought broadcasting

14. Classification of psychotic disorders

A 28-year-old woman presents in the GP surgery. She is over-talkative and over-familiar with you. It is difficult to get a full history, but it seems for the last 4 weeks she has been elated and experiencing voices telling her that her mother was a descendant of the Virgin Mary and that she is a female 'second coming'. This was the result of an experiment by the Nazi party who genetically engineered her grandparents. She believes that remnants of the Nazi party are now controlling her arms and legs, which results in her alternately trying to hug you and then kicking out at the desk. What is the most likely diagnosis?

A. Hebephrenic schizophrenia
B. Induced delusional disorder
C. Paranoid schizophrenia
D. Schizoaffective disorder
E. Schizoptypal disorder

15. Antipsychotics

Which of the following is the least likely to be a side effect of antipsychotic treatment?

A. Akathisia
B. Convulsions
C. Hypotension
D. Renal failure
E. Tachycardia

ANSWERS

Subtypes of schizophrenia

1 A   Classifying schizophrenia into subtypes is by no means simple in psychiatry. The term schizophrenia encompasses a heterogenous group of disorders, and as yet there has been no system of classification that has adequately been able to predict development of specific subtypes or reliable prognosis. That said, our current classification systems have divided schizophrenia into various types, and it does appear that, within limits, there is some utility to these categories. Hebephrenic schizophrenia (A) (sometimes referred to as 'disorganized' schizophrenia), is characterized by the predominance of thought disorder and affective symptoms. Social withdrawal is common. The affect is often fatuous and childlike. Delusions and hallucinations are often present, but are usually fragmented and are not the most striking feature. Negative symptoms tend to develop early and quickly, and for this reason this subtype is considered to have a poor prognosis. Catatonic schizophrenia (B) is characterized best by psychomotor disturbances, or catatonic behaviour. Catatonia is another complex concept which appears to have heterogenous aetiologies. In this subtype, there may be marked psychomotor retardation, with stupor, or florid over-activity. There are often unusual symptoms such as automatic obedience, in which people will follow a command without questioning, or the opposite (negativism). In severe cases, people may take on odd postures for long periods, or the limbs may be moved into positions and will remain there (waxy flexibility). Hallucinations and delusions may be present but again do not dominate the picture. For some unknown reason, catatonia appears to be much less common than in the middle part of the last century. Paranoid schizophrenia (C) is often thought of as the 'classical' subtype, and is dominated by delusions and hallucinations. Thought disorder is less common (although this is also contentious). Residual schizophrenia (D) refers to late-stage schizophrenia in which the syndrome of 'positive' symptoms (delusions, hallucinations, thought disorder) are replaced by predominately 'negative' symptoms (apathy, social withdrawal, avolition, blunting of affect, poverty of speech, self-neglect). Simple schizophrenia (E) is defined by ICD-10 as 'the insidious development of oddities of conduct, inability to meet the demands of society, and decline in total performance'. There are usually no overt psychotic symptoms.

Epidemiology of schizophrenia

2 C   Traditionally, the lifetime prevalence has always been quoted as 1 per cent, although most recent studies would suggest it is lower than this at around 0.4 per cent (with, obviously, some range around this).

Regardless, this means the answer could only realistically be (C). Incidence rates are reported as lower (because of the chronic nature of the disease), usually between 0.17 to 0.54. Apart from a few exceptions, the prevalence of schizophrenia tends to be fairly standard across countries, with little overall sex differences.

Genetics of schizophrenia

3 E Schizophrenia is undoubtedly a disease with both genetic and environmental substrates. It is generally held that the genetic component accounts for approximately 50 per cent of susceptibility. Although there is some debate around this (more recent studies suggest heritability up to around 80 per cent, although there is large heterogeneity), (E) would be the only really feasible answer. There is undoubtedly an increased risk (B) of schizophrenia between identical twins, that is beyond that of sharing an 'environment'. The risk of 1 in 100 (C) is approximately the risk in the general population (although see the question above; the prevalence may well have been overestimated in earlier studies). The risk of 1 in 10 (D) could be estimated to be the risk of developing schizophrenia if you have one first degree relative with the disease.

Antipsychotics (1)

4 C Neuroleptic malignant syndrome (NMS) (C) is a medical and psychiatric emergency. It often presents to accident and emergency or general practice so you must be familiar with recognizing it and the fundamentals of treatment – without treatment it has a mortality of up to 30 per cent. NMS occurs as a complication of antipsychotic medication use (and occasionally other psychotropics) and is thought to be the result of dopamine blockade in the hypothalamus (pyrexia) and nigrostriatal pathway (extrapyramidal symptoms such as tremor and rigidity). Peripheral blockade can cause changes in skeletal muscle contractility, which may exacerbate stiffness and cause muscle breakdown (with the consequent risk of rhabdomyolysis and renal failure). It must be treated as an emergency (although the syndrome is on a spectrum, and only mild or subclinical features may manifest) and appropriate referral is essential. As far as medical treatment is concerned, the offending antipsychotic must be immediately discontinued. Supportive treatment to ensure cardiovascular stability is the priority. Severe pyrexia may require other specialized cooling treatments. Some patients may actually require mechanical ventilation. It is unclear why some people develop NMS and others do not. It may be triggered on commencing treatment with antipsychotics, increasing dose or other environmental factors such as dehydration or exhaustion. Acute dystonias (A) are also associated with antipsychotic use, but refer to acute muscular spasms. They occur as the result of dopamine blockade in the nigrostriatum. Examples include torticollis and oculogyric crises. They can be extremely painful and frightening and must also be managed as an emergency with anticholinergics. Malignant hyperthermia (B) is a rare autosomal dominated inherited disorder. It produces symptoms similar to NMS but occurs after exposure to inhaled anaesthetics such as halothane and depolarizing muscle relaxants. Serotonin syndrome (D) may easily be confused with NMS, although the rigidity does not occur. It arises as the result of central serotonin release, usually because of serotonergic medications (e.g. selective serotonin reuptake inhibitors (SSRIs)). It is generally less severe than NMS although supportive treatment is also often required. The tyramine reaction (E), sometimes also known as the 'cheese reaction', is the result of ingesting tyramine in patients taking monoamine oxidase inhibitors.

Antipsychotics (2)

5 A Aripiprazole (A) is a relatively newer antipsychotic. It appears to have less propensity to weight gain than other 'second-generation' antipsychotics (such as olanzapine) as well as a lower incidence of extrapyramidal side effects such as acute dystonias, although it does have its own side effect profile, notably nausea and insomnia. Out of the list, this would therefore be the best choice. Clozapine (B) is an extremely effective antipsychotic but is reserved for treatment-resistant schizophrenia because of its side effect profile. In this man, therefore, you would want to have trialled at least one (and probably two) other antipsychotics before moving to clozapine. Olanzapine (C) is one of the most commonly used second-generation antipsychotics. It is effective in treating positive symptoms, but has a marked propensity to cause weight gain and may worsen diabetic control. This would clearly be undesirable in this case. Oral haloperidol (D) would still be likely to cause acute dystonia – the patient is clearly very sensitive to these. Extrapyramidal side effects may be caused by either oral or intramuscular formulations. Sertraline (E) is an SSRI, a class of antidepressant, and would therefore not be an appropriate choice of drug in this case.

Schizophrenia and the Mental Health Act

6 C While you would be unlikely to need in-depth knowledge of the MHA, many doctors (not just psychiatrists) may be called upon to use these Sections of the Act and it is a good idea to have some basic knowledge about the various ways that people are detained. Section 3 (C) is used to detain people for up to 6 months for treatment. It should not be used unless the person is known to services (and preferably to one of the professionals carrying out the assessment). According to the Department of Health's code of practice, Section 3 should be used when: 'the nature and current degree of the patient's mental disorder, the essential elements of the treatment plan to be followed and the likelihood of the patient accepting treatment on a voluntary basis are already established'. This is therefore the most appropriate Section – an established and successful treatment plan has been in place previously. He will not come into hospital voluntarily and his pattern of relapse is similar to previous episodes. While a Section 2 is arguably less restrictive (being for a shorter period of time), he has also had a recent previous admission under Section. Both Sections require two medical recommendations and an application by an Approved Mental Health Professional (AMHP). Section 2 (B) is used to detain people for a maximum of 28 days for assessment. This is most appropriate when the nature and degree of a person's condition are unclear and an initial phase of assessment is required to establish a longer-term treatment plan. Note it is sometimes mistakenly assumed that because a Section 2 is for assessment (not 'treatment') that you cannot prescribe drugs against the person's will. This is not the case as medications are often an integral part of an assessment, with the response to treatment being a very useful indicator of the nature and degree, as well as prognosis, of someone's condition. Section 135 (A) refers to a warrant permitting police to search premises and remove patients from those premises. It is required to enter someone's home when an assessment needs to take place and the patient refuses access. Applications for a Section 135 warrant must be made by the AMHP to a magistrate. Only the police may execute a Section 135 warrant and this must be accompanied by an AMHP and a doctor. Section 4 (D) is an emergency Section used to detain people fulfilling the requirements of the Act in terms of the nature and degree of the disorder and risk. It is used only in exceptional circumstances for emergency application for admission for assessment. It requires an application by an AMHP and only one medical recommendation, and is therefore used when two doctors cannot be found and delay to the assessment is likely to be highly undesirable. People may be detained for up to 72 hours on a Section 4, during which time a second recommendation must be secured in order to convert it to a Section 2. They should not be used unless absolutely necessary. Section 5(2) (E) is another 72-hour section and is the one you as the foundation year doctor are most likely to encounter. It is used for inpatients only (and therefore already would be inappropriate in this case) and is referred to as a 'holding power'. It can be used by any fully registered medical practitioner (i.e. F2 or above) in charge of a patient's care (or their deputy) to detain people for a full Mental Health Act assessment to be carried out, and only if it is not practicable to wait for the full assessment to be convened. However, you should never use a Section 5(2) without discussing with a psychiatrist first if possible.

Emergency management of acutely psychotic patients

7 C   Rapid tranquilization should only be used when non-pharmacological methods have failed and the risks to the patient or those around them are sufficiently high. Do not use rapid tranquilization without senior advice. This man is obviously unwilling to take oral medication, which makes (B) an inappropriate choice. Haloperidol decanoate (A) is a depot medication and would therefore not have an immediate effect, making this an inappropriate choice also. While lorazepam may be given as a slow intravenous injection (D), it is more likely to cause difficulties such as respiratory depression using this route, and on a mental health unit there are unlikely to be staff or equipment capable of monitoring this. Propofol (E) is used to induce anaesthesia so clearly would not be an appropriate medication. Lorazepam intramuscularly is a commonly used drug for rapid tranquilization, and this would be a reasonable starting dose. It is often combined with intramuscular haloperidol (not the depot formulation). Patients prescribed rapid tranquilization should be carefully monitored by nursing and medical staff to ensure there is no evidence of respiratory depression or other side effects. Before giving parenteral benzodiazepines, ensure the ward has a supply of flumazenil (a benzodiazepine antagonist).

Management of treatment-resistant schizophrenia

8 E   Clozapine has been known to cause neutropenia (E) or even agranulocytosis. This can lead to infection and sepsis, which would fit with the clinical picture here. This requires urgent treatment and the clozapine must be immediately stopped. This could also be neuroleptic malignant syndrome from the clinical picture, but the haematology does not particularly fit – you would expect to see raised leukocytes. There have been reports of eosinophilia (A) with the use of clozapine, but the exact mechanisms of this are complex and unclear. It is likely to be related to the side effects of myocarditis or colitis that can sometimes be seen with the use of clozapine. Either way, the clinical picture does not quite fit with this. Thrombocytosis (B) has been reported with clozapine but this would be unlikely to lead to this clinical picture. Similarly, anaemia (C) has occasionally been seen, but the clinical picture is closer to one of sepsis rather than anaemia. A low lymphocyte count (D) may be present as part of an overall decrease in all white blood cells with clozapine, but would be unlikely as an isolated abnormality.

Chronic schizophrenia

9 A   This symptom is tardive dyskinesia (TD), which generally occurs in those taking antipsychotics (particularly older depot antipsychotics) over many years. It is distressing as well as socially, if not physically, disabling.

There are numerous theories about why it occurs, although none has been universally proven. The best course of action in this case would be to try a gradual decrease in the depot medication (A), particularly as the man has been well for so long. This should be done with extreme caution and under regular medical supervision. Approximately 50 per cent of cases of TD improve. Decreasing the depot may cause an initial worsening of symptoms which should be explained to patients. Starting an anticholinergic (C) is absolutely the wrong thing to do, as these drugs may exacerbate TD, not alleviate it. This does point to the fact that TD is likely to have a different aetiology to parkinsonian side effects of antipsychotics. 'Second-generation' antipsychotics such as olanzapine (D) do seem to cause TD at a lower rate than older antipsychotics. However, in this case, the man is firmly against oral medication, and trying to impose this is merely likely to lead to non-compliance and a breakdown in the therapeutic relationship. One should never discontinue antipsychotics abruptly (E) unless there are compelling reasons to do so such as neuroleptic malignant syndrome. This can lead to all sorts of difficulties beyond the increased risk of a psychotic relapse, and may in fact worsen the dyskinetic symptoms. Although emotional support (B) should be offered to all patients where it is required or likely to benefit, the most appropriate management that is likely to be beneficial is medication review.

Prognosis in schizophrenia

10 E Curiously, having a rapid onset of symptoms (E) appears to confer a positive prognosis in schizophrenia. All of the other options are associated with a poor prognosis – being male (B), having no mood symptoms in the clinical picture (A), being younger at onset (C), and showing an initial poor response to treatment (D). Other poor prognostic markers include lack of social networks, being single, poor pre-morbid educational attainment, having predominantly negative symptoms and having a long duration of illness before treatment.

Other psychotic disorders

11 B This is a classic example of de Clérambault's syndrome (B), also sometimes known as 'erotomania', in which the sufferer, usually a single woman, becomes delusionally convinced that someone of 'exalted' (in current society usually famous) status has become infatuated with them. The delusion is often meticulously constructed, as the sufferer can explain why the object of their affection cannot reveal their feelings, although obviously the explanations are often outlandish or bizarre. The syndrome can cause considerable problems for the targeted person. Note this is not the same as stalking, although some stalkers will suffer with this syndrome. It is often, but not always, part of the picture of a schizophrenic illness. Capgras syndrome (A) is another of the delusional misidentification syndromes, in which the sufferer believes that a person close to them has been replaced by a double (or 'doppelganger'). It is also often part of schizophrenia, but may also be seen in organic brain disease such as dementia. Folie à deux (C) is also known as 'induced delusional disorder'. It is a rare phenomenon whereby two people in a close relationship (thereby already excluding this as an answer for this question!) develop the same delusional beliefs. It occurs more commonly if the pair have lived together for many years and away from the rest of society. Othello syndrome (D), as the name would suggest, is a syndrome of pathological jealousy. Unlike de Clérambault's, it is more common in men. The core of the syndrome is that the sufferer believes their partner is being unfaithful, despite their being no evidence for this. The syndrome is important to be able to recognize because of the potential for violence. Sufferers will often go to extreme lengths to try to prove the infidelity, and their subsequent failure usually only serves to increase the belief of their partner's ability to deceive. Querulant delusions (E) refer to patients with beliefs that lead to sustained and excessive complaints and litigations against authorities. They often end up in lengthy and tangled legal battles.

Side effects of antipsychotics

12 C This is likely to represent hyperprolactinaemia (C), which is a relatively common side effect of many antipsychotics, and by no means limited to the older antipsychotics. It is caused by dopamine blockade of the tuberoinfundibular pathway which regulates prolactin secretion. Symptoms of raised prolactin include gynaecomastia and sexual dysfunction. It is a significant side effect that must be treated seriously. Ignoring it may lead to poor compliance and, in the long term, sustained prolactin levels may lead to osteoporosis. Alpha-blockade (A) from antipsychotic use may lead to sexual dysfunction but would not explain the gynaecomastia. Drug-induced hepatitis (B) would be an unusual finding with haloperidol but it has been reported. Also, these symptoms would be unlikely to be the ones causing hepatitis to present. New-onset diabetes (D) is unlikely to cause sexual dysfunction at early stages, and gynaecomastia would only develop in the context of chronic kidney disease. This is therefore an unlikely option, especially as haloperidol is far less likely than some of the newer antipsychotics to cause problems with blood sugar. Prostatic hypertrophy (E) is a recognized cause of erectile dysfunction, but there is no reason to suggest that this would be a problem in a young man. Antipsychotics may worsen the symptoms of prostatic hypertrophy if they have significant anticholinergic effects (which haloperidol does not particularly), but this would not explain things adequately in this case.

Diagnosis of schizophrenia

13 B This question refers to the ICD-10 diagnosis of schizophrenia, and should not be mistaken with first-rank symptoms, which is a common mistake 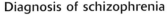 made. Grandiose delusions (B) are more commonly associated with mania, and as such are not specified in ICD-10 for the diagnosis of schizophrenia. Some delusions in schizophrenia, however, can sometimes appear to have a grandiose characteristic, such as believing that the CIA are targeting the individual using brain waves – this would more accurately be described as a 'persecutory delusion'. Formal thought disorder (A), including neologisms (new words being used), metonyms (existing words used in unusual ways) and tangential thinking (unusual connections made between thoughts) are relatively common in schizophrenia, particularly in the acute stages of the illness. Running commentary (C) is when one or more hallucinatory voices comment continuously on what the patient is doing, for example, 'he's walking to the shop now, turning left, over the road, why does he look so stupid when he does that?'. It is strongly suggestive of schizophrenia. For a diagnosis according to ICD-10, the symptoms must have been present for most of the time for a period of at least 1 month, or at some time on most days (D). Thought broadcasting (E), in which the sufferer believes that their thoughts are being transmitted so others can hear them, is also relatively common in schizophrenia. Similar symptoms include thought insertion and thought withdrawal and are sometimes collectively known as symptoms of thought alienation.

Classification of psychotic disorders

14 D This appears to be a schizoaffective disorder (D) of the manic type. The nature of these disorders is a topic of some debate, but according to ICD-10 they occur when both schizophrenic (in this case delusions of passivity in terms of being controlled by the Nazi party as well as auditory hallucinations) coexist with a diagnosable affective disorder (in this case clear manic symptoms). Both must be present within the same episode for the diagnosis to be made. This is not a classic presentation of hebephrenic schizophrenia (A) in which delusions and hallucinations are fleeting and not predominant, but a shallow and inappropriate affect tends to dominate the clinical picture. Disorganized behaviour and speech are also more prominent. An induced delusional disorder (B) is another term for a 'folie à deux' in which a delusion appears to be 'passed on' from someone with a psychotic belief to someone close to them, usually in an isolated relationship from the rest of the world. An example would be an isolated couple in which the wife wrongly believes she is pregnant and this belief is then shared by the husband. While many of the symptoms would be consistent with paranoid schizophrenia (C), such as auditory hallucinations, patients tend to have more paranoid delusions. The affective symptoms are also very pronounced and occur at the same time. Schizotypal disorder (E) is considered by some to be a personality disorder. It is characterized by eccentric behaviours and beliefs that may mimic schizophrenia but without any definite psychotic symptoms. Again, the exact nature of this disorder is unclear.

Antipsychotics

15 D There is almost no evidence for antipsychotics causing renal failure (D), although of course if they precipitate neuroleptic malignant syndrome then this may lead to renal failure through rhabdomyolysis. Also, most antipsychotics are metabolized hepatically, so dose adjustment even in renal disease is usually not indicated (although there are exceptions such as amisulpride). Akathisia (A), or restlessness, is certainly a recognized and common side effect of antipsychotics, particularly those with a propensity for extrapyramidal side effects. Convulsions (B) can occur with antipsychotic use as they tend to lower the seizure threshold. Clozapine significantly reduces seizure threshold, and seizures are a very real possibility for those taking this drug. Hypotension (C) occurs in antipsychotics with adrenergic blockade properties and is usually dose related. These medications should be titrated initially to prevent sudden hypotension and collapse, particularly in the elderly. Tachycardia (E) is also a recognized side effect of antipsychotics. It may be a portent of other more serious cardiac abnormalities with antipsychotic use, such as cardiac arryhythmias and prolonged QT interval, which may lead to sudden cardiac death.

SECTION 27:
AFFECTIVE DISORDERS

Questions

QUESTIONS

1. Subtypes of depression

A 35-year-old woman complains of low mood after the death of her husband in a car accident. She does not speak and remains immobile for long periods. What is the most likely diagnosis?

- A. Seasonal affective disorder
- B. Dysthymia
- C. Atypical depression
- D. Depressive stupor
- E. Post-partum depression

2. Differential diagnoses of depression

A 45-year-old female has had persistent mild depressive features since her late teens. She sometimes experiences loss of energy and tearfulness. She believes her low mood began after she was abused by her step-father as a teenager. She has no other symptoms. What is the most likely diagnosis?

- A. Depressive episode
- B. Recurrent depressive disorder
- C. Dysthymia
- D. Cyclothymia
- E. Bipolar affective disorder

3. Neurological differential diagnosis

What is the most likely condition causing a depressive episode in a 76-year-old man with a history of smoking and hypertension?

- A. Multiple sclerosis
- B. Parkinson's disease
- C. Huntington's disease
- D. Stroke
- E. Spinal cord injury

4. Endocrine causes of low mood (1)

A 35-year-old female visits her GP complaining of low mood and weight loss. On questioning she also experiences fatigue which is exacerbated by pain in her legs. Blood tests reveal high potassium. Which of the following is most likely to cause her depression?

- A. Cushing's disease
- B. Addison's disease
- C. Hypothyroidism

D.   Primary hyperparathyroidism
E.   Premenstrual tension syndrome

5. Infectious causes of low mood

A 43-year-old female visits her GP complaining of a 4-week history of fever, fatigue, low mood and lower back pain. She had visited China in the previous month and mentioned she was drinking plenty of goat's milk as this was the only type of milk available. What is the most likely infective cause?

A.   Hepatitis C
B.   Infectious mononucleosis
C.   Herpes simplex
D.   Brucellosis
E.   Syphilis

6. Organic causes of low mood

A 35-year-old woman has had a low mood for 2 months associated with fever, fatigue and joint pain. She has a rash on her face which gets worse with exposure to the sun. What is the most likely cause of her low mood?

A.   Pancreatic cancer
B.   Systemic lupus erythematosus (SLE)
C.   Rheumatoid arthritis
D.   Porphyria
E.   Pellagra

7. Iatrogenic causes of low mood

Which of the following is most likely to cause depression?

A.   Methyldopa
B.   Atenolol
C.   Ibuprofen
D.   Prednisolone
E.   Amlodipine

8. Endocrine causes of low mood (2)

A 25-year-old woman visits her GP complaining of low mood, fatigue and weight gain. She is observed to be wearing several layers despite its being a warm day. On examination she is found to have a pulse rate of 55. What is the most likely underlying diagnosis?

A.   Cushing's disease
B.   Hypocalcaemia
C.   Addison's disease

D. Hypothyroidism
E. Diabetes mellitus

9. Psychiatric disorders of elevated mood

A 45-year-old woman is taken to see a GP by her husband. He mentions that his wife has been irritable for the past 2 weeks. She is not sleeping well and on examination she has pressure of speech and mild elation. She is not hallucinating and there is no evidence of delusional thinking. What is the most likely diagnosis?

A. Hypomania
B. Mania
C. Cyclothymia
D. Agitated depression
E. Bipolar affective disorder

10. Features of mania

A 25-year-old man with bipolar disorder is seen on the psychiatric ward by a medical student. Taking a history is not easy, as the patient continually wants to speak. The patient is difficult to interrupt. What feature of mania is demonstrated by this patient?

A. Elevated mood
B. Poor concentration
C. Flight of ideas
D. Pressure of speech
E. Impaired judgement

11. Infective causes of mood disorders

A 25-year-old man is seen in accident and emergency with an elevated mood and mild signs of meningism. He has a low grade fever and a bulls eye rash is seen on his left lower arm. What is the most likely diagnosis?

A. HIV
B. Lyme disease
C. Encephalitis
D. Neurosyphilis
E. Meningococcal septicaemia

12. Classification of mood disorders

According to the International Classification of Diseases, which of the following is a core feature of depression?

A. Anergia
B. Diurnal variation of mood
C. Loss of appetite

D.   Suicidal ideation

E.   Waking early

13. Antidepressants

Which of the following antidepressants is not a serotonin specific reuptake inhibitor (SSRI)?

A.   Citalopram

B.   Fluoxetine

C.   Mirtazapine

D.   Paroxetine

E.   Sertraline

14. Risk factors for low mood

Which of the following is a significant risk factor for depression?

A.   Education to degree level

B.   Male gender

C.   Obesity

D.   Older age

E.   Social isolation

15. Thought content in mood disorders

Which of the following statements is most consistent with a diagnosis of psychotic depression?

A.   The bank has said I'm bankrupt and are going to sell all my clothes

B.   I have developed a special computer program which will cure people of depression

C.   The Queen is hiding in the police station and controls my movements through the radio

D.   I'm worried I have got cancer and will die soon

E.   The prime minister was on the radio last night and told the country how much he was in love with me

16. Risk factors for suicide

Which of the following is the most significant risk factor for completed suicide?

A.   Female sex

B.   Older age

C.   Previous suicide attempt

D.   Obsessive–compulsive symptoms

E.   Unemployment

17. Psychological symptoms in low mood

Which of the following symptoms is a recognized psychological symptom of depression?

A. Diurnal variation of mood
B. Nihilism
C. Loss of libido
D. Decreased appetite
E. Early morning waking

ANSWERS

Subtypes of depression

1 D Depressive stupor (D) is a rare presentation of depressive disorder. It can be characterized by mutism and akinesis (lack of movement). Depression with severe psychomotor retardation can lead to dehydration and pressure sores and should be treated urgently. Seasonal affective disorder (A) is characterized by the same psychiatric and biological symptoms that depressive patients face but is associated with the change of season. Depression will be worse in autumn and winter but will usually resolve in the warmer months. Patients may experience a lack of energy, difficulty waking in the mornings and overeating. Dysthymia (B) consists of chronic low grade mood symptoms not amounting to a depressive illness. Symptoms of atypical depression (C) are the opposite of what is experienced in conventional depression. Patients may have symptoms such as weight gain, increased appetite and hypersomnia. Post-partum depression (E) indicates a depressive disorder that appears after giving birth.

Differential diagnoses of depression

2 C Dysthymia (C) is defined as a chronic low grade mood disorder. Symptoms are not severe enough for a diagnosis of depressive episode although discrete episodes of depression may occur in addition. For a diagnosis of a depressive episode (A), at least one core symptom (low mood, anhedonia and anergia) must be demonstrated for a minimum period of 2 weeks. The grade of depression can be classified as mild, moderate or severe, depending on the number and severity of symptoms. Recurrent depressive disorder (B) is associated with repeated episodes of depression but between episodes the patient is euthymic. Cyclothymia (D) is diagnosed where there is persistent instability of mood with a cycle of low grade elevated and depressed mood. This can be differentiated from bipolar affective disorder (E) which is characterized by discrete episodes of mania or hypomania which may or may not be accompanied by episodes of depression.

Neurological differential diagnosis

3 D Stroke (D) is a major risk factor for the development of depression and occurs in approximately 30 per cent of patients. The patient has significant risk factors for cerebrovascular disease in terms of his long-term history of smoking and hypertension. Multiple sclerosis (A) is sometimes associated with depression or elevation of mood. Depression is common in Parkinson's disease (B) but may be missed due to the overlap of symptoms. Depression may be the presenting complaint in patients with Huntington's disease (C), preceding all other symptoms of this neurodegenerative condition. Disability due to spinal cord injury (E) is associated with depression, which may stem from physical factors such as chronic pain, or psychological factors such as loss of independence.

Endocrine causes of low mood (1)

4   B   The most likely cause is Addison's disease (B), caused by adrenocortical insufficiency. Symptoms include fatigue, joint/muscle pain in the legs, skin tanning and hyponatraemia and hyperkalaemia. As well as the biological symptoms of Addison's disease, the condition may present as depression with other manifestations of the disease appearing later. Cushing's disease (A) results in high circulating cortisol levels and is associated with irritability, aggression and depression. Signs and symptoms of Cushing's include centripetal obesity, cervical fat pads, plethoric facies and bruising. Signs and symptoms of hypothyroidism (C) include cold intolerance, bradycardia, weight gain and depression. Hypothyroidism can also mimic depression with symptoms such as forgetfulness, low energy and an inability to concentrate. Primary hyperparathyroidism (D) results in an increased production of parathyroid hormone as well as an elevated blood calcium level, leading to the symptoms of moans (depression), groans (abdominal symptoms), stones (kidney stones) and bones (osteoporosis). Premenstrual tension syndrome (E) (menstrual cycle disorders), is characterized by low mood, irritability and stress, associated with alterations in the balance of sex hormones.

Infectious causes of low mood

5   D   Brucellosis (D) is a contagious zoonosis transmitted via unpasteurized goat's milk or contact with infected animals. The infection induces fevers, headaches, fatigue, pain and depression. Hepatitis C (A) is a viral infection transmitted by intravenous drug use, sexual contact and exposure to infected blood products. As well as the generalized symptoms of fever, appetite loss and nausea, depression can ensue. It is hypothesized that the association with depression may be a due to a direct effect of the virus on neuronal pathways. Infectious mononucleosis (B), a viral disease caused by the Epstein–Barr virus, is characterized by symptoms such as fever, sore throat, fatigue and depression. Herpes simplex (C) infection may sometimes cause depressive symptoms. Syphilis (E) is a sexually transmitted disease that may lead to neurological involvement. Neurosyphilis is associated with several psychiatric conditions including psychosis, dementia, mania and depression.

Organic causes of low mood

6   B   SLE (B) is a multiorgan autoimmune disease associated with anti-nuclear antibodies. The classic manifestation is joint pain and a butterfly shaped malar rash on the face. Neurological involvement can cause headaches, seizures and/or depression. Depression is commonly associated with pancreatic cancer (A) and low mood is sometimes the first symptom of this condition. Rheumatoid arthritis (C) is a chronic inflammatory condition with primarily small joint involvement sometimes associated with depression. Patients do not usually develop a rash. In porphyria (D) there is a deficiency of enzymes in haemoglobin metabolism. Neurological involvement can cause anxiety, hallucinations and/or depression. Patients usually present with abdominal rather than joint pain. Pellagra (E) is caused by deficiency of vitamin B3 (niacin). Sensitivity to sunlight predominates the symptom cluster, which includes dementia and diarrhoea.

Iatrogenic causes of low mood

7 A Corticosteroids (D) such as prednisolone, hydrocortisone and dexamethasone are associated with mania but may also cause depression. The side effects of methyldopa include depression, suicidal ideation and nightmares. Some beta-blockers which cross the blood–brain barrier, such as propranolol, may cause depression but atenolol (B) does not. Ibuprofen (C) is a non-steroidal anti-inflammatory drug and is rarely associated with depression. Amlodipine (E) is a calcium-channel blocker, indicated for the treatment of hypertension. Depression is an occasional side effect of calcium channel blockers.

Endocrine causes of low mood (2)

8 D Hypothyroidism is associated with fatigue, weight gain and cold intolerance. On examination the patient may be bradycardic and have slow-relaxing reflexes. Low circulating thyroxine is associated with depression and should be further investigated with thyroid function tests (D). Cushing's disease (A) may be associated with depression (and other psychiatric disorders) and is characterized by centripetal obesity, cervical fat pads, plethoric complexion and bruising, but not cold intolerance or bradycardia. Hypocalcaemia (B) is rarely associated with depression. Addison's disease (C) can be associated with depression but not cold intolerance or bradycardia. Diabetes mellitus (E) can be associated with depression but would usually be associated with weight loss in a woman of this age.

Psychiatric disorders of elevated mood

9 A Hypomania (A) is associated with elevated mood (elation) and/or irritability which interferes with activities of daily living but is not severely disruptive or associated with psychotic symptoms. Mania (B) occurs over a time-course of at least a week and is defined by a significantly elevated mood which has a noticeable effect on work and social activities and is often associated with psychotic features (mood-congruent delusions and/or hallucinations). Cyclothymia (C) is persistent instability of mood, not a discrete episode.

Agitated depression (D) may present with an irritable mood and anxiety, but not elation. A diagnosis of bipolar affective disorder (E) can be made if there has been a history of two more affective episodes at least one of which must include elevated mood.

Features of mania

10 D Pressure of speech (D) in mania is the result of pressure of thought. The speech of a patient become increasingly difficult to interrupt as the patient wants to portray all of his/her thoughts. Speech is rapid and is worse with increased severity of mania. Manic patients may have an elevated mood (A) which may manifest as being over-cheerful or irritable. Manic patients find it difficult to maintain focus on one thing which leads to poor concentration (B). Flight of ideas (C) occurs when patients thoughts move from topic to topic, although there is usually a connection between the ideas. Mania often leads to impaired judgement (E).

Infective causes of mood disorders

11 B Lyme disease (B) is an infectious disease caused by bacteria belonging to the genus *Borrelia*, transmitted to humans via tick bites. Early symptoms will include fever, headache, fatigue and mood changes. An expanding rash known as erythema chronicum migrans (bulls eye rash) appears at the site of the tick bite and is strongly suggestive of the diagnosis. People with HIV (A) infection may develop manic symptoms. Symptoms of encephalitis (C) may include headache, fever and confusion, hallucinations, cognitive decline and mania. Neurosyphilis (D) is a sexually transmitted disease, associated with several psychiatric conditions including psychosis, mania and depression. People with meningococcal septicaemia (E) are acutely unwell and have a generalized erythematous rash.

Classification of mood disorders

12 A The three core features of depression are anergia (loss of energy) (A) anhedonia (loss of enjoyment) and low mood. At least one feature must be present for at least 2 weeks. Biological features include change in appetite (C) and weight, change in sleep pattern (classically waking early (E)), loss of libido and diurnal variation of mood (B), where the mood is worse in the morning. Psychological features of depression include feelings of guilt, hopelessness, and suicidal ideation (D).

Antidepressants

13 C Mirtazapine (c) is a noradrenergic and specific serotinergic antidepressant with a tetracyclic structure. Mirtazapine is often used second line. It differs from SSRIs (A, B, D, E) in that it does not usually cause nausea or weight loss and induces sleep.

Risk factors for low mood

14 E Risk factors for depression include having a family history, female gender (B), childhood abuse, poverty and social isolation (E). Being older (D) does not increase risk of depression and higher education may be protective (A). Obesity (C) is a risk factor for dementia but not depression as such.

Thought content in mood disorders

15 A Psychosis is an infrequent complication of depression although may be seen quite commonly in psychiatric settings. Delusions in depression are usually 'mood congruent', i.e. are understandable in the context of being depressed. Examples include delusions of poverty or low self-worth (A). Delusions in mania are frequently grandiose (B). Bizarre delusions, especially with passivity (C) or thought alienation, are suggestive of schizophrenia. Option (E) is suggestive of de Clérembault's syndrome which usually occurs in mania or schizophrenia, rarely depression. It is important to distinguish delusions from non-delusional ideation (D) which is not held with subjective certainty.

Risk factors for suicide

16 C Approximately 1 per cent of people who attempt suicide will kill themselves in the following year making this (C) the most significant risk factor. Suicide is always more common in men (A). Although rates used to rise in older age (B), more recent data suggest this is no longer a risk factor. Unemployment (E) is associated with increased risk but obsessive–compulsive disorder (D) may be protective.

Psychological symptoms in low mood

17 B Nihilism (B) is a psychological feature of depression characterized by an overwhelming feeling of hopelessness and negativity which may amount to delusional intensity. Other psychological features include persistent low mood, loss of enjoyment (anhedonia), hopelessness, guilt, poor concentration, irritability, low self-esteem, and suicidal thoughts. Diurnal variation of mood (A) where the patient usually feels worse in the morning is regarded as a biological feature as are loss of libido (C), and changes in appetite (D) and sleep (E).

SECTION 28:
ANXIETY AND
SOMATOFORM DISORDERS

QUESTIONS

1. Symptoms of anxiety

Which of the following is not a typical feature of anxiety?

    A. Constipation
    B. Dyspnoea
    C. Fear
    D. Palpitations
    E. Tremor

2. Diagnosis of anxiety disorders

A 46-year-old woman is referred to secondary psychiatric services by her GP. Over the last 6 months she has suffered multiple losses, including the death of her sister and a close friend. She lives alone with few social contacts. She has become extremely withdrawn, and is leaving the house less, stating that she gets 'terrified that I won't be able to get back to my house'. She reports that when she does go out, she feels breathless, sweaty and like 'she might faint and make a fool of myself'. What is the most likely diagnosis?

    A. Agoraphobia
    B. Generalized anxiety disorder (GAD)
    C. Obsessive–compulsive disorder (OCD)
    D. Panic disorder
    E. Social phobia

3. Management of anxiety disorders

A woman is diagnosed with agoraphobia. She is willing to try any form of treatment as her condition is very disabling. Which of the following management options would not be considered appropriate in the overall management of agoraphobia first line?

    A. Cognitive behavioural therapy (CBT)
    B. Exposure therapy
    C. Lorazepam
    D. Paroxetine
    E. Psychoeducation

4. Social phobia

Which of the following statements concerning social phobia is correct?

    A. Beta-blockers are of no therapeutic value in social phobia
    B. Genetic factors do not have a role in the aetiology of social phobia
    C. It only arises as the result of a particularly stressful social episode

    D.   Men are less likely to report symptoms of social phobia than women

    E.   Social phobia most commonly manifests before puberty

5. Generalized anxiety disorder

Which of the following statements regarding generalized anxiety disorder (GAD) is incorrect?

    A.   GAD is more common in women than men

    B.   GAD may be mistaken for a physical disorder

    C.   GAD may be triggered by stressful events

    D.   Physical disorders may be mistaken for GAD

    E.   The presence of major depression excludes a diagnosis of GAD

6. Theories of anxiety

Which of the following statements regarding theories of anxiety is correct?

    A.   Cognitive theories propose that anxiety is the result of distorted thinking, such as catastrophizing and labelling

    B.   Freud believed that anxiety was the result of conscious conflict

    C.   Neurobiological theories implicate dopamine as the most commonly involved neurotransmitter

    D.   Psychoanalytic theory argues that secure attachment is a primary cause of anxiety

    E.   The adaptive theory of anxiety states that anxiety is a maladaptive process

7. Obsessive–compulsive disorder (1)

Which of the following statements regarding OCD is correct?

    A.   OCD affects women and men equally

    B.   OCD is the most common anxiety disorder

    C.   The fear of contamination is a common compulsion

    D.   The compulsions in OCD cannot be resisted

    E.   The obsessive thoughts in OCD do not usually feel unpleasant

8. Obsessive–compulsive disorder (2)

Which one of the following statements regarding OCD is incorrect?

    A.   Antidepressants do not have a role in the management of OCD

    B.   Preventing patients from performing compulsions is a mainstay of behavioural therapy

    C.   Streptococcal infections may precipitate OCD in children

    D.   People with OCD know the intrusive thoughts are their own

    E.   Tourette's syndrome and OCD are interrelated disorders

9. Somatoform and dissociative disorders

Which of the following statements regarding somatoform and dissociative disorders is correct?

A. Amnesia may be a form of dissociation
B. Body dysmorphic disorder involves a psychotic belief about one's body
C. Cultural differences are not important in the diagnosis of somatoform disorders
D. Hypochondriasis implies there is nothing wrong with the patient
E. Multiple personality disorder has a prevalence roughly equal to that of schizophrenia

10. Post-traumatic stress disorder

A 42-year-old man is involved in a serious road traffic accident caused by a drunk driver. He is hospitalized for several weeks. Following discharge, friends and family notice that he is not going out, has become withdrawn and appears frightened and anxious all the time. He reluctantly agrees to see his GP. Which of the following would not be consistent with a diagnosis of post-traumatic stress disorder (PTSD)?

A. Diminished startle response
B. Flashbacks of the accident
C. Hypervigilance
D. Poor concentration
E. Reluctance to drive

ANSWERS

Symptoms of anxiety

1 A   The symptoms of anxiety can be classified in numerous ways, but are commonly thought of as psychological and somatic. The somatic, or physical, symptoms of anxiety are primarily the result of autonomic arousal and include gastrointestinal symptoms (dry mouth, epigastric discomfort and diarrhoea, not constipation (A)), respiratory (shortness of breath (B), hyperventilation), cardiovascular (palpitations (D), tachycardia) and genitourinary (urgency of micturition, impotence, occasionally menstrual disturbances). Other common symptoms include tremor (E), headache and sleep disturbances. The psychological symptoms of anxiety include intense worries or fear (C), irritability, hypersensitivity to noise and poor concentration. The focus of the thoughts or fears depends on the nature of the anxiety problem and is discussed further below. There may also be avoidance of the anxiety-provoking stimulus/stimuli.

Diagnosis of anxiety disorders

2 A   This is a fairly difficult question, at least in part because anxiety disorders often overlap. It is important, both from a prognostic and management point of view, to accurately identify the type of anxiety disorder, as well as exclude any other co-morbidities, such as depression, which is common in anxiety disorders. As a rule, try to identify the source of the anxiety-provoking stimulus. In this case, it appears to be a fear of leaving the house and being outside, driven by negative thoughts such as 'I might faint or not be able to get home'. This is extremely suggestive of agoraphobia (A), where the fear focuses on being out of the house, on public transport, in crowds, or other situations that the sufferer views as difficult to escape from. There is nearly always avoidance (e.g. going out less), and 'anticipatory' anxiety, where the thought of leaving the house brings on symptoms of anxiety. GAD (B) is characterized by so-called 'free-floating' anxiety, where there are persistent symptoms of anxiety (excessive 'worry' being particularly common) that are not restricted to any particular stimulus. Sufferers tend to be excessively apprehensive about a widespread range of things. Distinguishing between depression is often difficult. It is worth noting that while the two often coexist, they are undoubtedly separate entities in their own right. OCD (C) would not typically present in this way. There are further questions about OCD later in this section. Panic attacks are common in agoraphobia when people are exposed to the offending stimuli, but this is not the same as panic disorder (D). In the latter, the predominant picture is one of recurrent episodic panic attacks, in which there is usually intense fear of imminent doom, going mad or 'losing control'. Physical symptoms such as a feeling of choking are also common and hyperventilation is almost always present. Panic disorder arguably has the biggest overlap with agoraphobia. Social phobia (E) is a disorder that consists primarily of excessive worry about social situations, such as speaking in public and feeling 'scrutinized'. Alcohol misuse is often co-morbid in this disorder, as people may use alcohol as a relaxant in social situations. Sometimes there is a particular fear of losing control of the bladder or bowels or vomiting in public.

Management of anxiety disorders

3 C Benzodiazepines are often used in the short-term management of anxiety and, despite concerns over their potential for dependence and abuse, they continue to be extensively prescribed. Overall, they should be avoided where possible but may be prescribed in short bursts for severe anxiety, although with caution and preferably with specialist advice. Regardless of this, lorazepam (C) would not be an appropriate choice of benzodiazepines because of its short duration. Diazepam, with a longer half-life, would be a more appropriate choice. CBT (A) is now the mainstay of treatment for many anxiety disorders, including agoraphobia. It seeks to identify automatic negative thoughts and feelings and link them with unwanted behaviours and also identifies more helpful patterns of thoughts and actions. Exposure therapy (B) is a form of CBT in which the sufferer is gradually 'exposed' to the anxiety-provoking stimulus in a safe and graded fashion. This would perhaps begin by standing with the front door open for increasing lengths of time, while thoughts and feelings are examined. The length and degree of exposure is then gradually increased. Paroxetine (D) is a selective serotonin reuptake inhibitor (SSRI). Although the SSRIs have a confusing array of licenses for different conditions, they all appear to have a beneficial effect in anxiety disorders. Paroxetine has a license for panic disorder so would be a suitable choice here (there is no SSRI with a specific license for agoraphobia). Note that SSRIs do not have an immediate effect and may worsen symptoms in the first few days. Patients should be warned that it may be a few weeks before any benefit occurs. It is now commonly accepted that a dual approach of CBT and medication may be the most superior treatment option, but of course this will not necessarily work for everyone and, most importantly, treatment should be targeted to the needs of the individual. Psychoeducation (E), while a rather vague term, is a critical part of managing anxiety disorders. Common conceptions in sufferers are that they are going mad or may even 'die' from their fear and worry. It is extremely important that the nature of anxiety is fully explained to patients. Without this priming, it is far less likely that other treatments will be effective.

Social phobia

4 D While the epidemiology of social phobia suggests that men are approximately as likely as women to suffer with social phobia, they are less likely (D) to report symptoms or seek professional advice (as for many other mental health problems). Beta-blockers (A), while they do not have any role in tackling the source of social phobia, are often used for symptomatic relief in unavoidable stressful social situations, such as family gatherings, presenting something at work etc. They should only be used, however, as part of the overall management of social phobia which should include psychological interventions. Genetic factors do play a role in social phobia (B), and possibly even more so than other anxiety disorders. Both population and twin studies confirm this. It is now thought that avoidant personality disorder is aetiologically related to social phobia although more work needs to be carried out on this. While most cases of social phobia are triggered by a significant anxiety-provoking social situation, it may also develop in the absence of such a 'critical' event (C). Social phobia usually manifests in the late teens or in the third decade (E). However, as stated above, there is growing recognition of its likely relationship to certain personality types and disorders.

Generalized anxiety disorder

5 E Anxiety and depression are both very common, and both are risk factors for the other. While the symptoms may overlap, particularly in milder cases, this does not imply that one diagnosis 'trumps' the other (E). GAD is one of the most common psychiatric diagnoses, with prevalence rates usually quoted in the region of 3 per cent of adults, although when ICD-10 criteria are used it appears to lead to higher prevalence rates than using DSM-IV criteria. It is thought to affect more women than men, even when accounting for lower consultation rates in men (A). GAD is often mistaken for a physical disorder, particularly in the elderly (B). These patients may be started on potentially harmful medications, such as antihypertensives, rate-controlling drugs etc. A thorough history should help prevent this. The converse, of course, is also true (D). Perhaps the most quoted (although by no means the most common) is the patient presenting with 'anxiety' who actually has a phaeochromocytoma. Many disorders, including hyperthyroidism, hypoglycaemia and cardiac arrythmias, may mimic the symptoms of anxiety. Equally, anxiety may be triggered by physical symptoms, or excessive worry about physical health. Just because GAD is 'generalized' this does not mean that it may not be triggered by a particularly stressful life event (C), and in fact this is often the case.

Theories of anxiety

6 A   There are numerous theories of anxiety, but you should be familiar with the basics of the more common theoretical viewpoints. Cognitive theory has been studied extensively in anxiety (A), and looks at the distortions in cognitive processes that people with anxiety appear to hold. These include catastrophizing ('If I go outside, I'm sure I'll have a heart attack') and labelling ('I am just an awkward, boring person'). The fact that CBT is such an effective treatment for anxiety disorders also provides indirect evidence of the role of cognitive distortions in anxiety. Freud believed that anxiety was the result of intrapsychic, unconscious conflict (B). Broadly speaking, he believed that anxiety occurs when the ego is overwhelmed by different types of conflict or excitation. Most neurobiological studies of anxiety implicate non-dopaminergic pathways (C), particularly noradrenaline, GABA and serotonin. Dopaminergic pathways may be involved in certain anxiety disorders, e.g. OCD. Secure attachment would not lead to anxiety disorders (D) in psychoanalytic theory. Childhood attachment problems, conversely, may lead to the resurgence of anxiety problems in adulthood, particularly around separation. The adaptive theory (E) states that anxiety exists as an evolutionary advantage, commonly referred to as the 'fight or flight' response. The Yerkes–Dodson law may be considered an extension of this, where performance plotted against anxiety results in a bell-shaped curve – up to a point, some anxiety may increase performance.

Obsessive–compulsive disorder (1)

7 A   OCD, unlike most other anxiety disorders, seems to affect men and women equally (A). The mean age of onset is in the third decade, although there is often a considerable lag of some years before people present for assessment, often because of poor understanding of the nature of the disorder. OCD is probably one of the less common anxiety disorders (B), although it is now thought to be much more common than previous estimates, with figures nowadays at around 2–3 per cent for lifetime prevalence. The fear of contamination is very common in OCD sufferers, but this is an obsessive thought, not a compulsive behaviour (C). Obsessional thoughts consist of recurrent and intrusive words, images, ideas and beliefs that are usually always unpleasant for the sufferer, causing anxiety and distress. They must interfere with the sufferer's ability to carry out their everyday life. Compulsions represent repetitive behaviours (e.g. hand washing) or mental acts (e.g. counting) usually in response to an obsessional thought. The sufferer feels compelled to carry them out in order to reduce the anxiety provoked by the obsessive thought, although there seldom appears to be any rational connection between the compulsion and how it may reduce the obsessive anxiety. Generally, OCD sufferers attempt to resist compulsive acts as they realize they are maladaptive. However, resistance usually ends in increasing anxiety and eventually sufferers will succumb to the behaviour. So, in this sense, compulsive acts may be both resisted and not resisted (D). The obsessive thoughts in OCD are nearly always unpleasant, or certainly strange and unusual (E).

Obsessive–compulsive disorder (2)

8 A Antidepressants, particularly SSRIs, form the mainstay of the pharmacotherapy of OCD (A). They have significant anti-obsessional properties. The tricyclic antidepressant clomipramine has also been used to treat OCD as it has a potent serotonergic reuptake blocking action. Also, depression is a common co-morbid condition in OCD which will warrant its own assessment and management. Although it may appear counterintuitive and even cruel to prevent patients from carrying out their rituals, this is the most common psychological approach to treating the condition and is known as exposure and response prevention (B). It is a form of CBT. Beta-haemolytic streptococcal infections in children can occasionally lead to an autoimmune reaction known as 'PANDAS' – Paediatric Autoimmune Neuropsychiatric Disorders Associated with Streptococcal infections (C). The neuropsychiatric consequences include obsessive–compulsive symptoms and tic disorders. People with OCD could be said to have 'insight' into their intrusive thoughts and compulsions (D), they know their beliefs are the result of their own mind, and usually see the thoughts and behaviours as unhelpful or even ridiculous, despite still feeling compelled to follow them. The exception to this is OCD in children, where they often do not have this insight. There appears to be some commonality in the pathogenesis of both OCD and tic disorders. It is thought that this is related to basal ganglia changes (E).

Somatoform and dissociative disorders

9 A These disorders are difficult to understand and research into them is only just beginning to uncover any meaningful answers. Their classification, diagnosis and management is generally regarded to be unsatisfactory. However, there can be no doubt that psychological factors can lead to physical symptoms and vice versa. Broadly speaking, dissociation refers to a loss of integration between consciousness, memory, perception, identity and bodily movements. There are different forms this may take, with amnesia being one of them (A). Of course, amnesia may also have a very obvious, neurological basis following, for example, head trauma. Body dysmorphic disorder is classified as part of hypochondriacal disorders. It involves the persistent preoccupation that one's own body is in some way disfigured or otherwise abnormal. However, this is considered to be an overvalued idea and is not psychotic (B). One of the problems with the classification and aetiology of somatoform disorders is the wide way in which they may be culturally explained (C). Culture plays a huge part in how these 'symptoms' are understood; for instance, 'trance states' may be seen as abnormal in Western societies, but in others may be perceived as entirely normal, or even revered. One commonly encounters this kind of disparity in patients from Asian backgrounds complaining of pain 'all over the body' which does not appear to have a 'physical cause' in Western terms. Hypochondriasis occurs when sufferers have a persistent preoccupation with having a physical disorder for which no physical 'cause' can be found. However, this does not mean that there is nothing 'wrong' with the patient, as hypochondriasis represents a way of conveying some kind of psychological distress, albeit not in a way that modern medicine has traditionally understood (D). Multiple personality disorder is classified as a dissociative disorder. Despite widespread presence in the media, it is extremely rare and poorly understood (E). It is often used mistakenly as a way of defining schizophrenia in lay terms.

Post-traumatic stress disorder

10 A Post-traumatic stress disorder, while not as poorly understood as the somatoform disorders, is still often missed or even misdiagnosed. It actually has relatively well-defined and circumscribed clinical features, which follow a catastrophic or hugely stressful event. Patients suffering with PTSD show an exaggerated sensitivity and level of psychological arousal, which may present as an exaggerated startle response (A), poor sleep and concentration (D), and irritability or anger. Hypervigilance (C) will also often be present. There is nearly always some form of remembering the event, usually in vivid nightmares or flashbacks (B). If sufferers are put in a situation that reminds them of the event, this will cause extreme distress. This is partly why those with PTSD exhibit avoidance (E) of similar situations, in this case, driving again.

SECTION 29:
OLD AGE PSYCHIATRY

QUESTIONS

1. Neuropathology and dementia

Which of the following findings on a MRI scan would be most consistent with a diagnosis of early Alzheimer's disease?

    A.   Caudate atrophy
    B.   Cerebellar atrophy
    C.   Frontal atrophy
    D.   Hippocampal atrophy
    E.   Periventricular white matter lesions

2. Management of dementia

Which of the following modes of action of currently available pharmacological agents are thought to target some of the symptoms of dementia?

    A.   Drugs which decrease the levels of serotonin in the brain
    B.   Drugs which increase the levels of dopamine in the brain
    C.   Drugs which increase the levels of acetycholine in the brain
    D.   Drugs which decrease the levels of histamine in the brain
    E.   Drugs which increase the levels of GABA in the brain

3. Differential diagnosis of dementia

A 79-year-old married woman comes to see her GP with her husband. The husband reports his wife has a history of several months of deteriorating memory and is now forgetting names and faces. He also explains that at times she seems much more lucid, but there are occasions when she becomes very forgetful and confused, sometimes saying there are people sat in the living room with them, which the patient and her husband find distressing. More recently she has developed a tremor in her left hand. What is the most likely diagnosis?

    A.   Alzheimer's disease
    B.   Lewy body dementia
    C.   Parkinson's dementia
    D.   Pick's disease
    E.   Vascular dementia

4. Dementia and depression in older age

Which of the following features would suggest a diagnosis of depression rather than dementia in a patient presenting with memory loss?

    A.   Delusions
    B.   Fluctuating conscious level
    C.   Low mood

D. Poor verbal fluency
E. Excessive worry over memory loss

5. Depression in older age (1)

Which of the following statements most accurately reflects depression in older age?

A. Anxiety states are uncommon in depressive disorders in older age
B. Depression in older age is not associated with deliberate self-harm
C. Depression is less common in residential homes than in the general community
D. Old age is a risk factor for depression
E. Somatization is a common presentation of depression in old age

6. Depression in older age (2)

A 90-year-old woman is admitted to the psychiatric inpatient unit with severe depression. She has the following medical history: end-stage chronic renal failure, hypertension, type 2 diabetes controlled with oral hypoglycaemics, and has had a stroke 3 years ago leaving her with some slight speech slurring. Which of the following statements is false?

A. A serotonin specific reuptake inhibitor (SSRI) antidepressant would be a safe choice
B. Benzodiazepines should not be prescribed routinely for this patient
C. Electroconvulsive therapy (ECT) would be contraindicated because of the stroke
D. Lithium would not be the first line option
E. The patient's diabetes will impact on the course and prognosis of her depression

7. Depression in older age (3)

An 84-year-old man is brought in to the psychiatric unit with a diagnosis of severe depression with psychotic symptoms. He has had three previous admissions with very similar symptoms. During his admission he begins voicing his desire to leave the ward, claiming that the devil is possessing all of the staff and patients, and that he is next. He claims that if he isn't allowed to leave, he will do whatever he can to escape the devil, even if this means ending his life. He has had to be moved away from the door after trying to follow visitors out of the ward. What would be the most appropriate course of action?

A. Detain him under common law for his own safety
B. Do nothing as staff have been able to coax him back on to the ward
C. Place him on Section 3 of the Mental Health Act
D. Request an immediate Deprivation of Liberty Safeguard ('DOLS') assessment under the Mental Capacity Act
E. Use intramuscular rapid tranquilization to alleviate his distress and keep the ward safe

8. Mania in older age

Which of the following statements most accurately reflects manic syndromes in older age?

A. All manic elderly patients should be detained under the Mental Health Act

B. Bipolar disorder resolves in later life

C. In bipolar disorder beginning in old age, most would have had episodes of depression before a manic episode

D. Unipolar mania (i.e. mania occurring without episodes of depression) is more common than bipolar disorder in older age

E. Unlike depression, physical co-morbidity does not have an impact on manic syndromes in the elderly

9. Hallucinations in older age

An 80-year-old woman with a past medical history including hypertension, diabetes and macular degeneration is admitted to accident and emergency complaining of frightening images of birds swooping around her flat day and night. At first she thought they were real but now realizes they could not be. She has no past psychiatric history and apart from being very tearful about the images, there is nothing else of note in the mental state. What is the most likely diagnosis?

A. Charles Bonnet syndrome

B. Cotard's syndrome

C. Ekbom's syndrome

D. Fregoli's syndrome

E. Rett's syndrome

10. Psychotic symptoms in older age

A 74-year-old widowed woman, previously fit and well with no past psychiatric history, presents to her GP to 'have it out once and for all about these bloody neighbours'. She says for the last month her neighbours have been spying on her and are leaking radiation through her ceiling which is making her cough incessantly. On examination she does indeed have a severe cough and has lost weight since her last appointment 3 months ago. Otherwise she looks fairly healthy and well kempt, with an Mini-Mental State Examination (MMSE) of 29/30. Which of the following statements is the most accurate?

A. Antipsychotics are likely to have a rapid and successful effect

B. Rehousing is likely to be the most effective treatment

C. The cough is a delusional elaboration of her other symptoms

D. The most likely diagnosis is an early dementia

E. The most likely diagnosis is very late-onset schizophrenia-like psychosis (VLOSLP)

11. Alcohol misuse in older age

Which of the following statements concerning alcohol misuse in older age is the most accurate?

    A. Alcohol dependence almost always begins in earlier life
    B. Alcohol dependence is easier to spot in elderly people
    C. Genetic factors do not have an influence on alcohol misuse in older age
    D. Heavy alcohol use may lead to dementia
    E. The male:female ratio is much lower in older people with alcohol misuse than in the young

12. Anxiety disorders in older age

Which of the following statements concerning anxiety in older age is the most accurate?

    A. Cognitive behavioural therapy (CBT) is less effective in older age than in younger patients
    B. Inpatient management of anxiety is the most successful setting for treatment
    C. Men are more likely to develop anxiety disorders than women in older age
    D. Poor physical health is not associated with the onset of anxiety disorders
    E. Worries over physical health are more common in older adults with anxiety

13. Unusual causes of cognitive impairment

A 71-year-old man, previously fit and well, presents to his GP with his wife who states he has 'lost his marbles' over the last 2 months, with worsening memory loss. He scores 21/30 on the MMSE, losing points mainly on recall as well as dysphasia. His wife has also noticed that he has lost weight. Routine blood tests show the following:

$$Na^+: \quad 129\,mmol/L$$
$$K^+: \quad 4.4\,mmol/L$$
$$\text{Adjusted } Ca^{2+}: \quad 3.1\,mmol/L$$

What is the most likely diagnosis?

    A. Addison's disease
    B. Cerebral malignancy
    C. Cushing's disease
    D. Hyperthyroidism
    E. Primary hyperparathyroidism

14. Ethical considerations in older age

A 90-year-old woman is in hospital with late-stage colon cancer which has metastasized. She has been remarkably well all her life before being diagnosed with cancer. She lost her husband 3 years ago but has a supportive family. On the ward, she develops a chest infection. The consultant wants to start her on antibiotics, but she says she does not want them. The consultant asks for a psychiatric opinion, worried that she is depressed. However, the psychiatrist reports she is not depressed and is fully competent to make this decision and is choosing how to die as she wishes. What ethical concept is best described here?

- A. Autonomy
- B. Beneficence
- C. Capacity
- D. Justice
- E. Non-maleficence

15. Use of medications in older age

Which of the following statements is true about medicines use in older age?

- A. Antipsychotics are the drugs of choice for behavioural disturbance in dementia
- B. Fat-soluble drugs, such as diazepam, will have a longer duration of action because of increased body fat in older people
- C. Lithium doses in older people should generally be lower because the liver cannot excrete it as efficiently
- D. Older people are less sensitive to the effects of benzodiazepines
- E. Tricyclic antidepressants (TCA) will not cause constipation in older people because of a general increase in gut motility

ANSWERS

Neuropathology and dementia

1 D Loss of volume in the hippocampus (D) has been consistently demonstrated in imaging studies in Alzheimer's disease (AD). It is also reduced relatively early in the progression of the disease. Specifically requesting hippocampal volumes when investigating AD is important as otherwise it may not be specifically reported. Other findings on neuroimaging include generalized cerebral atrophy and enlarged ventricles. The caudate nucleus (A) may be slightly smaller in AD but this would not be a particularly important finding and may occur in other forms of dementia. It would also be common in disorders such as Huntington's disease. Cerebellar atrophy (B) occurs late in AD, but is commonly seen in certain movement disorders, including Wilson's disease and Friedreich's ataxia, among others. Atrophy of the frontal lobes (C) may occur in AD, but it is usually a later finding. Primary degeneration at this site is more consistent with one of the frontotemporal dementias, such as Pick's disease. Periventricular white matter lesions (E) refer to lesions occurring in the non-cortical areas adjoining the ventricles as opposed to subcortical lesions. In this sense they usually refer to cerebrovascular lesions and are associated with cognitive dysfunction (i.e. in vascular dementia).

Management of dementia (I)

2 C Compounds which increase the functional levels of acetylcholine (C) in the brain appear to have some effect on cognition in dementia. The compounds currently available block the enzyme that breaks down acetylcholine in the synaptic cleft and are therefore termed acetylcholinesterase inhibitors. In some patients (but by no means all) they lead to improvements in activities of daily living, although they have perhaps less direct benefit on memory itself. The drugs are not curative. Drugs which deplete levels of serotonin (A) in the brain would not have an effect on the cognitive symptoms of dementia. In fact, there are no products currently licensed with this mode of action. Drugs of abuse such as ecstasy cause massive release of serotonin (leading to the 'high') but there is a subsequent depletion of available serotonin before stores are built back up, leading to the depressive symptoms commonly observed after its use. Drugs increasing dopamine levels in the brain (B) are used in disorders such as Parkinson's disease, where the neurochemical lesion is a loss of dopaminergic pathways in the substantia nigra. Note that an increase in functional levels of dopamine may lead to psychotic symptoms. Drugs which decrease the levels of histamine in the brain (D), commonly referred to as antihistamines, would not be expected to have a positive effect on cognition, and indeed may cause confusion, particularly in older age. Drugs which decrease the levels of GABA in the brain (E) are usually sedative. The benzodiazepines are the most commonly used. They would not have a positive effect on cognition.

Differential diagnosis of dementia

3 B This is typical history of a patient suffering with Lewy body dementia/dementia with Lewy bodies (DLB) (B). Lewy bodies are cytoplasmic inclusions that are associated with numerous disorders, including Parkinson's disease. It accounts for around 5–10 per cent of all dementias. There is a classic 'triad' of symptoms in DLB, consisting of visual hallucinations, a fluctuating cognitive impairment and parkinsonism. The fluctuations can be quite marked, with changes seen from day to day or even hour to hour. In this way DLB is often confused with delirium. The hallucinations are usually visual and complex. They are often distressing to the patient, but by no means always. It is not uncommon for patients to calmly state that other people are in the room, for instance sat round the dinner table with them and their spouse. Parkinsonism (which occurs within a year of onset of cognitive difficulties) tends to consist of rigidity and gait difficulties more than tremor. Patients also often have postural hypotension and a risk of falls. DLB has classically been thought to have a more aggressive course than Alzheimer's, but this could in part be due to how it has been treated in the past – it is now known that these patients have marked and often fatal reactions to antipsychotic agents which are generally contraindicated in patients with DLB. While psychotic symptoms do occur in AD (A), they are less frequent than in DLB (although there have been estimates of them occurring in up to one-third of patients). Delusions tend to be encountered more than hallucinations. Parkinson's disease dementia (PDD) (C) occurs in approximately 30 per cent of people with Parkinson's disease, with a higher incidence with increasing age. In contrast to DLB, in PDD the onset of parkinsonism is over a year before cognitive difficulties. It is important to distinguish between PDD and depression, as the latter is also extremely common in PD. Generally, the cognitive profile is indistinguishable from that of DLB. Pick's disease (D) is often used interchangeably with the term frontotemporal dementia (FTD). The FTDs are often misdiagnosed, because they tend to present with significant personality and affective symptoms. There is probably a significant familial component and they can present relatively early in the fifth and sixth decades. The syndrome is characterized by 'frontal' signs such as disinhibition, aggression, antisociality, or the reverse picture of apathy. Memory tends to be preserved but with significant deficits on specific frontal lobe testing. Vascular dementia (E) may of course present in a wide variety of ways because of the possibility of cerebrovascular disease in any part of the brain. A fluctuating course is not typical of vascular dementia, although a 'step-wise' deterioration may be observed.

Dementia and depression in older age

4 E   This question addresses the overlap between dementia and depression and highlights how commonly the two are confused – wrongly diagnosing someone with dementia can have disastrous consequences, particularly if the patient is profoundly depressed. The term 'pseudodementia' is seldom used these days, and refers to depression 'masquerading' as dementia, although it does still have clinical value it highlights the importance of distinguishing between the two disorders. Depression in older age often presents with cognitive difficulties. Subjective and excessive worrying by the patient over their memory is not characteristic of dementia, and should prompt a more thorough search for other depressive symptoms. Insight is typically lost early in dementia (particularly Alzheimer's disease), with the majority of patients (although not all), having little insight into or worry over what may be significant cognitive difficulties. In depression, the patient may become extremely preoccupied with their 'memory'; poor cognitive function in depression is often the result of poor attention and concentration, and in-depth neuropsychological tests which can control for this should reveal no significant memory problems. Delusions (A) are a relatively common feature of both dementia and severe depression. The content of the delusions may be fairly similar, although dementia patients often suffer with delusions of theft and persecution, whereas patients with depression may have delusions with a more 'nihilistic' and bizarre quality, such as believing they are rotting or that the devil is punishing them. Fluctuating conscious level (B) is not characteristic of either dementia or depression and should prompt investigation for an acute confusional state (delirium). Low mood (C), while a hallmark of depression, is not enough to diagnose a depressive disorder. Low mood in itself is also common in patients with dementia, affecting possibly the majority of patients with dementia at some point. There are complex and poorly understood interactions between depression and dementia, on both a neuropathological and clinical level – expert assessment should always be sought. Poor verbal fluency (D) is a test that is often used to assess 'frontal lobe' functioning. However, it is also extremely reliant on attention and concentration. Typically patients are asked to name as many of a particular thing (such as animals, or words beginning with 's') in 1 minute. Poor performance on verbal fluency would not particularly distinguish between dementia and depression.

Depression in older age (1)

5 E   Somatization (E), or the displacement of psychological distress such as depression into physical complaints or symptoms, is common in the depressed elderly. This may be a result of older people tending to minimize their experience of sadness and that somatic complaints represent an alternative way of expressing their distress. Also remember that 'somatic' complaints may actually also represent real undiagnosed medical problems. Do not dismiss the depressed older person's complaints of stomach pain at the risk of missing an occult malignancy. Studies have shown that healthy older people are no more at risk of becoming depressed than healthy younger people (D). However, numerous factors that are associated with older age are associated with an increased risk of depression. Possibly the most important of these is medical co-morbidity, particularly chronic long-term illness. Anxiety states (A) are extremely common in depression in older age, and may in fact be the presenting feature. Deliberate self-harm (B) is societally often seen as an act of the younger generations – this is a dangerous misconception. Older people may also undertake acts of deliberate self harm and remember these may not be associated with depression, but may occur in the context of severe medical disability, pain or loneliness. In fact, when older people do engage in acts of self-harm, this is usually with a high level of suicidal intent and must be taken extremely seriously. Depression is certainly not less common in residential care settings (C) than in the general community. In nursing homes the rate may be up to three times that of the community.

Depression in older age (2)

6 C   ECT (C) is an important treatment for severe depression. It has a chequered history and many opponents. There are very few, if any, absolute contraindications to using ECT, and a stroke from 3 years ago would not be considered a barrier to treatment. Relative contraindications include heart disease, raised intracranial pressure and poor anaesthetic risk. SSRIs (A) are generally thought to be safe in renal impairment. However, it would be important to monitor renal function and urea and electrolytes, particularly as older people and those with renal impairment are at a higher risk of developing the syndrome of inappropriate antidiuretic hormone secretion (SIADH) from SSRIs, leading to hyponatraemia. Benzodiazepines (B) are not recommended for use in older age, and depression itself would certainly not be an indication for their use. They may cause increased confusion and falls. Lithium (D), while it may be appropriate in severe refractory depression, would not be first line in older age, and certainly not in someone with end-stage renal disease, as it is renally excreted and now thought to be directly nephrotoxic. The relationship between chronic disease, e.g. diabetes (E) and depression, is well established.

Depression in older age (3)

7 C This question requires you to have some knowledge about both the Mental Capacity Act 2005 ('MCA') and the Mental Health Act 2007 ('MHA'). It is important that all healthcare professionals have knowledge relevant to these acts as far as they may be required to use them – the MHA and the MCA are not just the jurisdiction of psychiatrists, and all doctors should know the fundamentals of assessing capacity as it is one of the cornerstones of informed consent. There are numerous guides available giving appropriate levels of information. Broadly speaking, the MCA should not be used to detain someone if they have a mental illness. It may be used to treat someone if that treatment is in their best interests and they lack capacity to decide that treatment themselves. However, if there is a clear indication that the person is suffering with a mental disorder, is refusing treatment and especially if they pose a risk to themselves or others, the MHA is likely to be the correct act to use. In this case, a Section 3 (C) of the MHA would be the most appropriate as the patient is known, and is presenting with similar symptoms to previous admissions. This allows for treatment for up to 6 months. Detaining 'under common law' (A) was used prior to the MCA coming into force to treat people lacking capacity. If someone has capacity, you cannot treat them against their will (although there are some unusual exceptions to this where the MHA may be used). One cannot do nothing in this case (B) as the man is at risk, both to himself and possibly others. Without any legal framework neither he nor those around him have access to appropriate safeguards (e.g. a tribunal). A Deprivation of Liberty Safeguards (DOLS) assessment (D) is part of the MCA and applies when someone's liberty is being deprived rather than restricted – this does not apply here. There is no evidence here that IM medication would be the most appropriate course of action (E). Nursing and other management techniques should be employed. IM medication should usually be a last resort and there is nothing in the vignette to say he will not take oral medication.

Mania in older age

8 C When 'late-onset' bipolar disorder occurs (C) (commonly taken to be above the age of 50), the manic phase tends to present latently, often many years following several depressive episodes. Not every manic elderly person should be detained under the Mental Health Act (A) – each individual must be assessed on a case-by-case basis. Bipolar disorder does not disappear later in life (B). In fact, it has been suggested by some that the frequency of episodes actually tends to increase in people with long-standing bipolar disorder as they get older. There is probably insufficient evidence, however, to be able to say this with much certainty. Unipolar mania (D) does occasionally occur but, as with younger patients, is fairly unusual. Physical co-morbidity (E) most certainly does have an impact on the course of manic syndromes in older age, with many now supporting the diagnostic entity of 'vascular-mania' in a similar way to the emergence of 'vascular depression'. Mania in older age is highly correlated with neurological and cerebrovascular disease.

Hallucinations in older age

9 A   This is a very typical description of Charles Bonnet syndrome (A). This is a syndrome of complex, vivid visual hallucinations that occur in people with severe visual impairment (e.g. macular degeneration). Insight is retained and there are no other symptoms (unless there is a co-morbid diagnosis). It is usually self-limiting but there is no specific treatment as such, although explaining the cause of the symptoms is often reassuring. The other options are all eponymous syndromes related to psychiatry. Cotard's syndrome (B) is usually seen in psychotic depression, and is a delusional state in which the sufferer believes a part of their body (or their whole being) has ceased to exist. Ekbom's syndrome (C), or delusional parasitosis, is the delusional (not hallucinatory) belief that animals or insects are crawling below the sufferer's skin. It is a difficult syndrome to treat because of the fixity of patients' beliefs that their problem is a physical one. Sufferers may engage in highly dangerous methods to rid themselves of the 'parasites', such as digging them out with instruments or using highly corrosive cleaning materials on the skin. Fregoli's syndrome (D) is a form of delusional misidentification, in which sufferers believe that complete strangers are actually people well known to them in disguise. Rett's syndrome (E) is a dominantly inherited X-linked developmental disorder seen almost exclusively in girls and is associated with severe physical and learning disabilities.

Psychotic symptoms in older age

10 E   VLOSLP (E), despite its unwieldy name, is considered by many old age psychiatrists to be an extremely well-circumscribed syndrome, although the literature is still somewhat confusing. This used to be termed 'late paraphrenia' but this term is currently not in vogue and probably therefore best avoided. VLOSLP typically affects women more than men and sufferers often have no other personality or cognitive problems. Delusions can take any form, but it is very common for sufferers to describe 'partition delusions', in which solid structures become permeable to people or substances – in this case radiation from the neighbours. Unfortunately, the response to antipsychotics (A) tends to be relatively poor. There may be some success but they are unlikely to alleviate all symptoms. Sufferers tend to live alone and be extremely lonely, so befriending or more formal psychological intervention may offer some relief. Rehousing (B) is often attempted because of incessant complaints from sufferers, and usually before these patients have come to the attention of psychiatric services. However, it is almost always only a stop-gap measure, and symptoms usually reappear very quickly, even in a new home. The cough (C) may be an incidental finding but it is unlikely to be a delusional elaboration – coughs being a common symptom. It would be important not to overlook this, as it may represent something more sinister (particularly given the weight loss). There is little to suspect a dementia here (D), particularly given the relatively rapid onset and the high performance on MMSE.

Alcohol misuse in older age

11 D There are several misconceptions concerning alcohol use and misuse in older people. Moderate use, harmful use and dependence on alcohol are all seen in older age, and are not uncommon. Alcohol should routinely be asked about when assessing older people, and it is important that you learn the skills of how to do this. Alcohol dementia (D) is a complex phenomenon as it may be the result of different pathologies. Prolonged and heavy alcohol misuse is associated with irreversible cognitive problems. Alcohol use may predispose to cerebrovascular disease, head injury (and subsequent Alzheimer's disease) as well as having a directly toxic effect on the brain. Korsakoff's syndrome may also occur with prolonged use, which in itself is an amnestic syndrome. Alcohol dependence may certainly arise *de novo* in older people (A). It may be precipitated by stressful life events. However, this does not mean that genetics (C) do not play a role in the aetiology of alcohol dependence in older people, whether this is because of dependence from a younger age extending into older age, or arising *de novo*. Alcohol problems are often covert in older people (B). Cognitive problems may also lead to a poor recollection of alcohol use. The consequences of alcohol misuse may be concentrated upon (e.g. recurrent falls) rather than the alcohol use itself. There is still a male preponderance in alcohol problems in older age (E).

Anxiety disorders in older age

12 E Anxiety disorders in older age behave fairly similarly to anxiety disorders in younger patients. However, there are certain things to bear in mind. One is that, in a similar way to depression, anxiety in older people may focus around issues related to physical health (E). Also, while both CBT and antidepressants are effective (A), medication may need to be tailored to the individual with more care – SSRIs may cause gastrointestinal bleeding, for example, and tricyclics may exacerbate falls because of their anticholinergic effects. There would be no reason to treat anxiety disorders in older people as inpatients (B) unless there were compelling issues around risk – this is true regardless of age. The demographic distribution of anxiety disorders remains as it is for younger people, with a preponderance of diagnoses among women (C). Poor physical health most definitely would be a risk factor for developing an anxiety disorder. The physical health problem may directly exacerbate symptoms of anxiety (such as cardiac arrhythmias or respiratory disease) or increasing poor physical health itself may cause anxiety problems (D).

Unusual causes of cognitive impairment

13 B Cerebral malignancy (B) (whether primary or secondary) may present with memory loss and dysphasia. Frontal lobe tumours, because of their location, may lead to very few other localizing signs, so do not presume the absence of either soft or obvious neurological signs rules out the presence of brain malignancy. The biochemical abnormalities show hyponatraemia, hypercalcaemia and a normal potassium level. This would be consistent with brain malignancy, as many tumours may produce parathyroid-related peptide which will lead to hypercalcaemia, although this would commonly be from secondary metastatic disease in the brain from a haematological malignancy or solid tumour such as breast or lung. New presentation of hypercalcaemia should always prompt suspicion for malignancy. The hyponatraemia similarly results from inappropriate secretion of ADH (SIADH). This may result directly from an ADH-secreting tumour (or one secreting atrial natriuretic peptide), which again is often lung but may also be head and neck tumours. Unexplained weight loss should also raise the possibility of occult malignancy. Addison's disease (A), or primary adrenal failure, leads to a loss of all steroids produced from the adrenal cortex. It is commonly an autoimmune condition and therefore affects women far more than men. The typical biochemical pattern includes hyperkalaemia and hyponatraemia due to the loss of aldosterone, as well as hypercalcaemia. Memory loss is not often described, although depression and fatigue are certainly common. Cushing's disease (C) is associated with increased levels of circulating glucorticoids and low potassium. Weight loss would be very uncommon, with weight gain usually occurring in these patients. Depression and fatigue are more common than memory problems as such. Cushing's disease (not Cushing's syndrome, which is the term used to describe increased levels of circulating glucorticoids regardless of the cause) is caused by endogenous increased glucorticoid production, usually from an adrenocorticotrophic hormone-producing adenoma or other tumours. Hyperthyroidism (D) would be unlikely to cause memory problems, and the biochemical markers do not fit with this disease. Anxiety (or more specifically, the physical constellation of symptoms associated with anxiety) is a much more common manifestation of hyperthyroidism. Primary hyperparathyroidism (E) would certainly result in raised calcium, but would be unlikely to cause a low sodium.

Ethical considerations in older age

14 A Ethical questions seldom have 'one single best' answer but you are asked here to describe which best fits the description. Autonomy (A) refers to the ethical concept of the right to make one's own decisions. In patients with capacity to make the decision in question, autonomy must be respected. This is not the same as necessarily autonomy being followed, as there may be examples when other ethical considerations will override autonomy, such as when there is significant risk to the public etc. In this case, the woman is making a decision, with full capacity, that she does not want any further treatment. Beneficence (B) refers to acting in the best interest of the patient, or performing acts or making decisions to benefit the patient. In this case, it is not straightforward – who are we to decide in this case what is in the patient's best interests? She may, of course, be made much more comfortable if treated with antibiotics, but equally she may be profoundly distressed if she were treated when she did not want this. In fact, as the woman has been deemed to have capacity, it would be in direct contravention of the Mental Capacity Act 2005 to treat her against her wishes. Capacity (C), as we can see above, is central to this question. However, it is a legal concept rather than an ethical one per se. Justice (D) refers to 'fairness' for example balancing the needs of the individual against the wider needs of society etc. This is not particularly relevant here, although the needs of the family may need to be considered. However, it is important to note that if capacity continues, the needs of the family, while important to be known, would never 'trump' the decision of the patient. Non-maleficence (E) is almost analogous to the mantra of 'first do no harm' and refers to the obligation of practitioners to not do anything to bring about harm, pain or suffering. Again, this is not straightforward in this case. It could be argued that not treating her would cause significant pain, but equally the psychological distress felt by treating against her wishes may be much worse. Ethical questions are difficult, and there is often no one 'right answer'. It is often a complex balancing act, in which many people may be involved. You should never act beyond your competence in ethical decisions – always ask for help if needed.

Use of medications in older age

15 B As we age, there is a general increase in our body fat, with less body water. This leads to an increased volume of distribution. For drugs that are fat-soluble, such as diazepam (B), this means there will be a general increase in the duration of action. This is important when using these drugs as it will become easier to inadvertently overdose the patient. Antispsychotics (A) have been shown to increase all-cause mortality in patients with dementia and are therefore to be avoided wherever possible. Also, people with Lewy body dementia are particularly susceptible to antipsychotics and should definitely not be prescribed other than in exceptional circumstances. There are a range of alternative pharmacological and non-pharmacological interventions for behavioural symptoms of dementia. You will encounter this during your time in acute hospitals on a regular basis – do not start patients with dementia on an antipsychotic drug without seeking senior advice. Lithium (C) should be given at lower doses, but this is because of decreased renal function in older people – lithium is an inorganic ion and is not metabolized by the liver. Older people are generally much more sensitive to the effects of benzodiazepines (D) and they should be used extremely cautiously. They are much more likely to cause falls, respiratory depression or paradoxical excitation. There is a general decrease in gut motility in older people, not increase. TCAs (E) also decrease gut motility, meaning that there is a much greater incidence of constipation – you should always assess older people for constipation as a cause of confusion.

SECTION 30:
PERSONALITY DISORDERS

QUESTIONS

1. Diagnosis of personality disorder (1)

In the general diagnosis of personality disorder according to ICD-10, which of the following is not necessary for a diagnosis?

A. The behaviour must affect the ability to control impulses
B. The behaviour or way of interacting must be pervasive across different situations
C. The patterns of behaviour are associated with considerable distress
D. The patterns of behaviour arise in late childhood or adolescence
E. There must be no evidence of organic brain disease or injury as a cause of the disorder

2. Theories of personality

Regarding personality and its development, which of the following statements is false?

A. Body build is not a reliable way to assess personality type
B. Freudian theory states that normal personality development involves successfully passing through various stages of development
C. Idiographic personality theories state that every individual is unique
D. It is now generally accepted that personality can be described by three factors
E. The environment plays a large part in personality development

3. Risk assessment

Which of the following is least likely to predict dangerous behaviour?

A. Co-morbid mental disorder
B. Co-morbid substance abuse disorder
C. Juvenile delinquency
D. Pathological lying
E. Superficial charm

4. Management of personality disorders

A 22-year-old woman with a diagnosis of borderline personality disorder attends accident and emergency after saying she has taken an overdose of paracetamol following an argument with her mother. She is an outpatient at the local personality disorder service where she has a key worker. This is her fourth attendance in accident and emergency for similar reasons in the last 6 weeks. A full assessment reveals no evidence of depression. Her blood results reveal low levels of paracetamol. She does not want to die but cannot say she will not try and harm herself again. What would the most appropriate management be?

    A. Admit to inpatient unit

    B. Call for urgent Mental Health Act assessment

    C. Detain under Section 5(2) of the Mental Health Act (MHA) in the accident and emergency department

    D. Discharge from accident and emergency with follow-up from her key worker

    E. Remove patient and ban from further accident and emergency attendances

5. Diagnosis of personality disorder (2)

A 29-year-old man is arrested for aggravated assault on a former girlfriend. It is his ninth offence of a similar nature. The court asks for a psychiatric opinion. He is noted to be emotionally cold with an extremely reduced tolerance to frustration. He feels no remorse for his actions, blaming his girlfriend for 'putting it about'. What is the most likely diagnosis?

    A. Anankastic personality disorder

    B. Antisocial personality disorder

    C. Emotionally unstable personality disorder

    D. Histrionic personality disorder

    E. Schizoid personality disorder

6. Diagnosis of personality disorder (3)

A 68-year-old woman attends her GP following the death of her husband. She is tearful but 'doesn't want to bother the doctor'. The GP notices that she says yes to every suggestion and she says she does not know how to cope as her husband did everything for her except the cooking. The GP feels very helpless and somewhat irritated by the end of the conversation. What is the most likely diagnosis?

    A. Anankastic personality disorder

    B. Dependent personality disorder

    C. Emotionally unstable personality disorder

    D. Histrionic personality disorder

    E. Schizoid personality disorder

7. Diagnosis of personality disorder (4)

A 19-year-old man is referred to the local psychiatric community team as his new GP is worried he is schizophrenic. The letter states that he is 'extremely odd, and does not seem to have an emotional response to anything'. On assessment, he states he has only come to understand the 'psychiatric care pathway' a little more but does not feel he has any problems. He seems aloof and disdainful of the psychiatrist. He appears to have few hobbies except for inventing his own mathematical equations. What is the most likely diagnosis?

A. Anankastic personality disorder
B. Emotionally unstable personality disorder
C. Histrionic personality disorder
D. Schizoid personality disorder
E. Schizotypal personality disorder

8. Diagnosis of personality disorder (5)

A 52-year-old woman comes in to her GP with a swollen knee which appears to be osteoarthritic. During the assessment, however, she quizzes the GP on every little detail of what he is doing. She began the interview by saying how disappointed she was that the GP was running twelve and a half minutes late and that her schedule had been ruined as a result. She asked several times about minute details concerning the referral process. What is the most likely diagnosis?

A. Anankastic personality disorder
B. Anxious-avoidant personality disorder
C. Emotionally unstable personality disorder
D. Histrionic personality disorder
E. Paranoid personality disorder

9. Diagnosis of personality disorder (6)

A 23-year-old woman is referred to the pastoral services at her college because of concerns over her behaviour. She is reported to have episodic outbursts of rage towards her classmates, although she acts in a flirtatious and fawning way towards her male tutors. She has been admitted twice with impulsive self-harming attempts. She has become obsessed with one of the more popular girls in the class, adopting a similar dress sense and texting her often. When she was told by the girl to leave her alone, she became enraged. What is the most likely diagnosis?

A. Anxious-avoidant personality disorder
B. Emotionally unstable personality disorder
C. Histrionic personality disorder
D. Narcissistic personality disorder
E. Paranoid personality disorder

10. Management of personality disorder

Which of the following statements regarding management of personality disorder is correct?

A. Antidepressant medications have no role in the management of personality disorder
B. Antipsychotic medications have shown evidence of effectiveness in management of personality disorder

C. Dynamic psychotherapy is contraindicated in emotionally unstable personality disorder
D. Benzodiazepines are the drug of choice in borderline personality disorder
E. Group psychotherapy is ineffective in managing personality disorder

ANSWERS

Diagnosis of personality disorder (1)

1 A While many people with personality disorder do have difficulty with impulse control (A), it is not necessary for a diagnosis. ICD-10 specifies that the individual's inner experiences or behaviour must be manifest in more than one of the following areas (but not necessarily all).

- Cognition
- Affectivity
- Control over impulses
- Manner of relating to others.

This behaviour cannot be limited to one situation or stimulus, but must pervade across the individual's inner and social worlds and must be inflexible, maladaptive and dysfunctional (B). There must be distress, either to the individual themselves, their social environment, or usually both (C). The disorder must have arisen during late childhood or adolescence (D), and should be 'stable' and of long duration. Changes occurring within adulthood themselves do not qualify as personality disorders, but may represent personality change, usually as the result of severe and enduring stress. An organic cause cannot be responsible for the disorder (E) – there is a separate diagnostic category for 'organic personality disorder' – an example would be frontal lobe injury.

Theories of personality

2 D There are a bewildering number of personality theories and constructs. However, it is becoming increasingly accepted that five (not three) factors can adequately describe personality. These can be remembered with the mnemonic 'OCEAN' - Openness to experience, Conscientiousness, Extraverson/intraversion, Agreeableness and Neuroticism (D). Kretschmer originally described three body-types that he believed were associated with specific personality types (A). However, empirical research has not shown any reliable link between the two. Freud hypothesized that for normal personality development, an individual must successfully pass through various developmental stages of 'the libido', namely oral, anal and genital (B). Failure at one, e.g. anal, would result in personality difficulties in later life (in this case, obsessional traits). Idiographic personality theories are concerned with the uniqueness of every individual (C), compared to nomothetic theories in which personality is thought to be made up of differing degrees of stable factors, and individuals differ only in the amount of each of these factors that they possess. The environment as well as our genetic makeup of course are responsible for how our personality develops (E) – this has been backed up by numerous twin and other studies.

Risk assessment

3 A   While there are specific examples when co-morbid mental disorder (which excludes personality disorder) would increase dangerousness (e.g. the presence of violent command hallucinations, high levels of perceived threat in paranoid states), overall, very little violence is directly attributable to mental illness (A). People with mental illness are more likely to be the victims of violence than perpetrators of it. Co-morbid substance misuse is positively correlated with dangerousness (B). The aetiology of this relationship, however, is extremely complex. Juvenile delinquency (C) may predict a tendency towards psychopathy (which itself is related to dangerousness). This forms part of one of the most commonly used assessment tools for psychopathy, the Hare Psychopathy Checklist – Revised (PCL-R), as part of Factor 2 – 'Socially Deviant Lifestyle'. (D) and (E) are also part of the PCL-R for psychopathy, but fall into Factor 1 of the checklist – 'Aggressive Narcissism'.

Management of personality disorders

4 D   The most appropriate option is to discharge her with follow-up from her key worker (D). She is currently in a service designed specifically to cope with the difficulties people with personality disorder face. There is little evidence here that an inpatient admission would be helpful (A). People with borderline personality disorder often feel chronically abandoned and not listened to, so while admission may make both the clinician and patient feel safer, it is seldom useful in the long term. People with personality disorder often use admissions as justification for their behaviours. Firm boundaries coupled with thoughtful empathy are necessary to help these individuals. Again, like their being no justification for admission, there is no evidence for using the MHA (and indeed it is unlikely she would be detainable). Therefore (B) and (C) would not be appropriate – and in fact one could not use Section 5(2) in any case as this is only applicable to current inpatients, not to patients in accident and emergency. Banning the patient from accident and emergency (E) will only serve to confirm the woman's feelings of abandonment – the behaviour is likely to escalate rather than stop, and will just occur in another department where she is not known, which is potentially much more dangerous.

Diagnosis of personality disorder (2)

5 B   Antisocial personality disorder (B), also known as dissocial, psychopathic or sociopathic personality disorder, is commonly seen in forensic settings, and tends to affect men more than women. Aside from the features listed above, these individuals show gross disregard for social norms, cannot maintain meaningful relationships and usually have disordered development in childhood, often with diagnoses such as conduct disorder. This disorder is classified in Cluster 'B', a system adopted by DSM-IV (but not ICD-10). Cluster B disorders include those that are overly dramatic, emotional or with impulse control problems. Note that the other options are not explained further here as they are used in subsequent questions.

Diagnosis of personality disorder (3)

6 B   Dependent personality disorder is described here (B). These people often only come to attention when their spouses leave or die. They tend to allow others to take responsibility for them and will find it extremely hard to make decisions. They tend to not ask things of others but require large amounts of help and advice. This disorder falls into the DSM-IV Cluster 'C' category, which includes disorders characterized by anxiety or fear.

Diagnosis of personality disorder (4)

7 D   The vignette is describing someone with likely schizoid personality disorder (D). The name is possibly confusing, although it is thought by some to be connected to schizophrenia. However, these people do not have the psychotic symptoms that are the hallmark. Instead, they tend to be isolative, aloof and emotionally detached (although not in the violent way of antisocial personality disorder). They gain little pleasure from things except perhaps unusual intellectual activities, and usually have few friends or relationships. This is a Cluster 'A' disorder (characterized by odd or eccentric patterns of behaviour). Schizoid personality disorder should not be confused with schizotypal personality disorder (E). The latter has actually been taken out of the personality disorder section in ICD-10 and placed within the schizophrenia and related disorders category. These individuals present with symptoms of social anxiety as well as odd cognitive and perceptual experiences and beliefs that do not amount to delusions or hallucinations. They may have unusual speech patterns. This disorder is definitely felt to be related to schizophrenia.

Diagnosis of personality disorder (5)

8 A   This represents an anankastic personality type (A), also known as obsessive–compulsive personality disorder in DSM-IV. This is not the same as obsessive–compulsive disorder, although the two may give rise to some diagnostic difficulties. However, those with anankastic personality disorders tend to be preoccupied with rules and schedules. They are perfectionists and overly pedantic. They are usually quite rigid and may be stubborn and difficult to get along with as they can come across as extremely judgemental. This is also a Cluster 'C' disorder.

Diagnosis of personality disorder (6)

9 C This is a difficult question, as this may get confused with narcissistic traits (D) or with emotionally unstable traits (B). However, this description is very suggestive of histrionic personality disorder (C), in which individuals are prone to overly dramatic displays and occasional self-harm. They are faddish and attention seeking, often sexually. They have a shallow affect and cannot maintain relationships easily. They also tend to be obsessed with their physical appearance. In contrast, emotionally unstable personality disorder (B) does not present quite like this, although obviously self-harming behaviour is prevalent here also. There is also often considerable overlap between them, but emotionally unstable individuals tend to have intense but unstable relationships and go to great lengths to avoid being abandoned, while at the same time pushing people away. They feel chronically empty. Likewise, narcissistic individuals may share some of these characteristics, but the core of narcissistic personality disorder is an inflated sense of self-worth, often being pretentious and boastful. They crave attention as well as celebrity and believe they are above others. They are usually callous and show little regard for the feelings of others.

Management of personality disorder

10 B There are some small studies showing benefits of antipsychotic medication (B) over a wide range of symptoms in personality disorder. However, there is no consensus about who will benefit from these drugs, in what way, and for how long. Individuals with personality disorder may sometimes end up on a vast array of medications which is more likely to be symptomatic of the treating clinician's feelings of therapeutic impotence than any observable benefit to the individual. Antidepressants (A) similarly may have a role, particularly in terms of helping with impulse control. However, as with antipsychotics, the use of psychotropic medication alone is almost certain to be a failure without consistent and long-term psychological interventions. Dynamic psychotherapy (C) is certainly used for the management of many types of personality disorder, including emotionally unstable. Benzodiazepines (D) should be used with extreme caution in people with borderline personality disorder because of their potential for dependence. Group psychotherapy (E) has been used for many years in the management of individuals with personality disorder. One advantage of this method is that issues of transference are not limited to the therapist, but spread out amongst the group. The evidence suggests that on the whole cognitive behavioural therapy (CBT) is more effective than medication for generalized anxiety disorder (C). The effects of both are probably additive, with the most success being for a combined approach of CBT and SSRIs. While CBT is commonly conducted with just one client and therapist (E), there is no reason that family members may not be invited to sessions and in fact may even act as co-therapists in certain situations.

SECTION 31:
PSYCHOTHERAPIES

QUESTIONS

1. Theories of psychotherapy

In the structural model proposed by Freud, what is the term used to define the mainly conscious part of the mind that negotiates between the inner wishes and needs and the external world?

    A.   Genital stage
    B.   Ego
    C.   Id
    D.   Oedipus complex
    E.   Superego

2. Defence mechanisms (1)

A 42-year-old woman suffers a painful breakup with her long-term partner after finding him in bed with another man. She finds the situation, including telling her friends and family, extremely difficult. One year later she is asked how she is feeling. She denies any knowledge of seeing her partner being unfaithful and says 'oh, we just had our differences, you know, there's no hard feelings'. What is this form of defence mechanism called?

    A.   Denial
    B.   Idealization
    C.   Regression
    D.   Repression
    E.   Splitting

3. Defence mechanisms (2)

Which of the following represents a 'mature' (i.e. 'healthy') defence mechanism?

    A.   Acting out
    B.   Dissociation
    C.   Projection
    D.   Projective identification
    E.   Sublimation

4. Types of psychotherapy (1)

The following statement refers to which type of psychotherapy? A type of talking therapy, usually short-term and practical, that aims to change the way individuals think or behave with regards to themselves and others, by exploring erroneous patterns of thoughts, feelings and behaviours.

A. Cognitive behavioural therapy (CBT)
B. Counselling
C. Mindfulness therapy
D. Music therapy
E. Psychodynamic therapy

5. Types of psychotherapy (2)

The following statement refers to which type of psychotherapy? A model of therapy where the interactions and relationships between people are explored as opposed to the inner world of the individual.

A. Cognitive analytical therapy
B. Dialectical behaviour therapy
C. Eye movement desensitization and reprocessing
D. Play therapy
E. Systemic therapy

6. Cognitive behavioural therapy (1)

A 32-year-old woman is being seen for CBT to treat a depressive episode. During the initial assessment, she tells the therapy that 'to tell the truth, I'm just a bad person'. How might this statement be named in the CBT formulation?

A. Arbitrary inference
B. Catastrophizing
C. Core negative belief
D. Generalization
E. Minimization

7. Choice of psychotherapy

John, a 19-year-old male sculpture student comes to his GP complaining of problems with sleeping. Over the last few months he has been increasingly preoccupied with counting, and is now checking the light switches and other electrical items over and over again well into the night. He now feels compelled to turn the light switch on and off seven times before he can go to bed. He has never had problems before and this is causing him and his girlfriend considerable distress. What is the most likely effective treatment?

A. Art therapy
B. CBT
C. Family therapy for patient and partner
D. Psychoanalytic therapy
E. Watchful waiting

8. Cognitive behavioural therapy (2)

Which of the following statements regarding CBT is false?

    A.   CBT may be carried out without a full qualification in CBT
    B.   CBT may make reference to early childhood experiences
    C.   CBT is more effective than medication for generalized anxiety disorder
    D.   CBT is not useful in dementia
    E.   CBT may involve family members

ANSWERS

Theories of psychotherapy

1 B While many of Freud's ideas have fallen out of favour, it is indisputable that he provided psychiatry and the emerging field of psychotherapy with a new systematic way of viewing the mind and behaviour. Nearly all of the fundamentals of psychotherapy can be traced back to his work. His structural model sought to understand our instincts and drives and divided the mind into three parts: the id, the ego and the superego. The ego (B) refers to the mainly conscious part of the mind that composes rational thinking and balances the needs of the individual against the demands of the outside world. The id (C) refers to the mainly unconscious part of the mind that contains innate instincts such as sexuality and aggression. It is not a term widely used in psychiatric literature these days. The superego (E) is analogous to what we might call 'conscience' and contains our moral rules. Freud believed it developed from our identification with authority figures and is part conscious, part unconscious. The genital stage (A) is one of Freud's stages of early development that must be passed through successfully to avoid problems later in life. The other stages were anal and oral. It is his work on early development that has perhaps been the most abandoned in current psychoanalytic thinking. The Oedipus complex (D), in the strictest sense from Freud, took place between the ages of 3 and 5 and is concerned with the child's realization of their gender, their resentment of never possessing what the opposite parent has and their jealousy of the parental relationship. Freud's model was intensely phallocentric however, and it has been modified by current psychoanalytic theorists to include both genders.

Defence mechanisms (1)

2 D Denial and repression may often be confused. Defence mechanisms are fundamentally unconscious strategies employed by an individual to cope with reality and stress. They are not always maladaptive (see below). Denial (A) refers to a refusal to accept reality despite all logical evidence. It refers mainly to events that are currently occurring in the individual's life. Repression (D) involves the unconscious exclusion of painful desires, thoughts or fears. In this case, the woman has unconsciously hidden the memory of seeing her partner in bed with another man in order to avoid reliving the intense pain this caused her. Idealization (B) involves perceiving another individual as having more positive traits or qualities than they may actually possess. It is actually part of the complex defence of splitting (E), in which the individual perceives things as either all 'good' (idealization), or all 'bad' (devaluation). Splitting can often be seen in borderline personality disorder, but here it is often wrongly defined as the intentional action by individuals with borderline personality disorder of turning people (usually staff) against each other. Regression (C) is another defence mechanism whereby the individual reverts to an earlier stage of development in order to avoid stressful events. It is thought to occur in those stuck at a particular stage of psychosexual development. For example, someone stuck at the oral phase may react to stress by eating or smoking excessively.

Defence mechanisms (2)

3   E   Sublimation (E) refers to transforming negative emotions or situations into positive feelings or behaviours and is classified as a 'mature' defence mechanism. Many artists are considered to have used this defence mechanism in order to 'sublimate' their nihilistic feelings about themselves and the world. Acting out (A) refers to the enactment of strong feelings that may have been stirred up during therapy, but enacted outside the therapy session. It is often destructive, for example the therapeutic investigation of emotional abuse that had been previously repressed may lead to feelings of anger that may be taken out on people close to the individual. It is not 'cathartic' and is usually unhelpful and possibly disastrous for ongoing therapy. Dissociation (B) refers to the modification of one's personality or identity in order to avoid distress. In severe forms it may present as the controversial 'multiple personality disorder'. This may result in a dissociative disorder, such as dissociative amnesia or fugue. Projection (C) is a defence mechanism used to decrease anxiety by ascribing one's own thoughts, fears, attributes or emotions to the external world, usually another person, while denying them as one's own. For example, a woman really dislikes her male co-worker. However, instead of addressing this, she projects this feeling by the belief that the co-worker dislikes her while saying she herself does not have a problem with him. Projective identification (D) can be thought of as a 'self-fulfilling prophecy' whereby in projected emotions or feelings, the recipient begins to alter their behaviour in order to make the behaviour 'real'. Thus in the example above, the projective identification may lead to the co-worker actually starting to dislike the woman in question, whereas previously he may have had no problem with her.

Types of psychotherapy (1)

4   A   CBT (A) is now the most prescribed form of psychotherapy in the NHS. It developed from both cognitive and behavioural models. It is usually short-term and used to address a specific problem. It focuses on the 'here and now' to a much greater extent than psychodynamic psychotherapy. It is very pragmatic, aiming to alleviate suffering and develop coping strategies, rather than necessarily getting to the 'root' of problems, although the therapist will often try and uncover 'core beliefs' the individual may hold about themselves and the world. Counselling (B) is a supportive therapy that aims to give individuals a space to discuss their problems, without usually offering advice. This is not to say that counsellors are not highly skilled. However, they do not usually deal with severe mental illness or pervasive personality problems. Mindfulness therapy (C) is a relatively new modality of therapy that shares similarities with CBT but combines cognitive theories with mindfulness stress reduction, which has demonstrated efficacy in relapse prevention for major depression. It has been successfully trialled enough that the National Institute for Health and Clinical Excellence (NICE) have recommended it for those with three or more episodes of major depression. Music therapy (D) refers to numerous forms of therapy in which music is used in various ways to establish and explore a therapeutic relationship with the goal of improving psychological health. Psychodynamic therapy (E) is the most traditional form of psychotherapy, with its origins in the work of Sigmund Freud. At its basic level, psychodynamic (also known as psychoanalytic) therapy tends to be longer-term therapy, looking at deep-rooted problems as a result of past trauma or stresses, including in the individual's childhood development. There are numerous techniques employed in this method of therapy, including free association, dream interpretation and the analysis of the 'transference' of the individual.

Types of psychotherapy (2)

5 E   Systemic therapy (E), also known as family therapy, is an umbrella term for a group of models, theories and techniques in which the relationships between individuals (i.e. in systems) are explored. In this way the focus is very different from traditional psychoanalysis, although the two fields are in many ways seeing a growing trend of learning from each other. Family therapy incorporates many different theoretical models, but the fundamental principles are to address issues around relationships. Examples of types of family therapy include narrative therapy, solution-focused therapy and strategic family therapy. Cognitive analytical therapy (A) developed later than CBT and was intended to be used in a time-limited fashion to make treatment available in resource-tight environments like the NHS. It combines techniques (as the name implies) from both cognitive and analytical schools, and seeks to identify chains of events that maintain problems, such as self-harming. Dialectical behaviour therapy (B) is a model that has been developed for the treatment of borderline personality disorder. It combines elements of CBT along with elements of distress tolerance and mindfulness. It fundamentally seeks to redress the relationship between client and therapist, where the latter is seen as an ally in the individual's struggles rather than an adversary. Eye movement desensitization and reprocessing (C) is another relatively new technique used primarily in the treatment of post-traumatic stress disorder. While it still remains somewhat controversial, the premise of the technique is that distressing memories are relived while another stimulus is being applied (such as therapist-led lateral eye movements). In this way, the distressing memories are thought to be replaced by more positive memory networks. Play therapy (D) is a form of psychodynamic therapy employed in children, using creative and imaginary plan to explore intrapsychic distress.

Cognitive behavioural therapy (1)

6 C   Cognitive therapy seeks to address individual's false beliefs about themselves and the world around them. People with depression often suffer with these beliefs more than people without depression (although people with personality disorders will often also share some of these beliefs). This represents a core negative belief (C), which are central ideas about one's self and represent 'absolute truths' by the individual. Core beliefs can of course also be positive, but these tend to disappear with the onset of disorders like depression. Arbitrary inference (A) is a type of cognitive distortion in which the individual jumps to a conclusion without having the necessary evidence. For example, 'if my friend doesn't pick up the telephone, it must be because they don't like me'. Catastrophizing (B) is another distortion in which the individual focuses on the worst possible outcome. For example, 'I overcooked the potatoes, the dinner is ruined and everyone will laugh at me'. Generalization, another distortion (D), occurs when the individual takes one example or incident and applies it to wide generalizations, for example, a man arriving 5 minutes late for his therapy session, stating 'I'm forever being late, I'm hopeless'. Minimization (E) is a distortion in which positive or successful outcomes by the individual are minimized (and 'poor' outcomes conversely are usually maximized). For example, 'so what that I got 89 per cent on my test, it was only a fluke'.

Choice of psychotherapy

7 B   CBT (B) is the most evaluated and recognized form of psychotherapy for obsessive–compulsive disorder (OCD). One of the core concepts of CBT in OCD is challenging the idea of 'magical thinking' in which OCD sufferers believe that they will either have to act on their distressing thoughts or feelings or indeed that they have acted on them in the past. The treatment may also involve 'exposure and response prevention' therapy in which the individual is exposed to a stimulus that will provoke their obsessions but are prevented from performing their compulsions which would normally decrease their anxiety. Art therapy (A) would not be an appropriate choice here. Art therapy is not limited to those with artistic 'ability' but uses artistic expression as a complementary means of conveying emotions and distress to solely verbal communication. There is nothing in the vignette to suggest that the problems that John is experiencing are the result of discord within his relationship, and therefore family therapy would not be the first choice here (C). Of course, OCD may lead to relationship difficulties and this must also be addressed. Involvement of partners and other close relations in therapy may be an extremely useful way of 'externalizing' the problem so the individual is not 'blamed' for the behaviours. While John may have deep-seated issues that have precipitated his OCD, there is less evidence that psychodynamic therapy is an effective treatment, and it is certainly likely to be more costly and more time consuming. If there was evidence of previous maladaptive patterns of behaviour or relationships then it may become a more viable option. Watchful waiting (E) is certainly not the right thing to do in this case, as there is obvious distress. Of course, a full assessment is needed to confirm the diagnosis before forging ahead with treatment, but delaying will almost certainly not improve the situation. Psychoeducation (D), in which OCD is gently and fully explained to the patient, is often a useful adjunct to other treatments.

Cognitive behavioural therapy (2)

8 D Certain cognitive and behavioural techniques may be very useful in dementia (D), both for people with dementia and their carers. It should not be assumed that cognitive impairment will automatically exclude people with dementia from benefiting from these therapies and techniques. CBT is often employed by mental health professionals without a full qualification under supervision from a qualified CBT therapist (A). This is an important part of training and as long as there is adequate supervision it is an acceptable and beneficial form of treatment. Many mental health professionals employ CBT 'techniques' in their everyday management and engagement with patients without this constituting 'therapy' as such. It is a common misconception that CBT does not make reference to early experiences (B). Although the basis of therapy is not to relate current methods of interaction with those from childhood, the CBT therapist may look at earlier experiences when trying to discover 'core beliefs' that the client holds about themselves. The evidence suggests that, on the whole, CBT is more effective than medication for generalized anxiety disorder (C). The effects of both are probably additive, with the most success being for a combined approach of CBT and selective serotonin reuptake inhibitors. While CBT is commonly conducted with just one client and therapist (E), there is no reason that family members may not be invited to sessions and in fact may even act as co-therapists in certain situations.

SECTION 32: PSYCHOSEXUAL, SLEEP AND EATING DISORDERS

QUESTIONS

1. Male sexual dysfunction disorders

A 25-year-old man recently married having abstained from sex until marriage. He reports becoming very anxious during sexual intercourse and is gripped by a 'fear of failure'. Consequently he finds himself monitoring his performance and as a result he cannot maintain an erection. What is the most likely diagnosis?

- A. Sexual aversion disorder
- B. Hypoactive sexual desire disorder
- C. Premature ejaculation
- D. Erectile dysfunction
- E. Orgasmic disorder

2. Psychiatric drugs causing sexual dysfunction

A 49-year-old man has been successfully treated for anxiety and depression. He is struggling to reach an orgasm during sex although his sexual desire is normal. What is the most likely cause of his current problem?

- A. Citalopram
- B. Trazodone
- C. Lithium
- D. Chlorpromazine
- E. Clonazepam

3. Paraphilias

A 35-year-old man is picked up by the transport police after reports that he had been rubbing his erect penis against several female passengers on a train. The female victims were unknown to the offender. What is the most likely diagnosis?

- A. Exhibitionism
- B. Voyeurism
- C. Frotteurism
- D. Sexual masochism
- E. Transvestic fetishism

4. Causes of insomnia

A 62-year-old female with a history of rheumatoid arthritis complains that when she attempts to sleep, she feels an urge to move her legs due to uncomfortable sensations. Movement does ease the distress. What is the most likely diagnosis?

- A. Obstructive sleep apnoea
- B. Periodic limb movement disorder

C. Restless legs syndrome
D. Nocturnal eating syndrome
E. Nocturnal leg cramps

5. Insomnia

A 23-year-old medical student is nearing her final examination. She feels as though she should study as much as possible and consequently has been revising into the early hours of the morning, drinking up to six cups of coffee per day as well as an energy drink. She has little difficulty getting to sleep but wakes intermittently during the night. She does not wake refreshed and feels tired the next day. There are no other symptoms. What is the most likely diagnosis?

A. Inadequate sleep hygiene
B. Environmental sleep disorder
C. Depression
D. Adjustment sleep disorder
E. Limit setting sleep disorder

6. Causes of hypersomnia

A 20-year-old male patient is taken to see a GP by his father. The patient has had three distinct periods of binge eating coupled with long periods (lasting up to 18 hours) of sleep over the past 3 months. Each attack lasts a few days or so and then spontaneously resolves. What is the most likely diagnosis?

A. Post-traumatic hypersomnia
B. Narcolepsy
C. Insufficient sleep syndrome
D. Depression
E. Kleine–Levin syndrome

7. Circadian rhythm sleep disorders

A 45-year-old businessman, who travels regularly as part of his work, visits the corporate physician complaining of difficulty in getting to sleep as well as daytime fatigue and reduced performance during presentations. He also has periodic headaches that are relieved by paracetamol. What is the most likely diagnosis?

A. Shift work disorder
B. Time zone change syndrome
C. Irregular sleep-wake syndrome
D. Delayed sleep phase syndrome (DSPS)
E. Advance sleep phase syndrome

8. Parasomnias

A 20-year-old female student visits her GP complaining of suddenly waking with a 'feeling of falling'. What is the likely diagnosis?

    A. Rhythmic movement disorder
    B. Somniloquy
    C. Nocturnal leg cramps
    D. Hypnic jerks
    E. Somnambulism

9. Diagnosis of eating disorders

Which of the following features would indicate a diagnosis of anorexia nervosa rather than bulimia nervosa?

    A. Fear of fatness
    B. Amenorrhoea
    C. Being at least 15 per cent below the expected weight
    D. Recurrent episodes of overeating
    E. Self-induced vomiting

10. Complications of eating disorders

Which of the following is not a recognized complication of sustained anorexia nervosa?

    A. Bradycardia
    B. Heart failure
    C. Hypercholsterolaemia
    D. Parotid gland enlargement
    E. Thrombocytosis

ANSWERS

Male sexual dysfunction disorders

1 D   Erectile dysfunction (ED) (D) is defined as the inability to develop or maintain an erection during sexual intercourse. Factors that can contribute to ED include previous negative sexual experiences contributing to performance anxiety. Use of recreational drugs, alcohol, stress and fatigue can also cause ED. Sexual aversion disorder (A) is characterized by a depressed sexual desire. Hypoactive sexual desire disorder (B) is a milder form of aversion disorder, associated with a lack of interest in sex. Premature ejaculation (C) is a condition in which a male ejaculates too soon, leading to diminished sexual pleasure. Orgasmic disorder (E) is characterized by a persistent or recurrent difficulty in achieving an orgasm following a normal excitation phase of sex. This may manifest as a delayed orgasm or an absence of orgasm altogether.

Psychiatric drugs causing sexual dysfunction

2 A   Citalopram (A) is an antidepressant drug that has a selective serotonin reuptake inhibition mechanism. It is indicated for the treatment of major depression. Side effects related to sexual dysfunction include a delayed ejaculation and anorgasmia. Trazodone (B) is a 5HT2a receptor antagonist. It is associated with priapism but rarely causes delayed ejaculation. Priapism is a medical emergency as ischaemic changes can result in impotence or, in serious cases, gangrene of the penis. Lithium (C) is a mood stabilizer used in the treatment of mania. Side effects of the drug specific to sexual dysfunction include diminished sexual interest as well as erectile dysfunction. Chlorpromazine (D) is a typical antipsychotic is associated with causing priapism. Clonazepam (E) is a benzodiazepine indicated in the treatment of anxiety disorders, mania and parasomnias. It is associated with loss of libido.

Paraphilias

3 C   Frotteurism (C) is defined as the paraphilic activity of touching and rubbing against another person's body for sexual pleasure. Frotteurs are usually males and the action is usually committed in a crowded public arena, for example on public transport. Exhibitionism (A) is characterized by indecent exposure of genitals in a public place. The penis may be erect or flaccid. Voyeurism (B) includes watching others have sex or undress. Mechanisms of voyeurism include using hidden cameras and peep-holes. Sexual masochism (D) is defined as the pleasure of receiving pain through sexual acts. Transvestic fetishism (E) is associated with attaining sexual arousal from cross-dressing. In transvestic fetishism there is no link to gender identity disorder.

Causes of insomnia

4 C Restless legs syndrome (C) (Wittmaack–Ekbom syndrome) is characterized by uncomfortable, often painful sensations in the legs, that is relieved by movement. The condition is either idiopathic or familial in most cases. It is associated with a number of medical conditions including rheumatoid arthritis, uraemia and iron deficiency anaemia. Obstructive sleep apnoea (A), usually associated with obese patients, features periods of upper airway obstruction during sleep causing apnoea (no longer than 90 seconds). It is associated with loud snoring and daytime fatigue. Periodic limb movement disorder (B) is most common in the elderly and is characterized by repetitive limb movements during sleep. The result is excessive daytime sleepiness. Nocturnal eating syndrome (D) is primarily a paediatric condition associated with excessive late-night consumption of food. The disorder has been linked to depression and anxiety. Nocturnal leg cramps (E) result in defined periods of painful muscular tension in the foot or calf which wakes the patient. The condition is associated with diabetes, pregnancy and arthritis.

Insomnia

5 A Inadequate sleep hygiene (A) is associated with factors that do not allow a good quality of sleep. These include high levels of caffeine consumption and frequent late nights. There is also a concurrent negative effect on the following day's productivity. Environmental sleep disorder (B) is caused by aspects of the surroundings that are not conducive to sleep. For example, lights, noise, heat and cold will reduce the ability to sleep. Depression (C) can cause sleep disorder, especially early morning wakening, but would be associated with other symptoms of depression. Adjustment sleep disorder (D) is associated with stress, conflict or environmental change, for example changing jobs. It is usually only temporary and once anxiety is diminished, sleep quality is restored. Limit setting sleep disorder (E) is primarily a paediatric condition that occurs when a caregiver imposes strict bedtime rules to a child with subsequent refusal by the child.

Causes of hypersomnia

6 E Kleine–Levin syndrome (E) is characterized by distinct periods of extreme somnolence and excessive hunger. Males are far more affected than females. Other symptoms which may manifest include sexual disinhibition, confusion, irritability, euphoria, hallucinations and delusions. Post-traumatic hypersomnia (A) may occur after there has been trauma to the brainstem or posterior hypothalamus. Although hypersomnia may occur, head trauma is more often associated with insomnia. Narcolepsy (B) features a classical tetrad of symptoms: (often brief) periods of sudden deep sleep, cataplexy (sudden bilateral loss of muscle tone), sleep paralysis and hypnagogic (onset of sleep) hallucinations. Insufficient sleep syndrome (C) is defined as the failure to obtain sufficient nocturnal sleep to support daytime activities. It is associated with professions that have unsociable working hours, such as doctors and long-distance lorry drivers. Although atypical depression (D) may be associated with hypersomnia and hyperphagia, the pattern would be more prolonged than a few days and other depressive symptoms would be evident.

Circadian rhythm sleep disorders

7 B   Time zone change syndrome (B) is characterized by difficulty initiating and maintaining sleep as well as daytime fatigue. Feelings of apathy and irritability may also ensue. Physical symptoms may manifest as altered appetite, muscle aches or headaches. Shift work disorder (A) occurs in patients who conduct shift work; patients who constantly change day/night shift patterns are particularly susceptible to insomnia or hypersomnia. Patients may present with physical symptoms rather than a sleep disorder. Irregular sleep-wake syndrome (C) is characterized by sleeping at irregular times. The disruption of the circadian rhythm leads to insomnia and frequent naps during the daytime. Medical associations include: Alzheimer's disease, head injury and hypothalamic tumours. DSPS (D) occurs when sleep begins late, leading to difficulties in waking up. Patients may adapt to the condition by taking evening or night jobs. Advance sleep phase syndrome (E) is the opposite of DSPS with early sleep occurrence and early awakening. It is more common in elderly patients.

Parasomnias

8 D   Hypnic jerks (D) (sleep starts) occur at the onset of sleep and are associated with contractions of the limbs, neck or body. When wakened by the jerks there is a characteristic feeling of falling into space. Rhythmic movement disorder (A) is characterized by the repetitive movement of the head before sleep and is sustained into sleep. It is most common in young children and prevalence declines with age. Somniloquy (B), also known as sleep talking, is primarily a condition of childhood. It is associated with the utterance of words or sounds during sleep with no distinguishable meaning. Nocturnal leg cramps (C) causes the sufferer to awaken due to painful muscular tension in the foot or calf. The condition is associated with diabetes, pregnancy and arthritis. Somnambulism (E), or sleep walking, causes patients to arise during sleep and execute activities usually performed during the day.

Diagnosis of eating disorders

9 D   Bulimia and anorexia nervosa, while distinct conditions, share certain features in common. However, the hallmark of bulimia nervosa is recurrent episodes of overeating, or 'bingeing', involving the consumption of large quantities of food over a short time (D). This is followed by efforts to control weight, often by vomiting, using appetite suppressants and periods of starvation. A fear of fatness (A) occurs in both anorexia and bulimia. Amenorrhea (B), while it may occur in bulimia, is a diagnostic criteria for a anorexia nervosa. Equally, having a low weight (C) is a feature of both disorders (but not diagnostic for bulimia, in which weight may be normal or even increased). For a diagnosis of anorexia, sufferers must be at least 15 per cent below expected body weight. Self-induced vomiting (E) is very common in bulimia nervosa, but equally occur in anorexia in an attempt to control weight.

Complications of eating disorders

10 E A low platelet count may be found in anorexia nervosa, but not an increased count (E). There may also be a pancytopenia. Bradycardia (A), as well as a host of other arrhythmias, are a common complication of anorexia nervosa. The aetiology is multiple, but includes hypokalaemia. Heart failure (B) may also occur in anorexia, both as a result of the disorder and occasionally as a result of refeeding, although the reason for this is not completely understood. Hypercholesterolaemia is a surprising finding in anorexia nervosa, but is by no means uncommon. The exact mechanism is still unclear (C). Parotid enlargement occurs as a result of nutritional deficiencies as well as purging behaviour (D).

SECTION 33: SUBSTANCE MISUSE DISORDERS

QUESTIONS

1. Substance misuse disorders (1)

A 26-year-old male sees his GP. He recently fell and broke his wrist while drunk and is seeing his GP for a follow-up appointment. He has lost his job as he was found drinking vodka from a water bottle. The patient insists his recent problems are down to 'bad luck' and not alcohol. What is the most likely diagnosis?

A. Acute intoxication
B. Dependence syndrome
C. Harmful use
D. Withdrawal state
E. Psychotic disorder

2. Substance misuse disorders (2)

A 40-year-old regular cocaine user was made redundant as an advertising executive 2 weeks ago. He presents with a 6-day history of low mood, anhedonia, irritability and increased appetite and has been feeling generally fatigued. What is the most likely diagnosis?

A. Withdrawal state
B. Complicated withdrawal
C. Amnestic syndrome
D. Residual disorder
E. Depression

3. Dependence syndrome

A 52-year-old confused man is brought to accident and emergency by ambulance after being found on the ground with a head injury. He is known to have alcohol dependence. On examination the patient is obtunded, ataxic and has bilateral weakness in his lateral recti ocular muscles. What is the likely diagnosis?

A. Wernicke's encephalopathy
B. Alcohol withdrawal
C. Korsakoff's syndrome
D. Intoxication
E. Delerium tremens

4. Complications of alcohol (1)

A 21-year-old university student is at a union event on a Friday night. He becomes aggressive and gets into a fight with a stranger over a spilt drink. What is the most likely diagnosis?

A. Alcohol-induced amnesia
B. Alcohol intoxication

    C.   Harmful drinking
    D.   At-risk drinking
    E.   Alcohol dependence

5. Complications of alcohol (2)

A 42-year-old man with alcohol dependence has gone to extreme lengths to prove his belief that his wife is having an affair with the gardener. The patient has admitted to placing secret surveillance cameras in the home he shares with his wife. What is the most likely diagnosis?

    A.   Alcoholic hallucinosis
    B.   Alcohol induced psychotic disorder
    C.   Othello syndrome
    D.   Alcoholic dementia
    E.   Korsakoff's syndrome

6. Sudden focal neurology

A 34-year-old man with a long history of alcohol dependence is admitted to a hospital ward. Two days later the patient is found to be quadriplegic and can only communicate 'yes' and 'no' using eye signals. What is the most likely diagnosis?

    A.   Wernicke–Korsakoff syndrome
    B.   Peripheral neuropathy
    C.   Marchiafava–Bignami disease
    D.   Central pontine myelinolysis
    E.   Alcoholic polymyopathy

7. Cardiopulmonary complications of alcohol misuse

A 26-year-old Asian man has been drinking a bottle of whisky a day for 10 years. He has had a cough for 6 weeks, with haemoptysis and night sweats. What is the most likely diagnosis?

    A.   Dilated cardiomyopathy
    B.   Tuberculosis
    C.   Atrial fibrillation
    D.   Pneumonia
    E.   Stroke

8. Gastrointestinal complications of alcohol misuse

A 45-year-old woman who lost her family in a road traffic accident 10 years ago has been dependent on alcohol since. She presents to her GP with difficulty swallowing. She is referred to a gastroenterologist who reports the presence of columnar epithelium in the lower oesophagus. What is the most likely diagnosis?

    A.   Alcoholic liver disease
    B.   Acute gastritis

C. Barrett's oesophagus
D. Mallory–Weiss tear
E. Chronic pancreatitis

9. Alcohol-associated psychiatric disorders

A 30-year-old city executive presents with alcohol dependence. On further questioning it emerges he has always been very anxious about having to give presentations to his colleagues. When he is required to speak in front of them, his heart races, he begins to sweat profusely and feels an urge to leave the stage. He has been drinking vodka in order to suppress these symptoms. What is the most likely diagnosis?

A. Social phobia
B. Depression
C. Psychotic disorder
D. Generalized anxiety disorder
E. Morbid jealousy

10. Hallucinations

A 30-year-old banker presents to accident and emergency. He is agitated and continuously scratches his skin, complaining there are 'insects crawling all over him'. His blood pressure is raised and an electrocardiogram reveals a tachyarrhythmia. What is the most likely cause of his symptoms?

A. Heroin
B. Cocaine
C. LSD
D. Caffeine
E. Benzodiazepines

11. Persecutory delusions

A 48-year-old man is seen by his community psychiatric nurse. On questioning he shows evidence of persecutory delusions despite treatment with risperidone. The patient has a history of long-term drug misuse. What is the most likely causative drug?

A. Barbiturates
B. Magic mushrooms
C. Glue sniffing
D. Heroin
E. Cannabis

12. Alcohol cessation

A 45-year-old man presents to his GP because he has recently become worried about his drinking. He says that drinking red wine can be 'beneficial' and drinks four bottles over the course of the week. He is otherwise well but now thinks he should cut down his drinking. What is the next appropriate step in management?

    A.   Education and advice
    B.   Referral to Alcoholics Anonymous
    C.   Disulfiram
    D.   Acamprosate
    E.   Risperidone

13. Management of alcohol withdrawal

A 40-year-old man is brought into accident and emergency. He is extremely agitated and confused about both time and day and provides a very unfocused history. He is sweating and tachycardic. Later that evening he complains that tiny birds are attacking him. What is the next appropriate step in management?

    A.   Oral chlordiazepoxide
    B.   Oral haloperidol
    C.   Oral thiamine
    D.   IV chlordiazepoxide
    E.   IV diazepam

ANSWERS

Substance misuse disorders (1)

1 C Harmful use (C) arises when substance misuse is continued over a long period (at least 1 month) by a patient, despite damage to the user's physical or mental health. The patient's occupation and family are often severely affected, with the damage being played down by the patient. There is insufficient information to diagnose dependence syndrome (B). Acute intoxication (A) occurs due to the immediate effect of consumption of a specific substance and the direct effects which result. Withdrawal state (D) is the physical dependence on a drug and the associated features which occur during abstinence. Severe withdrawal can be complicated by delirium, for example, delirium tremens in alcohol withdrawal. Psychotic disorder (E) as a result of alcohol use is usually characterized by auditory hallucinations and sometimes paranoid thinking.

Substance misuse disorders (2)

2 A When a patient is dependent on a drug, a period of abstinence may lead to withdrawal symptoms (A). Features are specific to individual drugs and can include both physical symptoms (e.g. appetite change and fatigue) and/or psychological symptoms (e.g. anxiety and depression). Withdrawal symptoms are relieved by reinstatement (starting drinking again). Complicated withdrawal (B) occurs when the withdrawal state is associated with delirium, seizures or psychotic features. Amnestic syndrome (C) is associated with chronic loss of memory. There is often difficulty learning new material as well as time perception. Residual disorder (D) occurs when symptoms of withdrawal persist despite continued abstinence. Depression (E) would have a history of at least 2 weeks.

Dependence syndrome

3 A Wernicke's encephalopathy (A) is seen in patients with alcohol dependence and is caused by thiamine (vitamin B1) deficiency. It is characterized by the triad of ataxia, confusion and ophthalmoplegia (most often involving the lateral rectus). Alcohol withdrawal (B) occurs in the acute setting, a day or two after the person last had a drink. Symptoms can be divided into physical (coarse tremor, sweating, insomnia, vomiting and tachycardia) and psychiatric (visual, tactile or auditory hallucinations or illusions. Korsakoff's syndrome (C) is a later complication following Wernicke's encephalopathy and is characterized by amnesia with a normal level of consciousness. Intoxication (D) is characterized by mood changes and disinhibition. Delirium tremens (E) is a medical emergency that usually occurs approximately 24–72 hours into abstinence and is characterized by confusion, hallucinations, affective changes, tremor, autonomic disturbance, seizures and delusions.

Complications of alcohol (1)

4 B The symptoms experienced as a result of alcohol intoxication (B) is dependent on the blood alcohol concentration (BAC). At a low BAC alcohol causes elevated mood and disinhibition, with an increased BAC leading to slurred speech, ataxia, aggressiveness and eventually unconsciousness. Alcohol-induced amnesia (A), also known as alcoholic palimpsest, typically involves short-term anterograde memory loss with the patient unable to recall events during a specific time window. Harmful drinking (C) occurs when a patient continues to drink despite continued damage to their mental and/or physical health. At-risk drinking (D) is the stage when the user is at increased health risk due to situational factors, e.g. pregnancy or drink driving. Alcohol dependence (E) is characterized by increased tolerance and withdrawal features on abstinence, amongst other features.

Complications of alcohol (2)

5 C Othello syndrome (C), also known as pathological or morbid jealousy, is a disorder which can occur as a result of either current or previous alcohol abuse although it occurs in other psychiatric disorders. The patient holds delusional beliefs that his/her partner is being unfaithful and may adopt extreme methods to prove this, e.g. hiring private detectives or planting secret cameras. The syndrome is associated with an increased risk of homicide towards the partner. Alcoholic hallucinosis (A) is characterized by auditory hallucinations. Alcohol-induced psychotic disorder (B) may occur as a result of long-term alcohol misuse. It differs from Othello syndrome as classically delusions are grandiose or persecutory. Alcoholic dementia (D) results in widespread cognitive difficulties due to the toxic effect of alcohol. Korsakoff's syndrome (E) is an amnestic syndrome which results in severe anterograde amnesia.

Sudden focal neurology

6 D Central pontine myelinolysis (D) occurs due to severe damage to the myelin sheath of neurons in the pons. The most common cause in alcoholics is over-rapid correction of hyponatraemia. Symptoms include a pseudobulbar palsy and quadriplegia. Wernicke–Korsakoff syndrome (A) is characterized by neuronal degeneration in the mammillary bodies secondary to thiamine deficiency in heavy drinkers. Wernicke's encephalopathy is defined by the classic triad of confusion, ophthalmoplegia and ataxia. Korsakoff's syndrome is characterized by chronic anterograde amnesia. On examination, peripheral neuropathy (B) is typically characterized by sensory loss in the lower extremities, absent tendon reflexes and weakness of the affected limbs. Marchiafava–Bignami disease (C) is a progressive neurological condition characterized by corpus callosum demyelination associated with chronic alcoholism. Presentation is variable and often non-specific: sudden stupor, coma or seizures, dementia, incontinence, aphasia, apraxia. Long-term alcohol misuse can lead to myopathy (E). Common symptoms are weakness, stiffness and cramps.

Cardiopulmonary complications of alcohol misuse

7 B   Long-term alcohol abuse can lead to suppression of the immune system, putting users at risk of *Mycobacterium tuberculosis* infection (B). Characteristic features include low grade fever, night sweats, weight loss and haemoptysis. Dilated cardiomyopathy (A) is associated with alcohol dependence and the patient will present with symptoms such as breathlessness, pulmonary oedema and/or arrhythmia. Atrial fibrillation (C) can be caused by excessive alcohol consumption or 'binge drinking'. Alcohol abusers are at increased risk of pneumonia (D) for the same reasons as TB: a suppressed immune system. The most common pathogens responsible are *Klebsiella* and *Streptococcus pneumoniae*. Symptoms will include high fever, purulent cough, pleuritic chest pain and shortness of breath. Stroke (E) is very unlikely at this age.

Gastrointestinal complications of alcohol misuse

8 C   Barrett's oesophagus (C) arises from long-term distal oesophageal exposure to alcohol which causes squamous epithelium to undergo metaplasia, resulting in the formation of columnar epithelium. It is diagnosed on endoscopy after the patient complains of long-standing heartburn. There is a risk that the Barrett's oesophagus may progress to adenocarcinoma. Alcoholic liver disease (A) exists as a spectrum of liver pathology: it begins with fatty change and progresses to alcoholic hepatitis in heavy drinkers. Cirrhosis may arise in alcoholics after 10–30 years of persistent use. Acute gastritis (B) is defined as the inflammation of the stomach mucosa and is caused by excessive alcohol consumption. Epigastric pain, nausea, vomiting and loss of appetite are characteristic features. Mallory–Weiss tears (D) arise as a result of an alcoholic binge which triggers a vomiting episode. Continued vomiting can cause an oesophageal tear associated with haematemesis. Alcohol is the most common cause of chronic pancreatitis (E). Chronic pancreatitis is characterized by epigastric pain which radiates to the back (relieved on sitting forward), steatorrhoea (fatty stools) and diabetes.

Alcohol-associated psychiatric disorders

9 A   Alcohol has anxiolytic properties and, as a result, patients with anxiety syndromes such as social phobia (A) may self-medicate to relieve the symptoms. Furthermore, dependent patients who undergo alcohol withdrawal may experience anxiety and panic symptoms. Alcohol is a depressant and when combined with social consequences of excessive use, can result in depression (B). Long-term alcohol use can cause a psychotic disorder (C) to develop, characterized by hallucinations and delusions. Hallucinations are usually auditory but may be visual. Delusions are primarily grandiose or persecutory in nature. Symptoms are transient and resolve with abstinence of alcohol. Generalized anxiety disorder (D) tends to have less focused and situationally dependent symptoms. Morbid jealousy (E) is associated with alcohol dependency and will manifest as a delusion that a partner is unfaithful. There may be associated impotence as well as a high risk of violence towards the partner.

Hallucinations

10 B Acute psychological effects of cocaine (B) are increased alertness, euphoria, irritability, delusions and hallucinations. Cocaine users may also experience the sensation of insects crawling on their skin, known as formication. Physical effects of cocaine are tachycardia, hypertension and arrhythmias. Heroin (A) induces initial euphoria followed by sedation. Physical signs will include pin-point pupils, bradycardia, respiratory depression and constipation. There are few psychiatric sequelae associated with its use. Characteristics of LSD (lysergic acid diethylamide) (C) intoxication include depersonalization, illusions, synaesthesia and visual hallucinations. Caffeine intoxication (D) can lead to headache, anxiety, confusion, tremors, irregular heart beat, nausea and vomiting. Benzodiazepines (E) are central nervous system depressants and may lead to drowsiness, confusion and reduced anxiety.

Persecutory delusions

11 E Long-term cannabis use (E) has been linked to increasing the risk of schizophrenia. Patients with the Val-Val polymorphism of the gene coding for catechol-O-methyl transferase are highly susceptible to developing schizophrenia after chronic cannabis use. Chronic barbiturate users (A) may show signs of increased irritability and aggressiveness as well as fatigue. Magic mushrooms (B) contain active chemicals such as psilocybin and psilocin which cause visual disturbances. Chronic glue sniffing (C) can lead to irreversible brain damage, memory defects and mood disorders. Heroin (D) rarely causes psychiatric symptoms.

Alcohol cessation

12 A A 750 mL bottle of 12 per cent wine is around nine units; therefore this patient is drinking 36 units of alcohol per week. This level of drinking may be associated with a small increased risk of harm. Men are advised not to drink more than 21 units per week and four units per day. Early interventional advice within the GP setting can lead to a reduction in alcohol consumption and reduce the risk of progression to heavier drinking. Alcoholics Anonymous (B) offers long-term support for people with alcohol dependence. Disulfiram and acamprosate are both used in maintenance of abstinence in people who have been alcohol dependent. Antipsychotics (E) have no place in the management of this scenario.

Management of alcohol withdrawal

13 A The patient is suffering from delirium tremens due to alcohol withdrawal. Delirium tremens usually presents 24 hours to 1 week after drinking cessation and patients may experience marked confusion, visual and auditory hallucinations with autonomic instability (sweating, a raised pulse and blood pressure). Oral chlordiazepoxide (A) is the most appropriate drug to use in this situation. It reduces the severity of symptoms and reduces the risk of seizures. IV chlordiazepoxide (D) or diazepam (E) would only be used if the oral route was unavailable. Any person presenting with alcohol withdrawal should also receive high dose intravenous thiamine, not oral thiamine (C) which is poorly absorbed. Antipsychotics (B) should be used only if psychotic symptoms are persistent.

SECTION 34:
PSYCHOPHARMACOLOGY

QUESTIONS

1. Classes of psychiatric drugs (1)

Which of the following is an atypical (second-generation) antipsychotic drug?

    A. Chlorpromazine
    B. Isoniazid
    C. Lithium
    D. Olanzapine
    E. Trazodone

2. Classes of psychiatric drugs (2)

A 29-year-old man is seen by a psychiatrist and commenced on venlafaxine. What class of drug is this?

    A. Monoamine oxidase inhibitor
    B. Noradrenaline reuptake inhibitor
    C. Selective serotonin reuptake inhibitor (SSRI)
    D. Serotonin and noradrenaline reuptake inhibitor (SNRI)
    E. Tetracyclic antidepressant

3. Classes of psychiatric drugs (3)

Which of the following drugs is not used as a mood stabilizer?

    A. Carbamazepine
    B. Lamotrigine
    C. Lithium carbonate
    D. Sodium valproate
    E. Trimipramine

4. Indications of psychiatric drugs (1)

Which of the following would be the most appropriate choice in the first line management of new-onset schizophrenia?

    A. Clozapine
    B. Lithium carbonate
    C. Pimozide
    D. Quetiapine
    E. Sertraline

5. Indications of psychiatric drugs (2)

Which of the following would not be an appropriate choice in the prophylaxis of bipolar disorder?

A. Carbamazepine
B. Diazepam
C. Lithium
D. Olanzapine
E. Sodium valproate

6. Indications of psychiatric drugs (3)

Which of the following would be the most appropriate choice of drug for the management of a 55 year old with postoperative delirium who has become extremely agitated?

A. Amitriptyline
B. Haloperidol
C. Lithium carbonate
D. Temazepam
E. Zuclopenthixol acetate (Acuphase)

7. Side effects of psychiatric drugs

Which of the following is most likely to cause tardive dyskinesia in a middle-aged man with schziophrenia?

A. Aripiprazole
B. Clozapine
C. Flupentixol decanoate
D. Lithium carbonate
E. Trazodone

8. Mode of action of psychiatric drugs

Which of the following primarily acts to increase levels of acetylcholine in the brain?

A. Aripiprazole
B. Carbamazepine
C. Diazepam
D. Donepezil
E. Haloperidol

9. Contraindications of psychiatric drugs

Which of the following drugs is contraindicated in myasthenia gravis?

A. Chlorpromazine
B. Citalopram
C. Galantamine
D. Procyclidine
E. Pyridostigmine

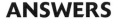

ANSWERS

Classes of psychiatric drugs (1)

1 D   Olanzapine (D) is an atypical or second-generation antipsychotic. These drugs are the usual first line choice for treating psychotic illnesses such as schizophrenia and generally cause fewer extrapyramidal side effects compared to older antipsychotic drugs. However, they are not without side effects and most are associated with weight gain and metabolic changes. Chlorpromazine (A) is an example of a 'typical' or first-generation antipsychotic, and in fact was the first drug specifically designed with antipsychotic properties. It is an antagonist at a wide range of receptors which accounts for some of the side effects observed with this drug. It has particularly potent anticholinergic effects. Isoniazid (B) is an anti-tuberculous agent which has incidental antidepressant activity. Lithium carbonate (C) is an inorganic ion that has antimanic properties as well as being used in the prophylaxis of bipolar disorder. Trazodone (E) is an antidepressant in the 'SARI' (serotonin antagonist and reuptake inhibitor) class. It also has prominent sedative and anxiolytic properties.

Classes of psychiatric drugs (2)

2 D   Venlafaxine (D) is an SNRI. It is used as a second line agent for treating depression. Monoamine oxidase inhibitors (A) are another class of antidepressants. They are seldom used in current practice because of their side effect profile as well as potential interaction with various tyramine-rich foods (commonly referred to as the 'cheese reaction'). Noradrenaline (or norepinephrine) reuptake inhibitors (NARIs) (B) include atomoxetine and reboxetine, also developed for the treatment of depression. SSRIs (C) are now the most commonly used class of antidepressants and include agents such as fluoxetine, sertraline and citalopram. They are generally well tolerated and are less lethal in overdose compared with older drugs. Tetracyclic antidepressants (E) include mirtazapine and mianserin.

Classes of psychiatric drugs (3)

3 E   Trimipramine (E) is a tricyclic antidepressant. Antidepressants must be used cautiously in patients with bipolar affective disorder as there is a risk of inducing a manic episode, although they are sometimes necessary in patients with depressive episodes as part of their bipolar disorder. Carbamazepine (A), lamotrigine (B) and sodium valproate (D) are all anti-epileptic agents used in the prophylaxis of bipolar disorder as well as the acute manic phase of the illness, although lamotrigine is thought to be more effective in treating depressive episodes than mania. Lithium carbonate (C) is an inorganic ion used in the treatment of mania, depression and the prophylaxis of bipolar disorder.

Indications of psychiatric drugs (1)

4 D Quetiapine (D) is an atypical, or second-generation, antipsychotic, which are recommended by NICE as first line agents in new-onset schizophrenia. There have been increasing concerns about these agents in terms of their metabolic side effects, and as a result there has been some resurgence in the use of older, typical antipsychotic drugs. Clozapine (A) is a powerful antipsychotic that is reserved for the treatment of treatment-resistant schizophrenia. It is associated with a significant risk of developing neutropenia or even agranulocytosis, which means the patient must have regular full blood count checks. Lithium carbonate (B) is used in bipolar disorder and affective psychoses, not typically in schizophrenia. Pimozide (C) is an older antipsychotic that is used very infrequently in current practice. It has been associated with unexplained deaths and should only be prescribed after an electrocardiogram (ECG). Regular monitoring with ECG is also recommended during treatment. It is associated with prolongation of the QT interval and should not be used with other drugs (such as tricyclic antidepressants) that may also prolong the QT, or with drugs that may cause electrolyte disturbances such as diuretics. Sertraline (E) is an SSRI used as an antidepressant. It does not have antipsychotic properties.

Indications of psychiatric drugs (2)

5 B Diazepam (B) is a benzodiazepine with various indications, such as relief of anxiety and as a sedative. It, like all the benzodiazepines, is associated with the development of tolerance and possible dependence so should only be used in short-term management. It does not have antimanic properties as such, but is often used to control agitation and other erratic behaviours during an acute manic episode. Carbamazepine (A) and sodium valproate (E) are both anti-epileptics used in the prophylaxis of bipolar disorder. Lithium (C) is an inorganic ion used in the treatment of mania, depression and the prophylaxis of bipolar disorder. Olanzapine (D) is an antipsychotic that is also effective in (and licensed for) the prophylaxis of bipolar disorder.

Indications of psychiatric drugs (3)

6 B Delirium is treated in various ways, and certainly not just pharmacologically. While in certain circumstances benzodiazepines may be used, generally an antipsychotic is the treatment of choice, such as haloperidol (B). Amitriptyline (A) is a tricyclic antidepressant. Given its anticholinergic properties it may actually worsen confusion and would therefore not be an appropriate choice. Lithium carbonate (C) is used for the prophylaxis of bipolar disorder and treatment of manic and depressive episodes. It does not have a role in the treatment of delirium. Temazepam (D) is a benzodiazepine and also a controlled drug. As stated above, while on some occasions benzodiazepines may be an appropriate choice for treatment of delirium, temazepam would not be the most appropriate one to choose from this class. A rare but important consequence of the use of benzodiazepines is paradoxical agitation. Zuclopenthixol acetate (E), trade name Acuphase, is a potent intramuscular antipsychotic medication. It is used in the management of extremely agitated patients who are not responding to the standard pharmacological treatments for rapid tranquilization. It should be used with extreme caution, only in specialist units and for short-term management.

Side effects of psychiatric drugs

7 C Tardive dyskinesia is a distressing complication of antipsychotic use. It typically comes on after many years of treatment (hence 'tardive') and is associated principally with the use of typical antipsychotic agents, and in particular depot medications, such as flupentixol decanoate (C). It is extremely difficult to treat once present. Aripiprazole (A) is a newer antipsychotic which appears to have a lower incidence of tardive dyskinesia than older agents (although of note it has not been licensed for a sufficient length of time to definitively state this). Clozapine (B) is a potent antipsychotic used in the management of treatment-resistant schizophrenia. Unlike other agents, it is actually thought to improve the symptoms of tardive dyskinesia. Lithium carbonate (D), an antimanic agent, and trazodone (E), an antidepressant, rarely cause tardive dyskinesia.

Mode of action of psychiatric drugs

8 D Donepezil (D) is an acetylcholinesterase inhibitor (AChEI), used to ameliorate the cognitive and non-cognitive symptoms of dementia. It works by increasing the functional amount of acetylcholine in the brain. Aripiprazole (A) is an antipsychotic that works as a partial dopamine agonist. Carbamazepine (B) is an anti-epileptic with mood stabilizing qualities. Diazepam (C) is a benzodiazepine. These drugs work as GABA agonists. Haloperidol (E) is another antipsychotic. It is thought to exert its antipsychotic effects by, as with other antipsychotic drugs, antagonizing dopamine.

Contraindications of psychiatric drugs

9 D Procyclidine (D) is an antimuscarinic (anticholinergic) agent used in Parkinson's disease as well as to treat the parkinsonian (extrapyramidal) side effects of antipsychotic medication. Myaesthenia gravis (MG) is an autoimmune neurological disorder caused by circulating antibodies against acetylcholine receptors at the postsynaptic neuromuscular junction. Any drugs that inhibit acetylcholine (such as anticholinergics) will worsen the symptoms of MG. Chlorpromazine (A) is a first-generation antipsychotic. It should be used with caution in patients with MG as it does have anticholinergic properties. However, it is not contraindicated as such. Citalopram (B) is an SSRI. It has potent effects at the 5-HT1A receptor but minimal activity at muscarinic receptors (although note not zero activity). Galantamine (C) is an AChEI used in the management of Alzheimer's disease. It increases the availability of acetylcholine so in theory should improve the symptoms of MG, although it does not have a license for this in the UK. Pyridostigmine (E) is another AChEI, but in this case is used in the treatment of MG and in fact is one of the mainstays of treatment.

SECTION 35:
CHILD PSYCHIATRY AND
LEARNING DISABILITY

QUESTIONS

1. Diagnosis of psychiatric problems in childhood (1)

A 4-year-old boy is brought into his GP by his parents. They are worried as he is constantly dropping things and trips often, sometimes causing injury. He does not show any affection towards his family and does not play well with others at nursery, although his older sister is a very warm child. He plays with dinosaurs by himself but completely ignores other toys. His speech is relatively normal. What is the most likely diagnosis?

    A. Asperger's syndrome
    B. Attachment disorder
    C. Childhood autism
    D. Conduct disorder
    E. Down's syndrome

2. Diagnosis of psychiatric problems in childhood (2)

A 12-year-old boy is referred to the child psychiatry service. His behaviour has become so aggressive that he has been excluded from school for assaulting fellow pupils and more recently teachers. He has smashed up several classrooms and the previous week the fire brigade were called as he set fire to his bedroom. He shows no remorse for the way he behaves. What is the most likely diagnosis?

    A. Attention deficit hyperactivity disorder (ADHD)
    B. Childhood disintegrative disorder
    C. Conduct disorder
    D. Oppositional defiant disorder (ODD)
    E. Tic disorder

3. Management of conduct disorder

Which of the following would be least appropriate for the first line management of conduct disorder?

    A. Cognitive behavioural therapy (CBT)
    B. Family therapy
    C. Methylphenidate
    D. Parent training
    E. Risperidone

4. Diagnosis of psychiatric problems in childhood (3)

Which of the following is not part of the diagnostic criteria for ADHD?

    A. Aggression towards peers
    B. Excessive motor activity

C. Inattention
D. Symptoms present in more than one setting
E. Symptoms present for at least 6 months

5. Diagnosis of psychiatric problems in childhood (4)

A 9-year-old boy is brought to the GP as he has started wetting the bed, despite being continent for the last 4 years. What is this symptom known as?

A. Cluttering
B. Encopresis
C. Enuresis
D. Pica
E. Trichotillomania

6. Diagnosis of psychiatric problems in childhood (5)

A 9-year-old boy is referred to the local child psychiatry service. For the past 18 months he has begun displaying odd speech, with outbursts of strange and sometimes obscene words. More recently he has begun grimacing and blinking excessively. He is unable to control this and it is causing him some distress. What is the most likely diagnosis?

A. Asperger's syndrome
B. Gilles de la Tourette syndrome
C. Hyperkinetic disorder
D. Lesch–Nyhan syndrome
E. Transient tic disorder

7. Management of psychiatric problems in childhood

An 11-year-old boy is diagnosed with Gilles de la Tourette syndrome. There is no evidence of any co-morbid diagnosis. What would the most appropriate management be?

A. Atomoxetine
B. Deep brain stimulation
C. Psychoanalytic therapy
D. Psychoeducation
E. Risperidone

8. Diagnosis of learning disability

Which of the following statements regarding learning disability is correct?

A. Epilepsy is over-represented in patients with learning disability
B. Mild learning disability is usually defined by an IQ between 35 and 49
C. The point prevalence of schizophrenia in people with learning disability is equal to that of the general population

    D.   Suicide is more common in people with learning disability than the general population

    E.   A person with learning disability cannot consent to treatment for medical conditions

9. Learning disability syndromes

Which of the following is not usually associated with learning disability?

    A.   Angelman's syndrome

    B.   Down's syndrome

    C.   Edwards' syndrome

    D.   Guillain–Barré syndrome

    E.   Hunter's syndrome

10. Down's syndrome

Which of the following statements regarding trisomy 21 is correct?

    A.   Alzheimer's disease is more common in people with Down's syndrome than the general population

    B.   Mosaicism is responsible for approximately 20 per cent of cases of Down's syndrome

    C.   Not all cases of trisomy 21 will result in learning disability

    D.   People with Down's syndrome cannot live independently

    E.   People with Down's syndrome have a lower incidence of anxiety than the general population

ANSWERS

Diagnosis of psychiatric problems in childhood (1)

1 A This pattern is typical of Asperger's syndrome (A), a condition which is still not fully understood, but shares similarities with autism in terms of qualitative abnormalities in social interactions as well as unusual or intense interest in a restricted range of behaviours or activities. Motor clumsiness is also common. Unlike autism (C), however, there is usually no language delay or marked cognitive difficulties, which are the other hallmarks of that disorder. The disorder usually persists into adolescence and adulthood and there is also an association with psychotic episodes. While the lack of warmth may lead one to think of an attachment disorder (B), the other symptoms would not be typical for such a diagnosis. Attachment disorders are considered elsewhere in this book. This history would not suggest a conduct disorder (D), in which there would typically be marked repetitive and resistant defiant or dissocial behaviours. Conduct disorders are also considered elsewhere in this book. There is nothing in the history to suggest Down's syndrome (E), in which there is usually severe development and language delay as well as a characteristic physical appearance and associated medical problems.

Diagnosis of psychiatric problems in childhood (2)

2 C This history strongly suggests a conduct disorder (C). These disorders have caused significant debate as to their aetiology, with many considering them to be a social rather than psychiatric problem. Regardless, they cause significant problems to society as well as the individual, and unless managed well, will almost inevitably lead to other problems in later life. There is a strong association with adult dissocial personality disorder (psychopathy). There are thought to be genetic, family and wider environmental factors involved in the aetiology of these disorders. This history is not typical of ADHD (A), in which the predominant symptoms are those of inattention or poor concentration, hyperactivity and fidgeting and impulsivity. While children with ADHD can be difficult to manage, there is not such a degree of violent and destructive behaviour as exhibited here. However, ADHD and conduct disorder are often co-morbid with each other. Childhood disintegrative disorder (B) is a type of pervasive developmental disorder sharing some characteristics with childhood autism. However, unlike autism, children usually have an initial period of entirely normal development, before a period of definite loss of previously acquired skills and social withdrawal. Perhaps the most difficult distractor here is ODD (D). While ODD may progress to a more frank conduct disorder, it usually manifests in younger children and is characterized by disobedient and disruptive behaviour, but without the frank aggression and violence seen above. Tic disorders (E), such as Gilles de la Tourette syndrome, usually have their onset in childhood. Tics are involuntary, rapid, recurrent non-rhythmic motor movements or vocal acts that serve no apparent purpose. They can sometimes be suppressed but usually only at great difficulty and with significant accompanying anxiety. Their aetiology is complex but is likely to be related to basal ganglia abnormalities.

Management of conduct disorder

3 E Risperidone (E) is an antipsychotic. These drugs should be used with extreme caution in children, and should really only be prescribed to target psychotic symptoms. They have the potential to cause significant harm if not monitored carefully, and they seem to lead to more severe side effects, such as extrapyramidal symptoms, than in adults. While there is some evidence of antipsychotics being effective in reducing aggression in conduct disorder, they would certainly not be a first line choice of treatment. CBT (A) has been used effectively in conduct disorder. There are a number of different approaches used that could be classed under the umbrella of CBT, such as problem-solving skills training. The goal of such therapies is for the child to develop alternative skills to approach situations that previously had resulted in aggressive or violent behaviour. Family therapy (B) is used in conduct disorder and will be particularly useful in cases where there are disordered family dynamics or difficulties in bonding and attachment within the family unit. Supporters of family therapy believe it is helpful in avoiding excessive blame being placed on the child for their behaviour. Methylphenidate (C) is a stimulant medication that has been successfully used as part of the management of conduct disorder. It is particularly effective when there is a co-morbid element of ADHD in the presentation. Note that medications should be combined with other forms of social and psychological therapy in the treatment of conduct disorder. Parent management training (D) is another effective treatment which is supported by the National Institute for Health and Clinical Excellence. It involves parents and therapists working together to develop specific and systematic strategies to cope with and change aggressive behaviours.

Diagnosis of psychiatric problems in childhood (3)

4 A Aggression (A) is not part of the diagnostic criteria for typical ADHD, although ADHD and conduct disorder are often co-morbid together. If aggression is significant in the presentation, then a diagnosis of conduct disorder should be considered. Excessive motor activity is one of the hallmarks of ADHD (B), including fidgeting, running or climbing excessively, leaving seats in class etc. Inattention (C) is the other major symptom cluster in ADHD, which may manifest in numerous ways such as appearing not to listen, making careless errors, not finishing tasks, forgetfulness etc. Symptoms must occur in more than one setting (D), e.g. school and home, for the diagnosis to be made. Symptoms must also be present for at least 6 months (E) for a diagnosis to be made according to ICD-10.

Diagnosis of psychiatric problems in childhood (4)

5 C   Enuresis (C) refers to involuntary voiding of urine either at night (nocturnal enuresis) or during the day (diurnal enuresis) or both. It may be primary, in which case the child has never achieved a period of being dry, or secondary (as in this case), when wetting begins after a period of being dry (usually given as at least 6 months). The latter is more commonly associated with psychological or emotional problems, while broadly speaking the former is often down to a developmental delay, a structural problem or other medical causes. Cluttering (A) is the symptom of rapid speech with a breakdown in fluency but no repetitions or hesitations (as compared to stammering). Encopresis (B) is the voluntary or involuntary voiding of faeces in inappropriate settings. It, like enuresis, may be the result of a wider emotional disorder, or may be secondary to the abnormal continuation of normal infantile incontinence. Pica (D) refers to the persistent eating of non-nutritive substances, e.g. sand, paint, or even faeces. Trichotillomania (E) is the specific disorder of pulling out one's own hair and is considered to be an impulse control disorder, with possibly some relationship to obsessive–compulsive disorder.

Diagnosis of psychiatric problems in childhood (5)

6 B   Gilles de la Tourette syndrome (B) is a chronic tic disorder in which both vocal and motor tics are present (as in this case). The onset is usually at around 7–10 years and tends to worsen through adolescence. The cause is not fully understood, but there are undoubtedly both genetic and environmental factors involved. Neuropathologically, there are thought to be dysfunctions in thalamic, basal ganglia and frontal cortical structures. Asperger's syndrome (A) is a developmental disorder predominantly associated with problems in social interaction, of which there is no mention in the above vignette. Hyperkinetic disorder (C) refers to a spectrum of disorders which includes ADHD. The core features of ADHD include excessive motor activity and restlessness. Lesch–Nyhan syndrome (D) is a rare X-linked recessive disorder that results in the inability to metabolize uric acid, leading to hyperuricaemia. There are numerous manifestations, including learning disability, striking self-injurious behaviour and odd movements that may resemble Huntington's chorea but equally may look like Tourette's. However, as there is no history given of developmental problems this would rule out this diagnosis here. This history does not represent a transient tic disorder (E) as it has been occurring for more than 1 year. Remember, for a diagnosis of Tourette's, both vocal and motor tics must be present. In a tic disorder it will be either one or the other.

Management of psychiatric problems in childhood

7 D Psychoeducation (D) for both the patient and their carers is critical in managing tic disorders, including Tourette's. The purpose is to explain the nature and course of the disorder to prevent deterioration in personal and family functioning. People with Tourette's are at high risk of co-morbid disorders such as depression and obsessive–compulsive disorder – screening for these is also critical and targeted therapy should be recommended if they coexist. Atomoxetine (A) is a stimulant usually used in ADHD. It has been successfully used for Tourette's syndrome but is probably only useful when there is co-morbid ADHD. Deep brain stimulation (B), is still a relatively experimental technique although it has been used for many years now. It involves the surgical implantation of a 'brain pacemaker' and has been used, with mixed success, in various movement disorders such as Parkinson's disease, and possibly affective disorders such as treatment-resistant depression. However, it is still highly experimental and there is an obvious risk of complications, and it would certainly never be used in a relatively straightforward case of Tourette's, and certainly not in a child. Psychoanalysis would not be indicated here (C) and there is no evidence that it is of use in tic disorders. Risperidone (E) is an atypical antipsychotic that has been used successfully in Tourette's syndrome. However, while this may be an option, there is nothing to suggest here that the disorder is of sufficient severity to warrant the use of antipsychotic medication in such a young patient. It would almost certainly be best in this case to try supportive and educational techniques in the first instance before trialling medication.

Diagnosis of learning disability

8 A People with learning disability, of whatever severity, are more likely to have co-morbid epilepsy (A), with some specific syndromes being noticeable, such as Lennox–Gestaut syndrome and autistic spectrum disorders. Mild learning disability is usually classified as occurring in people with an IQ of between 50 and 70 (B). Moderate learning disability is classified in the IQ range of 35 to 49, with severe learning disability at 34 and below. Obviously this classification is extremely arbitrary and the assessment and management of individuals requires much more sophisticated tools. Schizophrenia (C), like epilepsy, is over-represented in learning disability. Suicide is actually less common in people with moderate and severe learning disabilities (D), although the rates for those with mild learning disability have not been adequately established. Lack of means may play a part in this, as may poor understanding of lethality.

Note that self-injurious behaviours are common in learning disability, and increase with the severity of the disability. While capacity must be carefully assessed when consenting someone with learning disability for medical treatment, by no means does this mean that a learning disability automatically assumes incapacity (E). Remember capacity is decision specific and must be assessed each time a decision is required.

Learning disability syndromes

9 D Guillain–Barré syndrome is an ascending peripheral polyneuropathy caused by an immune response to certain foreign antigens, the most common being *Campylobacter jejuni*. There is no association with learning disability (D). Angelman's syndrome (A) results from inactivation of the maternally inherited chromosome 15 (also known as genomic imprinting). It results in severe learning disability, almost no use of language, ataxia and unusual behaviour such as frequent laughter and highly excitable behaviour. Down's syndrome, or trisomy 21 (B), is an extremely common form of learning disability. Edwards' syndrome results from trisomy 18 (C). Only 5–10 per cent of infants will live beyond their first year. In those that do, severe learning disability will be ubiquitous. Hunter's syndrome (E) is a lysosomal storage disease caused by a deficiency in the enzyme iduronate-2-sulfatase. Despite a wide phenotypic presentation, it is always progressive and severe. Learning disability is often, although not always, present.

Down syndrome

10 A Alzheimer's disease is over-represented in patients with Down's syndrome (A), and for those that survive to their sixth decade, at least 50 per cent of people will show clinical evidence of dementia. The reason for this is almost certainly that the amyloid precursor protein is encoded on chromosome 21, but other genes may also be important, such as superoxidase dismutase. Mosaicism, as opposed to nondisjunction in gametes causing trisomy 21, occurs for only 1–2 per cent of cases of Down's syndrome (B). While there is some variation in the clinical presentation of Down's syndrome, such as only around half presenting with congenital cardiac difficulties, all people with trisomy 21 will have some degree of learning disability (C). While many people with Down's syndrome will require significant support, often including residential placement depending on the degree of disability, many people with trisomy 21 will be able to live independently, although will nearly always require some support to do this (D). People with Down's syndrome are at a higher risk of most psychiatric disorders, including anxiety problems (E).

Index

Note: References give the page number for the question with the answers in italics. In a few cases, the reader will find no mention in a question of significant items referenced from an answer, despite the index giving the page number for that question.